UROLOGIC

Laparoscopic Surgery

NOTICE

Medicine is an ever-changing science. As new research and clinical experience broaden our knowledge, changes in treatment and drug therapy are required. The editor and the publisher of this work have checked with sources believed to be reliable in their efforts to provide information that is complete and generally in accord with the standards accepted at the time of publication. However, in view of the possibility of human error or changes in medical sciences, neither the editor nor the publisher nor any other party who has been involved in the preparation or publication of this work warrants that the information contained herein is in every respect accurate or complete, and they are not responsible for any errors or omissions or for the results obtained from use of such information. Readers are encouraged to confirm the information contained herein with other sources. For example and in particular, readers are advised to check the product information sheet included in the package of each drug they plan to administer to be certain that the information contained in this book is accurate and that changes have not been made in the recommended dose or in the contraindications for administration. This recommendation is of particular importance in connection with new or infrequently used drugs.

UROLOGIC
Laparoscopic Surgery

Editor

Raul O. Parra, M.D., F.A.C.S.

Professor and Chairman of Urology
St. Louis University School of Medicine
St. Louis, Missouri

Associate Editor

John A. Boullier, M.D., Ph.D.

Assistant Professor of Surgery
Division of Urology
St. Louis University School of Medicine
St. Louis, Missouri

McGRAW-HILL
HEALTH PROFESSIONS DIVISION

New York • St. Louis • San Francisco • Auckland
Bogotá • Caracas • Lisbon • London • Madrid • Mexico City
Milan • Montreal • New Delhi • San Juan • Singapore • Sydney • Tokyo • Toronto

UROLOGIC LAPAROSCOPIC SURGERY

1234567890 KGPKGP 98765

ISBN 0-07-048580-1

This book was set in Times Roman by *TopDesk Publishers' Group.*
The editors were *Martin J. Wonsiewicz* and *Mariapaz Ramos Englis*;
the production supervisor was *Clare Stanley*;
the text and cover designs were by *TopDesk Publishers' Group*;
the indexer was *TopDesk Publishers' Group.*
Project supervision was by *TopDesk Publishers' Group.*
Quebecor Printing/Kingsport Press was printer and binder.
This book is printed on acid-free paper.

Library of Congress Cataloging-in-Publication Date

Urologic laparoscopic surgery / editor, Raul O. Parra.
p. cm.
Includes bibliographical references and index.
ISBN 0-07-048580-1 (hardcover)
1. Genitourinary organs—Endoscopic surgery. 2. Laparoscopic surgery. I. Parra, Raul O.
[DNLM: 1. Surgery, Laparoscopic. 2. Urologic Diseases— surgery. 3. Urogenital Diseases—surgery. 4. Digestive System Diseases--surgery. WD 500 U58 1995]
RD571.U725 1995
616.4'6059—dc20
DNML/DLC
for Library of Congress 95-988

This book is dedicated to
Silvia, Suzanne, Andrew, and Gabriel

Contents

Contributors

The numbers in brackets refer to chapter(s) authored or co-authored by the contributor.

Charles H. Andrus, M.D., F.A.C.S.
Associate Professor of Surgery
Chief of Surgical Endoscopy
Department of Surgery
St. Louis University School of Medicine
St. Louis, Missouri
[3, 4, 5]

John A. Boullier, M.D., Ph.D.
Assistant Professor of Surgery
Division of Urology
St. Louis University School of Medicine
St. Louis, Missouri
[8, 10, 13]

Jorge Cueto Garcia, M.D., F.A.C.S.
Past President (Founder) of the Mexican and Latin American Associations of Laparoscopic Surgery (ALACE)
Surgeon of the American British Cowdray Hospital, Mexico, D.F.
Professor of Surgery, Escuela Medico Militar, Mexico, D.F.
Teapa No. 4
Lomas Chapultepec
Mexico, D. F.
[20]

James M. Cummings, M.D.
Assistant Professor of Urology
St. Louis University School of Medicine
St. Louis, Missouri
[2]

Sakti Das, M.D., M.S., F.R.C.S. (EDIN & C), F.A.C.S.
Chairman, Department of Urology
Kaiser Permanente Medical Center
Walnut Creak, California
[16]

Durga D. Gaur, M.D., M.S., F.R.C.S. (ENG.)
Consultant Urological Surgeon and Associate Professor of Urology
Bombay Hospital Institute of Medical Sciences
[17]

Paul G. Hagood, M.D.
Chief Resident, Division of Urology
St. Louis University School of Medicine
St. Louis, Missouri
[1, 12]

Jose M. Hernandez-Graulau, M.D.
Associate Clinical Professor of Surgery
University of Illinois School of Medicine at Peoria
Peoria Urological Associates
Peoria, Illinois
[6]

Santiago Isorna, M.D., Ph.D., F.E.B.U.
Professor Urology-University Las Palmas G.C.
Head of Department of Urology-Hospital N.S. del Pino
C/Angel Guimera, 93
Las Palmas-Canary Islands
Spain
[19]

M. Pilar Laguna, M.D.
Staff Urologist
Urology Service
IUNA - Fundacion Puigvert
Barcelona, Spain
Cartagena
[19]

Donald J. Mehan, M.D., F.A.C.S.
Professor of Surgery, Division of Urology
St. Louis University Health Sciences Center
St. Louis, Missouri
[9]

Michael E. Moran, M.D.
Clinical Assistant Professor of Urology
Capital District Urologic Surgeons
Albany Medical Center and St. Peter's Hospital
Albany, New York
[7, 11]

Raul O. Parra, M.D., F.A.C.S.
Professor and Chairman, Division of Urology
St. Louis University School of Medicine
St. Louis, Missouri
[4, 8, 10, 12, 13, 15, 18, 19, 20]

Marceliano Garcia-Perez, M.D.
Head of the Department of Urology
Valme University Hospital
Seville, Spain (E. U.)
Virgen De Lujan, 1 - 2°B
41011 Sevilla, Spain
[19]

Sidney Radomski, M.D., F.R.C.S. (C)
Assistant Professor
Department of Surgery, Division of Urology
University of Toronto
Toronto, Ontario, Canada
[11]

Alejandro Weber Sanchez, M.D.
President of The Mexican Assn. of Laparoscopic Surgery
Counselor of The Mexican Board of Surgery
Gabriel Mancera 341
Col. Del Valle, Mexico
[20]

Steve J. Shichman, M.D.
Associate Professor
Division of Urology, Department of Surgery
University of Connecticut Health Center
c/o Greater Hartford Urology, P.C.
Hartford, Connecticut
[8]

Nicholas Stroumbakis, M.D.
Urology Fellow
Memorial Sloan Kettering Cancer Center
Bayside, New York
[6]

R. Ernest Sosa, M.D.
Associate Professor Surgery/Urology
Director, Brady Stone Center
Director, Urologic Endoscopy
New York Hospital-Cornell Medical Center
New York, New York
[2, 8]

Dr. J. G. Valdivia-Uria
Professor and Chairman of Urology
Facultad de Medicina de Zaragoza, Spain
Urbanizacion Santa Fé C/Cuarta, No. 13
50411 Cuarte de Huerva
Zaragoza (Spain)
[14]

Catherine M. Wittgen, M.D.
Chief Resident
Department of Surgery
St. Louis University School of Medicine
St. Louis, Missouri
[4]

Foreword

This text is unique in that Dr. Parra has not merely edited it but also contributed to the majority of its chapters. As a result, there is no unnecessary repetition and yet there is a familiar and fairly constant presentation of the various techniques.

The book's first two sections deal with general laparoscopy and operative laparoscopy where individual techniques are highlighted. In the section on general laparoscopy, there is a fascinating chapter on the history and evolution of laparoscopic surgery. Many of the basic techniques in laparoscopy, such as the setup, the insertion of trocars, and laparoscopic suturing, are constantly changing. This book avoids an endless recital of techniques that may be outmoded by the time the book appears in favor of a review of the essentials involved in modern laparoscopy and the complications that may ensue. The discussion of the physiologic and anesthetic principles of laparoscopy is vitally important, particularly when one considers that many of these procedures are lengthy and are being carried out on elderly patients.

The second section is devoted to discussions of twelve urologic procedures that are performed laparoscopically. It is difficult to know the exact role that each of these will play in the future in any individual urologist's practice. For example, laparoscopic varicocelectomy may or may not be superior to older techniques. Pelvic lymphadenectomy, although attractive and initially advocated for all neoplasms of the bladder, prostate, and urethra, is being used less often. Eventually, its value will be more clearly defined. In contrast, the role of laparoscopic bladder and incontinence surgery seems to have expanded, and more laparoscopists are participating in this form of therapy. Another procedure, intraperitoneal drainage of lymphoceles, has been one of the most dramatic laparoscopic success stories. Patients can now be cured of the problem overnight with a gratifyingly dramatic response.

The future role of several other laparoscopic procedures is unclear because, although they are technically feasible, they are also technically demanding and take a greater length of time than any corresponding open procedure. Examples are laparoscopic nephrectomy, pyeloplasty, adrenalectomy, and ureterectomy. However, the mere fact that these procedures are tedious does not mean that they are any less indicated.

Once the basic instrumentation has been improved somewhat, I feel certain that the new operations will be embraced with greater enthusiasm by most urologists, with great benefit to patients in terms of reduced morbidity and convalescence time.

Technically, it is easier to do laparoscopic procedures in children, hence many pediatric urologists have become very enthusiastic laparoscopists. The value of laparoscopy in the boy with an undescended testis is incontrovertible.

Dr. Gaur made a significant contribution to the urologic literature with his technique of balloon dissection to create a working space within the retroperitoneum. This technique has allowed access to the kidney and ureter and, in some patients, facilitated the procedures significantly. As with all procedures, however, there are limitations to the retroperitoneal approach. For example, in obese patients with a large kidney, retroperitoneal endoscopic excision is technically difficult. Some people have advocated that with the use of a retroperitoneal approach, one can also do a small incision and remove the kidney as a combination of endoscopic and open surgery. In this fashion, the procedure may be accomplished with less morbidity for the patient. However, this technique has to be further evaluated.

The complexities of laparoscopic bowel surgery are clearly discussed in the final chapter, and I hope that these procedures will in due course be less technically demanding.

The content of this book is easily absorbed and logically enunciated. Moreover, Dr. Parra has illustrated his work with the same expertise with which he performs his surgery. I have no hesitation in recommending the book to all urology residents and practicing urologists, both those who are now laparoscopists and those who are new converts to this exciting field of urology.

Arthur D. Smith, M.D.
Chairman, Department of Urology
Long Island Jewish Medical Center
New Hyde Park, New York

Preface

Henry David Thoreau described new technology as "improved means to unimproved ends."

Laparoscopy in urology, after an initial phase of enthusiasm, has entered a period of declining interest. Is this the beginning of the end for laparoscopic surgery in urology? I believe not. It is instead the tempered evolution of any novel medical technique introduced to an arena replete with effective time-proven treatments.

All new technology should be examined critically prior to widespread implementation, but this rational sequence is very seldom accomplished in a controlled, unemotional or measured fashion. There are visionaries who with the best of interest vigorously apply new techniques within the context of sound critical academic pursuits. Unfortunately, there are also the entrepreneurs, who in search of a profitable gimmick, take advantage of the sensationalism associated with promising new, yet unproven, treatments for their own economic interest. Finally, there are the critics, the objective and the recalcitrant. The latter view any drastic change in their environment as an example of yet another unnecessary piece of technology in search of a disease. Closely watching, the former is the bulk of practicing physicians awaiting the results of conclusive clinical studies before deciding whether or not to include the new technology in their practice.

Within urologic laparoscopy we are witnessing both ends of the spectrum. A few individuals continue to apply laparoscopic surgery unconventionally, detracting from serious consideration of the method. Luckily, the majority of committed and interested urologic laparoscopic surgeons continue to work within the framework of scientific prudence. Indeed, present publications, including this text, place emphasis on the refinement of indications and proper guidelines for urologic laparoscopy. This continued scrutiny and fine tuning will eventually lead to thoughtfully applied and rewarding laparoscopic procedures. A case in point is the laparoscopic pelvic lymphadenectomy. Initially this procedure was enthusiastically, if somewhat indiscriminately, performed. However, experience has shown that when sound selection criteria are applied, few patients are appropriate candidates for laparoscopic staging, but those who are reap clear benefits in terms of decreased pain and a shorter convalescence.

In my opinion the ongoing process of defining the proper indications for this new technology is what has led to a seeming decrease in the use of laparoscopy in urology. I strongly believe this to be the correct approach and feel that, because we have embarked on this course, laparoscopic surgery in urology will not be a passing fad. It is here to stay, but only in those areas where a clear advantage over conventional surgery can be demonstrated.

Given this, the question arises as to who should perform laparoscopy. Anyone interested must make a serious commitment. Laparoscopic procedures should not be cavalierly undertaken nor should they be performed as an occasional adventure. Unlike our colleagues, the general surgeons, we lack an organ analogous to the gallbladder in which the advantages of the approach virtually forced the acquisition of laparoscopic skills. For the general practicing urologist, the opportunities to apply laparoscopic surgery are less frequent. The occasional lymphadenectomy and the even less common nephrectomy do not justify the effort and expense necessary to incorporate laparoscopy into his or her armamentarium. It is more likely that laparoscopy in urology will be carried out in referral centers where it will ultimately be more efficiently performed.

When I became interested in publishing this book two years ago, the goal was to create a lasting and practical reference. The process has proved tedious and difficult to consummate, because we have tried to identify the procedures and corresponding indications most likely to stand the test of time. At the same time we were compelled to monitor the meteoric day-to-day changes occurring in this modality with an eye to the significant and practical. Unfortunately, for many of these new procedures, adequate information is not available to predict their eventual durability. Despite this, we have included descriptions of these techniques, because, in the words of Dr. Owen Wagesteen: "The past never returns, but the character of the future can be determined, in part, by what is done in the present."

Raul O. Parra, M.D., F.A.C.S.

Acknowledgments

No book would be complete without taking time to acknowledge the efforts of those who have labored mightily behind the scenes to bring this effort to fruition. My secretarial staff, Mary Ann Barrale and Debra Forrest have been very faithful in working long hours to type manuscripts and coordinate communications amongst myself and the various authors. Without their diligence, kindness, and good humor none of these pages would have appeared today.

Dr. Boullier and I would also like to thank the other members of the faculty of the Division of Urology at St. Louis University not only for contributing to this book with manuscripts but also for being a source of ideas and gentle criticism when needed.

Finally, we would like to thank the contributors for their diligence in providing the material requested of them in a timely and clear fashion. Their insights into the area of urologic laparoscopy have also served to educate us in many ways.

UROLOGIC
Laparoscopic Surgery

SECTION ONE

General Laparoscopy

1

History and Evolution of Laparoscopic Surgery

Paul G. Hagood

Introduction

The Hippocratic injunction to "do no harm" is considered a relative term in modern medical practice. The physician realizes that every manipulation and treatment designed to do good must of necessity inflict some harm. In all surgical fields precedence suggests that some morbidity is an immutable trade-off for the greater good of the cure. Recently, advances in laparoscopy have allowed us to rethink the fixed realities of surgical morbidity.

Given the obvious advantages laparoscopy presents, the most pregnant question concerning the history of its development is, "Why not sooner?" The elegance of laparoscopy is apparent with the first view of the abdomen, but this view remained relatively unappreciated long after the inventions that made it possible were in existence. Surgeons may have envisioned laparoscopy as early as 1864.[1] Records that describe direct visual inspection of body cavities are as ancient as the Talmud.[2] A review of the time line detailing the significant inventions,

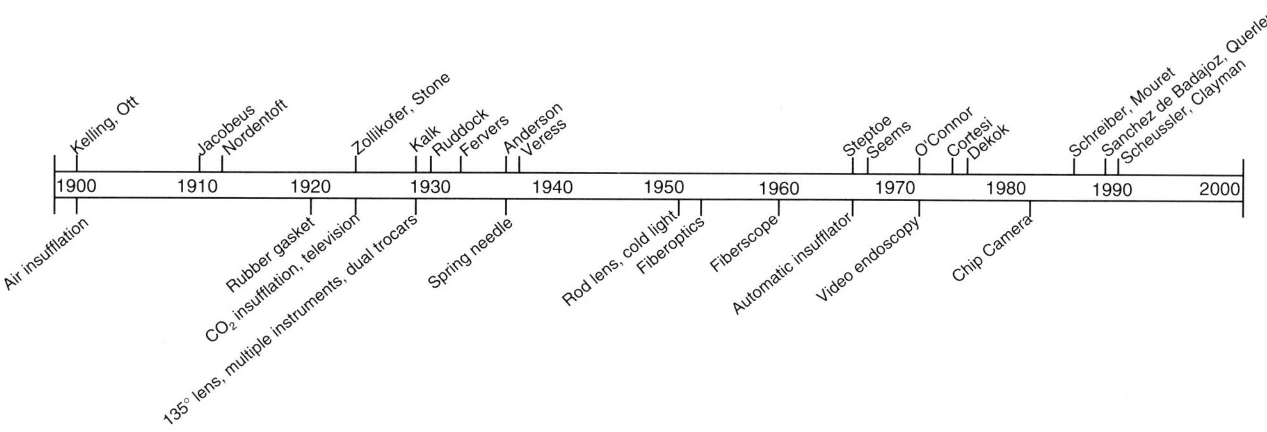

Figure 1-1 Laparoscopic time line. Top, medical innovators. Bottom, technical achievements.

diagnostic uses, and therapies attempted laparoscopically demonstrates that most of the landmarks were achieved early in the twentieth century, certainly by the 1940s (Fig. 1-1). The lack of acceptance of laparoscopy between 1941 and 1989 cannot reasonably be ascribed to a lack of technology. During this period little laparoscopy was attempted outside the gynecologic arena. Even among gynecologists, the use of the laparoscope was controversial. Although Rudduck had performed over 500 laparoscopic operations by 1930 and the first therapeutic intervention had been described in 1941,[3] 20 years later, in 1961, a report on a tubal ligation was still considered groundbreaking.[4] Of course there were considerable obstacles to overcome, and laparoscopy was more dangerous in its infancy. In response to the complications of laparoscopy, Decker devised the culdoscopic method of pelvic investigation in 1944.[5] Unfortunately, the practical effect of the introduction of culdoscopy was to dampen the minimal enthusiasm for laparoscopy for the next 20 years.[6] It would be imprudent, however, to blame the gynecologists for limiting the expansion of laparoscopy in these decades, when in fact they as a group were the only ones to show any concerted interest in the field.

The forces and genius that brought laparoscopy to its present state are well documented (the reader is directed to the excellent text by H. J. Rueter and M. A. Rueter and the outline by Gomel and Taylor), but it is doubtful they are completely understood or appreciated.[7,8] A review of the history of laparoscopy with its fitful starts and stops would be instructive in helping us to see its future. This history begins in antiquity with the founding of endoscopy.

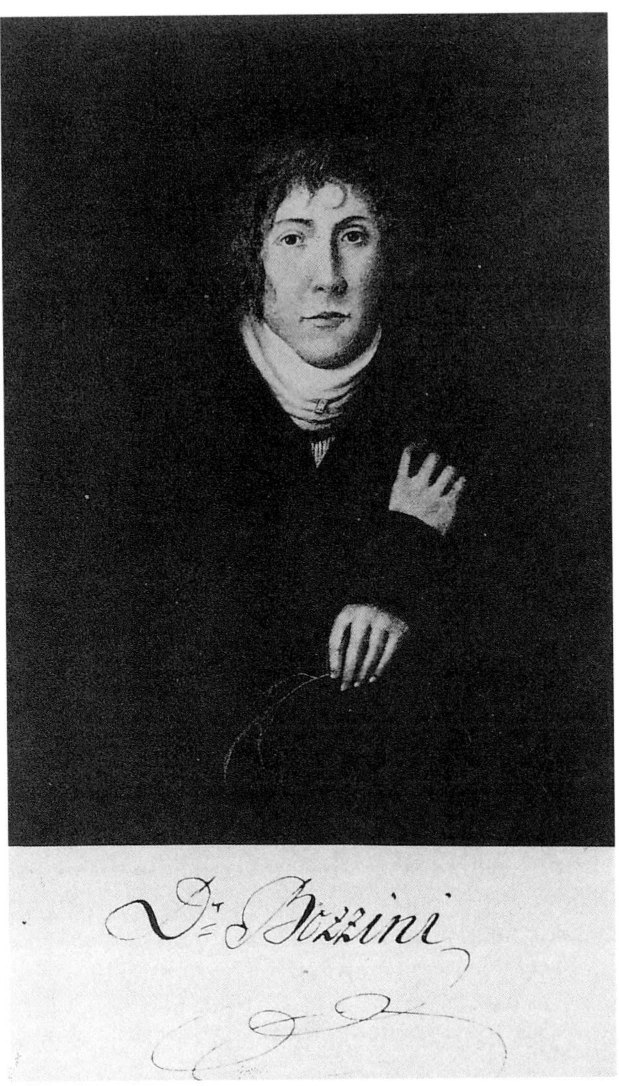

Figure 1-2 Dr. Philipp Bozzini.

Endoscopy

Hippocrates II (460–375 B.C.) wrote, "Then lay the patient backwards and look with the speculum to see where the rectum is affected."[6] The Talmud refers to a *siphopherot* made of lead, bent at its tip with a *mechul* (wooden mandarin) used for inspection of the vagina.[2] Numerous vaginal speculums dating back to the early first century A.D. have been discovered.[7]

The first lamp for endoscopy was a shielded burglar's lantern, employed by Arnaud in his full-time job as a gynecologist.[8] In 1805, Bozzini developed the first self-contained endoscope. This *Lichtleiter* was primitive, but it provided access to a hollow organ and enabled light to enter and exit a body cavity.[9] This brilliant and unconventional pioneer was officially reprimanded by the local medical society for undue curiosity, having been so bold as to place this instrument into the urethra of a patient and attempt direct bladder inspection.[8] Although he died at age 36 of typhoid fever, Bozzini's abbreviated career is generally considered the beginning of modern endoscopy[1,7,8] (Fig. 1-2).

Over the next 30 years numerous people experimented with various instruments, but the first endoscope that enabled the physician to actually see (a marked improvement) was invented by Antonin Jean Desormeaux in 1853[10] (Fig. 1-3). The design of this cystoscope (*l'endoscope*) was similar to those

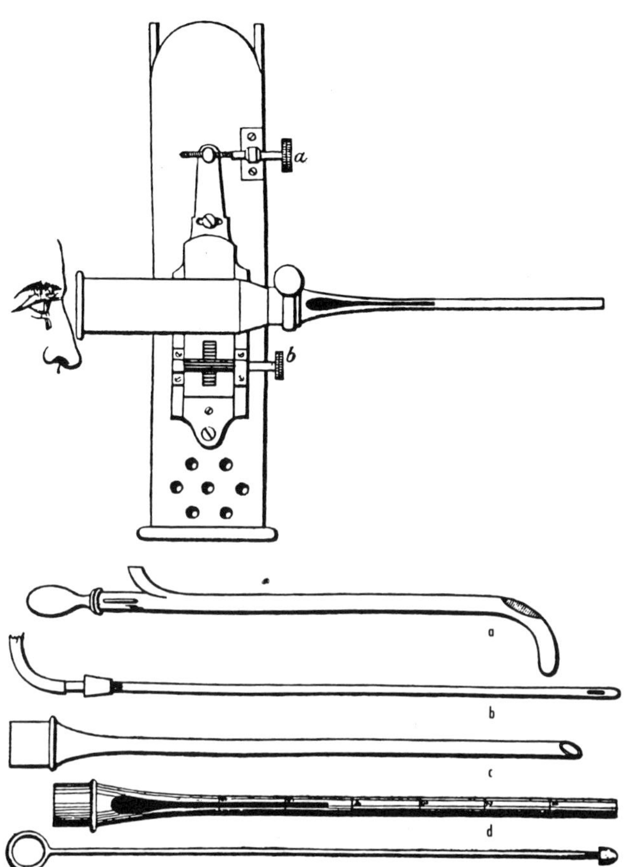

Figure 1-3 Endoscope of Dr. Francis Cruise after Desormeaux instrument.

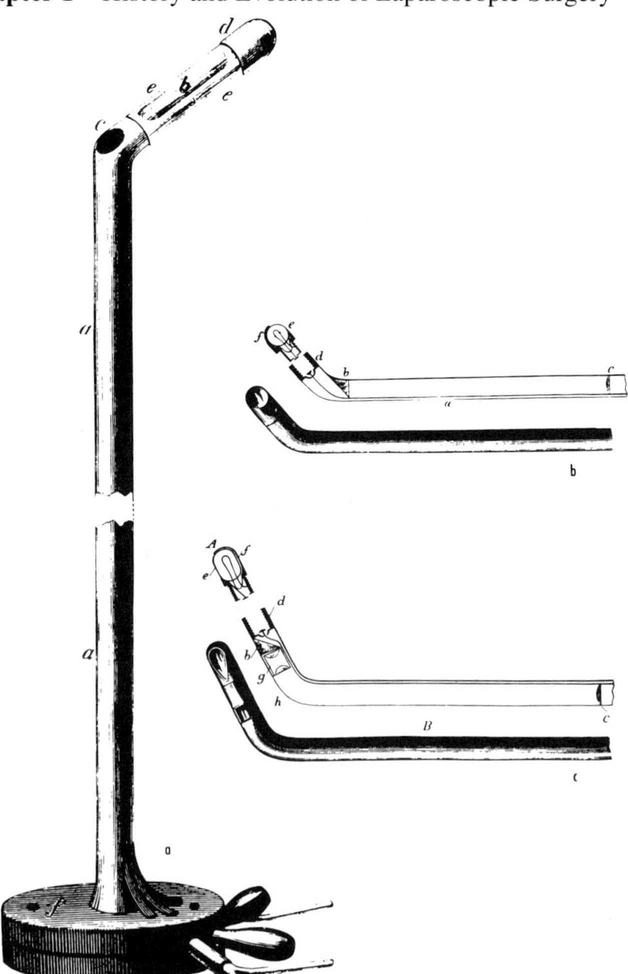

Figure 1-4 The Nitze cystoscope.

constructed by Pierre S. Ségalas in Paris and John D. Fisher in Boston some 20 years before.[11,12] The otoscope designed by Jean-Pierre Bonnafont in 1834 even more closely resembled the machine Desormeaux produced, so much so that strenuous objections were made at the medical academy to giving Desormeaux precedence.[7] Desormeaux went on to do extensive clinical work with endoscopy, presenting remarkable descriptions of various scopes with diagnostic and therapeutic interventions described. Cruise stated that although others (including Avery, Ségalas, and Haken) had preceded him, Desormeaux was an exception in that he was "most indefatigably" at the work of endoscopy.[1] There were more than a few skeptics though. As Furstenheim reported, when Desormeaux demonstrated stones in the bladder to ten physicians, there were always three or four who insisted they saw nothing.[13]

The true forerunner of the modern cystoscope was introduced by Max Nitze on October 2, 1877, before the National Medical College in Dresden[14] (Fig. 1-4). Nitze was the first to introduce glass optics for magnification. The creation of this instrument depended on industry, ingenuity, and serendipity. While cleaning a microscopic eyepiece, Nitze viewed the Matthäi-Church across the street and saw the image inverted and reduced. He recognized an immediate application of optics to the emerging field of endoscopy.[7] He also used a glowing platinum wire for illumination, after the manner of Bruck.[15] Because this new instrument required continuous water cooling, cystoscopy preceded other forms of endoscopy. Nevertheless, these technical limitations did not seem to dampen the enthusiasm of investigators in the latter half of the 19th century. Working in Ireland, Cruise stated with remarkable vision that "there is no part of the human body into which a straight tube can be placed where it will not be found of use."[1] With Edison's incorporation of a carbon filament into a vacuum tube in 1880,[16] the heat generated by the incandescent bulb was low enough to allow for close inspection of living tissue.[7] Mignon miniaturized the Edison lamp, making

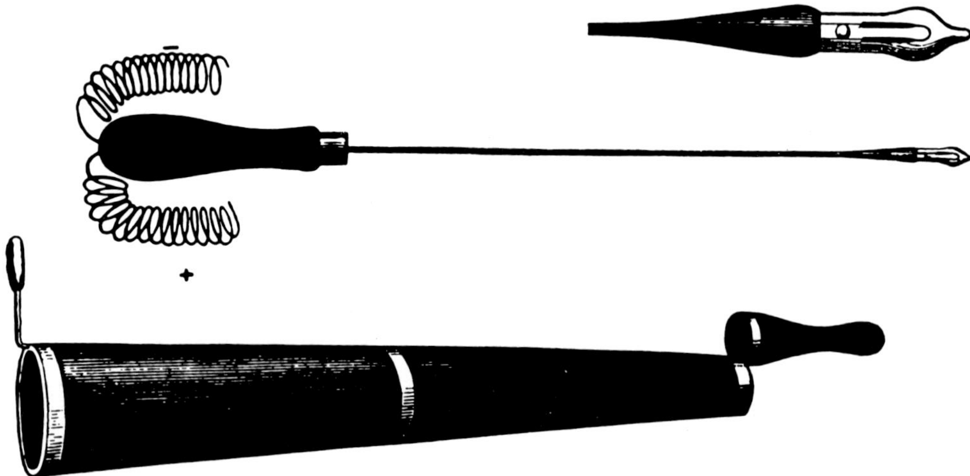

Figure 1-5 Newman's cystoscope with mignon lamp

it practical for endoscopy.[16] David Newman in Scotland is generally credited with being the first to incorporate a Mignon light into the endoscope.[17] Although some insist Dittel preceded Newman in affixing the light distally,[8] the illustration of Newman's cystoscope for females clearly demonstrates that the lamp is to be placed within the bladder (Fig. 1-5). Boisseau de Rocher introduced a Mignon lamp cystoscope in 1890 that offered the first double channel for ureteral catheterization. Even more important, he separated the optics from the sheath, paving the way for his own introduction of interchangeable lenses.[18,19] With these and many related inventions, the nineteenth century closed with intense interest in endoscopy. Laparoscopy of necessity arose from general endoscopy. It is probably not coincidence, then, that laparoscopy started in Dresden, where Nitze first worked.

Laparoscopy

Laparoscopy rose and fell in popularity, and rose again with the tides of larger, often unrelated surgical currents. Small incisions were the fad in the late nineteenth and early twentieth centuries, and surgeons such as "Button Hole Thompson" held sway.[7] Not only was the ability to operate through the smallest of incisions considered evidence of style and surgical grace, on a more practical level the patient's immediate survival and quality of recovery directly depended on the size of the incision and the speed and skill of the surgeon. The *Lancet* recorded lively polemics between noted surgeons on the propriety of various boutonniere incisions and endoscopy.[20] It is not surprising that it is within this era that laparoscopy was born.

Fenwick introduced a trocar cystoscope for suprapubic exam in 1889.[21] This was significant in that the natural orifice was not used for access. Cadaveric experiments with abdominal wall puncture exams of the bladder had been performed for some time, even dating back to the *Lichtleiter*.[7] Instrument or telescopic inspection of a body cavity without any natural orifice was performed in 1901 by two independent investigators. Kelling in Dresden used a Nitze cystoscope to view the abdomen of a dog.[22] Ott, working in Petrograd a few months prior, used a speculum and head lamp for illumination of the abdomen.[23] Kelling went on to complete many serious investigations of the technique in animals, but the first reports of clinical trials in humans were published by Jacobeus in Sweden some 10 years later.[24] Jacobeus had wide experience with the method and reported on thoroscopic and laparoscopic procedures performed as early as 1910.[25] By 1912 he had performed closed-cavity endoscopy with a Nitze cystoscope in over 100 patients. Following this he devoted most of his attention to thoroscopy. His report from 1923 also described the first bleeding complication requiring laparotomy.[8] From his body of work endoscopy and laparoscopy diverged.

Curiously, numerous investigators at this time described their independent development of laparoscopy. It was common for the American surgeons not to have heard of work going on in Europe. Orndoff in 1920,[26] Stone in 1924,[27] and Steiner in 1924[28] all presented their description of a "new technic" for abdominal examination. To their credit, their work was in fact original, each added to the technique, and all eventually learned of and openly acknowledged the work of the Europeans. In perspective, this phenomenon illustrates the relative lack of interest in the procedure at the time, as well as the difficulty all physicians have in surveying the available literature.

Significant contributions to the technique were made by C. Fervers in 1933 and Janos Veress in 1938. Fervers is often credited with recommending CO_2 as the insufflating agent,[25,29] although Zollifker probably introduced the idea in 1924.[30] Fervers was the first to actively and consistently engage in therapeutic laparoscopy, and he described the procedures of abdominal adhesiolysis and viscera biopsy with instruments of his own design. Veress in Hungary is credited with inventing the spring-loaded cannula still in use today (although prototypes had been suggested by Boesch earlier).[8,31] Kalk, a hepatologist, performed numerous exams and liver biopsies. His numerous and massive treatises described many instruments, and he was the first to propose the use of dual trocars. He also introduced the 135-degree foroblique lens in 1929.[32]

During this same period of time, remarkable discoveries were made that created modern surgery. Anesthesia, antibiotics, and antisepsis made elective surgery a reality. Antibiotics alone decreased the mortality of surgeries to tolerable levels in the middle of this century, and as a result complex surgeries never before realistically attempted became routinely possible. As the complexity of surgeries increased, the doctrine of surgical exploration expanded exponentially. The pendulum had swung away from the buttonhole incision.

In this middle era laparoscopy was promulgated by a dedicated few. The first therapeutic laparoscopies were introduced by the gynecologists, but it was almost 20 years from when the technology was first used to when it was even debated in a serious fashion. Anderson suggested a laparoscopic method of tubal fulguration in 1937 and even described instruments of his own design to accomplish this. It is uncertain, however, if he ever performed the operation.[33] Using electrocautery, Powers and Barnes performed tubal ligation as early as 1941.[3] Neuman and Frick, working with monkeys in 1961, demonstrated that a cystoscopic instrument could be adapted to act as a surgical clip applier to the fallopian tubes.[8] They recommended a culdoscopic approach to the tubes and had entered patients into a clinical trial when Palmer in 1962 reported the electrocautery fulguration of the fallopian tubes.[4] This generated considerably more attention than the 1941 communications. Although these reports should be considered milestones, few non-gynecologists seemed to understand their implications.

Significant technical improvements in endoscopic optics were made in the early 1950s. Specifically, the invention of the proximal light source by Fourestiere, Gladu, and Vulmiere[34] and the Hopkins[8] rod lens optics decreased the size of the telescope and significantly improved the image, eventually making the endoscope accommodating to more cavities and tools. The invention of the fiberoptic endoscope by Hirschowitz in 1960 would also prove essential for the development of laparoscopy.[35] From this point a long series of events would conspire to make laparoscopy attractive to surgeons at large. One was a technical achievement, one a diagnostic redefinition, and one a sociopolitical contrivance.

Therapeutic Laparoscopy

To a small degree therapeutic laparoscopy was delayed until Philo T. Farnsworth and John L. Baird's invention—the television—had become sophisticated enough to enable all members of the surgical team to participate in the operation. It is argued that the sterilizable miniature television camera has made therapeutic laparoscopy possible. It is doubtful, though, that the lull in laparoscopy resulted entirely from a lack of either invention or imagination. Television dates to January 27, 1926, when in J. L. Baird's laboratory the first wired transmission of a "televisor" image took place.[36] The tube image system developed by Farnsworth in the fall of 1927[37] was essentially the same system used for video arthroscopy in 1973[38] (Fig. 1-6). Obviously significant refinements were made along the way. Closed circuit television programs of endoscopic procedures were produced using Fourestiere's systems in 1959. A fiberscopic attachment to an 18-lb, three-tube camera was the first color video system used. By 1973 cameras were attached directly to the endoscopes, and by 1975 the tube cameras were as small as 2" × 2" × 8" and weighed 1.25 lb. Solid-state technology in 1981 produced the chip camera (CCD), dramatically reducing the size and weight of

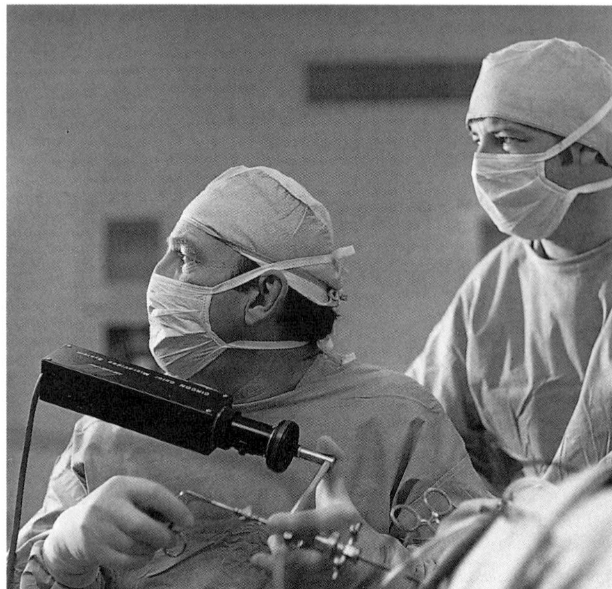

Figure 1-6 Dr. O'Connor performing first video arthroscopy

endoscopic cameras and ushering in the video revolution.[38,39] Of course it was not until 1989 that the revolution actually started. Considerable prejudice against laparoscopy limited the application of the technology.

Laparoscopy also waited on the decline of the doctrine of surgical diagnostics. By the middle 1970s advanced noninvasive methods of diagnosis had essentially eliminated the diagnostic laparotomy. As the need for diagnostic laparotomy waned, surgeons began to rethink surgical interventions and seriously investigate minimally invasive therapy. Most historians point to Semm's work in the late 1960s as the birth of modern laparoscopy and the concept of minimally invasive therapy.[8,25]

In large part the hesitancy to accept laparoscopy is based on the simple fact that laparoscopy does little to increase the efficacy of the surgical intervention. Laparoscopy decreases patient morbidity, but it does not offer a more accurate assessment of pelvic nodes,[40,41] a cleaner extirpation of a renal mass,[42] or a remarkably better success rate for varix ablation.[43] In fact, in most cases, the laparoscopic procedure is considerably more difficult for the uninitiated.[44,45] To overcome the inertia of this argument a considerable external social force had to be applied. More important than the television camera or non invasive diagnostics, consumer advocacy ushered in the modern era of laparoscopy.

The first laparoscopic cholecystectomy was not performed until 1987, by Philippe Mouret[46] in Lyon, France. This was done incidental to a laparoscopy being performed to monitor and assist a vaginal hysterectomy. For whatever reason, Mouret did not publish any reports on the procedure, but he introduced it to his colleague Dubois. Dubois then performed the operation in some 50 patients, wrote the first description and presented a film of the procedure at the Society of American Gastrointestinal Endoscopic Surgeons meeting in Louisville in 1989.[47] Not surprisingly the initial reaction was one of "shock and disbelief" in the surgical community. Widespread skepticism prevailed at the highest levels of the medical establishment. With censure considered by some, the initial reviews were "highly critical, incredulous and strongly sarcastic," reminiscent of Bozzini's experience.[48] Nevertheless, an energetic and enterprising surgeon, Eddie Joe Reddick, saw the presentation by Dubois, immediately duplicated the procedure, and presented it to the American public (and secondarily to the American surgical community) with great fanfare.[49]

Upon its debut, laparoscopic cholecystectomy attracted considerable attention in the lay press, and a myriad of nicknames such as "Nintendo"[50] and "Keyhole"[51] surgery were given to the technique. Waving newspaper clippings, patients were requesting a laparoscopic cholecystectomy within days of the announcement that it had been done by Reddick in Nashville.[52] In response to the tepid initial reaction by the medical establishment, Perissat and Vitale wrote, "One can be cynical about this explosion of interest in the new laparoscopic surgery, but the fact is that it is our patients who encourage us to move forward."[48] These parallel the sentiments of Cruise in 1865 when he wrote, "*Apropos* to the slight shown towards the endoscope, a long and amusing history might be written of the opposition which has greeted every improvement in the science and art of medicine from its earliest date. Frivolous objections avail nothing at the time they are advanced, and only afford material for merriment and ridicule in the future."[1] More remarkable than the convolutions in the introduction of the laparoscopic cholecystectomy is that in less than 5 years it has essentially replaced the open procedure, with nearly 80% of all cholecystectomies now being done laparoscopically.[48]

Urologic Laparoscopy

Progress in acknowledging the laparoscopic potential in urology followed the same course, although the time scale was markedly truncated. Schuessler, in private practice in Texas, startled the urologic community with the presentation of a common procedure, (pelvic lymphadenectomy), turned laparoscopic.[53] The first series of laparoscopic pelvic lymphadenectomies was published by Querleu for staging cervical cancer.[54] Shortly thereafter, Schuessler reported his initial experience.[53] Although laparoscopic explorations for undescended testis had been done previous to this report, its impact was marginal, with the procedure being dismissed as amenable to few patients with little other clinical applicability. Since Schuessler's report there has been an explosion of urologic procedures attempted laparoscopically and a deluge of reports and videos generated to document the progress. A list of recent urologic accomplishments is included in Table 1-1.

In a few cases the laparoscope will become the defining tool for the urologist, as it has for the cholecystectomy. Lymphocele drainage and revision of continuous ambulatory peritoneal dialysis (CAPD) catheters may be among the few procedures where the laparoscope exceeds any other technology.[55,56]

More often, though, it will become a refining tool. Parra demonstrated that not every patient is a candidate for a laparoscopic node dissection, but select patients will benefit greatly.[57] Jordan has shown convincingly that there is a definite but not all-inclusive role for laparoscopy in the diagnosis and treatment of undescended testis.[58] Laparoscopy has also been shown to be a legitimate alternative for the treatment of varicoceles, especially bilateral veins.[43] The utility of other procedures such as nephrectomy,[42] cystectomy,[59] and diverticulectomy[60] is still unknown, and these may remain oddities with only rare academic applicability.

The Future of Laparoscopy

Many reviewers emphasize the importance of emerging technology in the field of laparoscopy. On the immediate horizon are three CCD cameras; High Definition Video, Biplanar (3-D) systems, and Virtual Reality software.[38] Most important, the escape from analog equipment to complete digital systems

TABLE 1-1 Urologic Laparoscopic Highlights (Date of published report)

Cortesi (1976)[63]	Examination for intra-abdominal testes in adults
Wichham(1979)[64]	Retroperitoneoscopy for ureterolithotomy
Silber (1980)[65]	Examination for intra-abdominal testis in child
Hald(1980)[66]	Extraperitoneal pelviscopy for lymphadenectomy
Fuerst (1985)[67]	Laparoscopic exam of pelvic nodes with isosulfan blue
Sanchez de Badajoz(1990)[68]	Varix ablation
Querleu (1991)[54]	Pelvic lymphadenectomy, female
Schuessler (1991)[53]	Pelvic lymphadenectomy, male
Clayman (1991)[42]	Simple nephrectomy/Endobag
Schuessler (1991)[69]	Bladder neck suspension
McCollough (1991)[70]	Lymphocele marsupialization
Hagood (1992)[43]	Varix ligation
Parra (1992)[60]	Diverticulectomy
Lowe(1992)[71]	Partial cystectomy
Kozminski (1992)[72]	Laparoscopically assisted ileal conduit
Gaur (1992)[61]	Retroperitoneal nephrectomy
Kaoussi (1992)[73]	Ureterolysis
Nezhat (1992)[74]	Uretero-ureterostomy
Waterhouse (1992)[75]	Retroperitoneal lymphadenectomy
Clayman (1992)[7]	Nephroureterectomy
Schuessler (1992)[77]	Radical prostatectomy
Morgan (1992)[78]	Renal cyst marsupialization
Winfield (1993)[79]	Partial nephrectomy

will significantly boost resolution and recording, and (for better or worse) end product manipulation. The intent is to bring laparoscopy back to the surgeon, removing the technical wedge between him and the patient by making the camera as sensitive as the eye and the instruments as mobile as the hand.

Much work needs to be done in the surgical arena in terms of providing adequate exposure for complex cases and improving suturing and anastomosing techniques. Gaur's work in retroperitoneoscopy is exceptional and will be a source of many advances in the near future.[61]

Although some insist that virtually all procedures will be done laparoscopically by the 21st century,[62] we can never lose sight of the fact that laparoscopy is considerably more tedious and less exacting than traditional surgery in some cases. It is essential to remember that a decrease in morbidity is not always a justified trade-off for diminished efficacy and possibly increased mortality. More important, it remains to be seen if laparoscopy can introduce novel procedures and not just telescopic imitations of old practices.

Eventually, we anticipate that most urologists will feel as comfortable with laparoscopy as with any other technique available and will be able to use it when indicated, not just when feasible. As we mentioned before, laparoscopy does decrease patient morbidity. Much work needs to be done to refine the indications. Laparoscopy was truly born in our specialty, and we should be reluctant to yield any endoscopic procedure within our domain.

References

1. Cruise FR: The utility of the endoscope as an aid in the diagnosis and treatment of disease. *Dublin Qt J Med Sci* 39:329, 1865.
2. Kielleuthner L: Geschichte der Urologie. *Mu Med Wo Schr* 76:1652, 1929.
3. Power SH, Barnes AC: Sterilization by means of peritoneoscopic tubal fulguration: Preliminary report. *Am J Obstet Gynecol* 41:1038, 1941 .
4. Palmer R: Laparoscopic tubal fulguration. *Bull Féd Gynecol Obstet Langue Francaise* 14:298, 1962.
5. Decker A, Cherry T: Culdoscopy: A new method in diagnosis of pelvic disease. *Am J Surg* 64:40, 1944.
6. Toellner R: *Histoire de la medicine, de la pharmacie, de l'art dentaire t de l'art veterinaire.* Paris, 1978.
7. Rueter HJ, Rueter MA: *Philipp Bozzini and Endoscopy in the 19th Century.* Stuttgart: Max Nitze Museum, p 25, 1988.
8. Gomel V, Taylor PJ: Introduction, In *Laparoscopy and Hysteroscopy in Gynecologic Practice.* Edited by Gomel V, Taylor PJ, Yuzpe AA, Rioux JE, Chicago: Year Book Medical Publishers, p 1, 1986.
9. Bozzini P: Lichtleiter, eine erfindung zur anschauung innerre theile und krankheiten nebst der abbildung. *J Pract Arzneykunde u Wundarzneykunft* 24:107, 1806. Reprinted in Reuter HJ, Rueter MA: Philipp Bozzini and Endoscopy in the 19th Century. Stuttgart; Max Nitze Museum, p 142, 1988.
10. Desormeaux AJ: De l'endoscope et de ses applications au diagnostic et au traitement des affections de l'urethre et de la vessie. *Paris 1865.*
11. Segalas PS: Handworterbuch der ges chir und augenheilkunde. *Walther Jager Radius (Leipzig)* 1:614, 1839.
12. Hays, I: Instruments for illuminating dark cavities. *J Med Physic Sci (Philadelphia)* 14:409, 1827.
13. Fürstenheim E: Notizen über das endoskop und seime verwerthung besonders in krankheitien der harnwege. *Dtsch Klinik* 32:313, 1863.
14. Nitze M: Demonstration seines beleuxhtungssapparats der harnewege. *Verh Dtsch Ges Chir* 9:91, 1881.
15. Bruck J: *Das urethroskop zur durchleuchtung der blase und ihrer nachbarteile durch galvanisches gluhlicht.* Breslau, 1867.
16. McNeil I: *An Encyclopedia of the History of Technology.* New York: Rutledge Press, 1990.
17. Newman D: *Lectures on Surgical Diseases of the Kidney.* London, 1888.
18. De Rocher B: Perfectionnements a la cystoscopie. *Ann Mal Org. Genito-Urin* 8:65, 1890.
19. De Rocher B: Cystoscopie et catheterisme des uretes. *Ann Mal Org Genito-Urin* 10:413, 1892.
20. Thompson, H: Remarks on the use of the endoscope. *Lancet* 1:20, 1866.
21. Fenwick EH: *The Electric Illumination of the Bladder and Urethra.* London, 1888.

22. Kelling G: Zur coelioskopie. *Arch Klin Chir* 126:226, 1923.

23. Ott O: Die direkte beleuchtung der bauchhohle, der harnblase, des dickdarms und des utgerus zu diagnostichen zwecken. *Rev Med Tcheque* (Prague) 2:27, 1909.

24. Jacobeus HC: Kurze ubersicht über meine erfahrungen mit der laparoskopie. *Munch Med Wschr* 58:2017, 1911.

25. Gunning J: The history of laparoscopy. *J Reprod Med* 12:6, 1974.

26. Orndoff RH: The peritoneoscope in diagnosis of diseases of the abdomen. *J Radiol* 1:307, 1920.

27. Stone ZE: Intra-abdominal examination with the aid of the peritoneoscope. *J Kans Med Soc* 24:63, 1924.

28. Steiner OP: Abdominoscopy. *Surg Gynecol Obstet* 38:266, 1924.

29. Fervers C: Die laparoskopie mit dem cystoskop. *Medsche Klin* 29:1042, 1933.

30. Nadeau OE, Kampmeir OF: Endoscopy of the abdomen: Abdominoscopy. A preliminary study, including a summary of the literature and a description of the technique. *Surg Gynecol Obstet* 41:259, 1925.

31. Veress J: Neues instrument zur ausfuhrung von brust-oder bauchpunktionen und pneumothorax behandlung. *Detsch Med Wschr* 41:1480, 1938.

32. Kalk H: Erfahrungen mit der laparoskopie. *Zu-Klin Med* 111:303, 1929.

33. Anderson ET: Peritoneoscopy. *Am J Surg* 35:136, 1937.

34. Fourestier N, Gladu A, Vulmiere J: Perfectionnnements a l'endoscopic medicale: Realization bronchoscopique. *Presse Med* 60:1292, 1952 .

35. Hirschowitz BJ: A personal history of the fiberscope. *Gastroenterologie* 76:864, 1979.

36. Tiltman RF: *The Baird of Television.* New York: Arno Press, 1974.

37. Everson GA: *The Story of Television: The Life of Philo T. Farnsworth.* New York: Arno Press, 1974.

38. Miller F: Personal communications. VP Research and Development (emeritus), Circon Corp., Santa Barbara, CA.

39. Brehm J: Personal communications. VP Sales and Administration, Medical Dynamics, Inc., Englewood, CO.

40. Parra RO, Andrus C, Boullier J: Staging laparoscopic pelvic lymph node dissection: Comparison of results with open pelvic lymphadenectomy. *J Urol* 147:857, 1992.

41. Guazzoni G, Montorsi F, Berfamaschi F, et al: Open surgical revision of Laparoscopic pelvic lymphadenectomy for staging of prostate cancer: Impact of laparoscopic learning curve. *J Uro* 151:930, 1994.

42. Clayman RV, Kavoussi LR, Soper NJ, et al: Laparoscopic nephrectomy: Initial case report. *J Urol* 146:278, 1991.

43 Hagood PG, Mehan DJ, Worischeck JH, Andrus CH, Parra RO: Laparoscopic varicocelectomy: Preliminary report of a new technique. *J Urol* 147:73, 1992.

44. Sackier JM, Berci G: Diagnostic and interventional laparoscopy for the general surgeon. *Cont Surg* 37:15, 1990.

45. Parra RO, Hagood PG, Boullier JA, Cummings JM, Mehan DJ: Complications of laparoscopic urological surgery: Experience at St. Louis University. *J Urol* 151:681, 1994.

46. Cuschieri A, Dubois F, Mouiel R, Mouret P, et al: The European experience with laparoscopic cholecystectomy. *Am J Surg* 161:385, 1991.

47. Dubois F, Berthelots G, Levard H: Cholecystectomy par coelioscopie. *Presse Med* 18:980, 1989.

48. Perissat J, Vitale GC: Laparoscopic cholecystectomy: Gateway to the Future (Editorial). *Am J Surg* 161:408, 1991.

49. Reddick EJ, Olsen DO: Laparoscopic laser cholecystectomy: a comparison with mini-lap cholecystectomy. *Surg Endosc* 3:131, 1989.

50. Satava RM: Nintendo surgery (innovations in surgery). *JAMA* 267:2329, 1992.

51. Faivelson S: "Keyhole" cholecystectomy injuries prompt call for better training. *Med World News* 33:27, 1992.

52. Cowley G: Hanging up the knife: A novel surgical technique promises to save patients time, money and blood. *Newsweek* 115(7):58, Feb 12, 1990.

53. Schuessler WW, Vancaillie TG, Reich H, Griffith DP: Transperitoneal endosurgical lymphadenectomy in patients with localized prostate cancer. *J Urol* 145:988, 1991.

54. Querleu D, LeBlanc E, Castelain B: Laparoscopic pelvic lymphadenectomy in the staging of early carcinoma of the cervix. *Am J Obstet Gynecol* 164:579, 1991.

55. Parra RO, Jones JP, Hagood PG: Laparoscopic intraperitoneal marsupialization: Report on a new technic for lymphoceles. *Surg Laparosc Endosc* 2:306, 1992.

56. Brunk, E: Peritoneoscopic placement of a Tenckhoff catheter for chronic peritoneal dialysis. *Endoscopy* 17:186, 1985.
57. Parra RO, Andrus CH, Boullier JA: Staging laparoscopic pelvic lymph node dissection: Experience and indication. *Arch Surg* 127:1294, 1992.
58. Jordon J, Robey E, Winslow B: Laparoscopic management of the abdominal/trans-inguinal testis. *J Endourol* 6:143, 1992.
59. Parra RO, Andrus CH, Jones JP, Boullier JA: Laparoscopic cystectomy: Initial report on a new treatment for the retained bladder. *J Urol* 148:1140, 1992.
60. Parra RO, Jones JP, Andrus CH, Hagood PG: Laparoscopic diverticulectomy: Preliminary report of a new approach for the treatment of bladder diverticulum. *J Urol* 148:869, 1992.
61. Gaur, DD: Laparoscopic operative retroperitoneoscopy: Use of a new device. *J Urol* 148:1137, 1992.
62. Gomella LG, Strup S: The history of urologic laparoscopy: from cystoscope to laparoscope. In *Laparoscopic Urologic Surgery*. Edited by Gomella L, Kozminski M, Winfield H, New York, Year Book Medical Publishers, p 3, 1993.
63. Cortesi N, Ferrari P, Zambardae A, et al: Diagnosis of bilateral abdomen cryptorchidism by laparoscopy. *Endoscopy* 8:33, 1979.
64. Wickham JEA: The surgical treatment of renal lithiasis. In *Urinary Calculus Disease*. New York: Churchill Livingstone, p 145, 1979.
65. Silber SJ, Cohen R: Laparoscopy for cryptorchidism. *J Urol* 124:928, 1980.
66. Hald T, Rasmussen F: Extra peritoneal pelviscopy: A new aid in staging of lower urnary tract tumors: A preliminary report. *J Urol* 124:245, 1980.
67. Fuerst DE: Laparoscopic examination of the pelvic lymph nodes. *Urology* 26:482, 1985.
68. Sanchez de Badajoz E, Diaz-Ramirez F, Vara-Thorbeck C: Endoscopic varicocelectomy. *J Endourol* 4:317, 1990.
69. Schuessler WW, Vancailli TG: Laparoscopic bladder neck suspension. *J Laparoendosc Surg* 3:169, 1991.
70. McCullough CS, Soper NJ, Clayman RV, et al: Laparoscopic drainage of a post transplant lymphocele. *Transplantation* 51:725, 1991.
71. Lowe BA, Noy MJ, Strang E: Laparoscopic segmental cystectomy. *J Urol* 147:408A, 1992.
72. Kozminski M, Partamian KO: Case report of laparoscopic ileal loop conduit. *J Endourol* 6:(2):147, 1992.
73. Kavoussi LR, Clayman RV, Brunt LM, et al: Laparoscopic ureterolysis. *J Urol* 147:426, 1992.
74. Nezhat C, Nezhat F, Green B, Gonzalez G: Laparoscopic ureteroureterostomy. *J Endourol* 6:143, 1992.
75. Waterhouse RL, Stone NN, Schlussel RN: Laparoscopic retroperitoneal lymph node dissection for testicular cancer. *J Urol* 147:41A, 1992.
76. Clayman RV, Kavoussi LR, Firenshau RS, et al: Laparoscopic nephroureterectomy: Initial case report. *J Laparoendosc Surg* 1:343, 1991.
77. Schuessler WW, Kavoussi LR, Clayman RV. Laparoscopic radical prostatectomy: Initial case report. *J Urol* 147:246A, 1992.
78. Morgan C, Rader D: Laparoscopic unroofing of a renal cyst. *J Urol* 148:1835, 1992.
79. Winfield H, Donavan J, Godet AS, et al: Laparoscopic partial nephrectomy: Initial case report for benign disease. *J Endourol* 7:521, 1993.

2

Preoperative Preparation and Patient Selection

James M. Cummings
R. Ernest Sosa

Introduction

Careful patient selection, preparation, and adherence to basic surgical principles are essential to successful laparoscopic surgery. All candidates for endocavitary surgery should be carefully evaluated by a thorough history and physical examination, appropriate laboratory tests, and radiologic studies. Patients at high risk for a standard laparoscopic approach can undergo either an open operation or, if the surgeon's laparoscopic experience warrants it, a modified laparoscopic procedure.

Absolute Contraindications

Absolute contraindications for laparoscopy are listed in Table 2-1. Patients suffering from an infectious process afflicting the skin or integumental tissues of the abdominal wall such as cellulitis, impetigo, or frank abscess are at high risk for the introduction of intraperitoneal infection during access. However, if an appropriate antibiotic course effectively controls the infection, laparoscopy may be safely performed. If peritonitis is suspected on clinical grounds, under no circumstances should laparoscopy be entertained. In patients where signs and symptoms suggestive of intestinal obstruction exist, the entrance to the peritoneum is fraught with the risk of damaging dilated loops of bowel, with subsequent intraperitoneal contamination. Finally, individuals known to have a coagulation disorder such as hemophilia or other clotting factor defects should not be considered appropriate candidates for laparoscopic surgery despite the ability to temporarily correct the disorders. These patients are at risk for significant occult hemorrhage following release of the taponading effect of the pneumoperitoneum (Fig. 2-1).

TABLE 2-1 Absolute Contraindications

Infectious process of the skin or abdominal wall tissue
Active intraabdominal infections, "peritonitis"
Bowel obstruction
Uncorrectable coagulopathies

Relative Contraindications

The relative contraindications for laparoscopic surgery are listed in Table 2-2. For the novice laparoscopist the most acceptable patient for intervention is the thin, healthy individual with a virginal abdomen. Unfortunately, most urologic patients

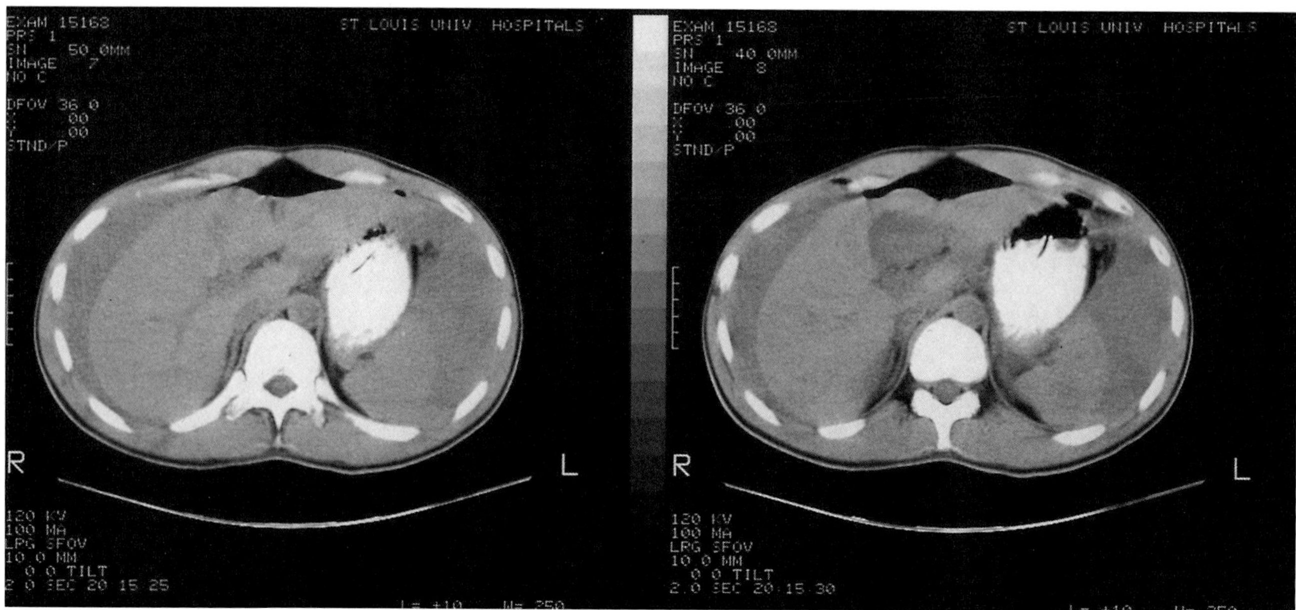

Figure 2-1 Abdominal CT of a hemophiliac patient following a laparoscopic varicocelectomy. Despite appropriate hematologic corrective measures preoperatively, massive intraperitoneal bleeding occurred.

who are candidates for laparoscopic surgery do not meet these criteria. Patients with a prior history of abdominal surgery, vascular aneurysms, tuberculosis, diverticulitis, appendicitis, and so on, are at greater risk for visceral and vascular injury during blind Veress needle and trocar insertion. Patients with vascular abnormalities such as portal hypertension present special problems with regard to hemostasis during access. Many of these patients can be successfully managed laparoscopically using an open trocar placement technique (Chap. 5). Additionally, establishing a pneumoperitoneum and inserting the trocars may be difficult in obese patients. However, new instrumentation has been developed to accommodate such individuals. Patients with a history of umbilical or urachal abnormalities such as Prune Belly Syndrome and prior umbilical hernia repair can present problems when not appreciated preoperatively. Communicating hydroceles can lead to the development of a significant pneumoscrotum that is best anticipated prior to surgery. In patients with unreducible inguinal or abdominal wall hernias the pneumoperitoneum may lead to vascular compromise of the incarcerated bowel. The physiologic challenges posed by laparoscopy differ in many ways from the challenges of open surgery. The increased intraabdominal pressure of insufflation diminishes venous return to the heart, thereby decreasing cardiac output and increasing intrathoracic pressure.[1-7] Ventilatory rates and volumes must be increased gradually to maintain the PCO_2 at a physiologically safe level. The resultant increase in intrathoracic pressure further diminishes the venous return to the heart. It is evident that patients with severe cardiac or chronic obstructive pulmonary disease are not good candidates for laparoscopy.[2] Likewise patients with a hiatal hernia do not tolerate extreme Trendelenburg positions when combined with the previously mentioned physiologic stresses posed by the pneumoperitoneum.

TABLE 2-2 Relative Contraindications

Previous abdominal/pelvic surgery
Vascular abnormalities
Previous intraabdominal inflammatory/infectious process
Obesity
Umbilical or urachal abnormalities
Communicating hydroceles
Unreducible inguinal or abdominal wall hernias
Cardiopulmonary disease
Hiatal hernia

TABLE 2-3 Patient Preparation

Routine Procedures (varicocele, lymphadenectomy)

- NPO past midnight
- May have oral medication with a sip of water day of surgery
- Stop all potential anticoagulants (aspirin, NSAIDs)
- CBC, Chem 18, PT and PTT, Type and Screen

Complex Procedures (nephrectomy, cystectomy, diverticulectomy) In addition to the above

- Clear liquid diet the day prior to surgery
- Mechanical bowel prep: Golitely 4L
  If radical perineal prostatectomy is planned erythromycin and neomycin base: 1 g of each PO at 1300, 1500, and 2100 h
- Type and cross × 2 units

Patient Preparation (Table 2-3)

The Preoperative Work-Up

In preparation for surgery patients are interviewed, examined, and tested to ensure that they are good surgical candidates. Although blood transfusions are seldom needed and conversion to laparotomy is not common, the surgeon as well as the patient should be prepared for such an eventuality. All patients should have blood typed and screened. Those scheduled for laparoscopic lymph node dissection and possible subsequent radical prostatectomy should have at least two units of blood available and may elect to bank autologous blood.

A decompressed bowel is essential for safe entry, good visibility, and exposure during laparoscopic surgery. Patients are asked to avoid gas-producing foods 1 to 2 days before surgery. A full mechanical and chemical bowel prep is advisable in instances where lysis of adhesions is anticipated, or if mobilization of the large bowel is planned to access the retroperitoneum. Bowel preparation can be mechanical only for briefer interventions. Oral solutions that can be taken by the patient at home the day before admission to the hospital are commercially available.

Medications

Patients are asked to stop medications with antiplatelet activity (aspirin, nonsteroidal anti-inflammatory drugs). All cardiac and other important drugs are taken the morning of surgery with a sip of water.

Informed Consent

It is the surgeon's obligation to inform the patient of the indications, alternative options, and possible risks of laparoscopy. The various options for management of complications and unexpected findings should be discussed beforehand. The patient should understand that conversion to open laparotomy may be necessary due to the inability to attain laparoscopic access (adhesions, properitoneal insufflation, obesity, etc.) or due to a complication that requires an open celiotomy for proper management. Accordingly, the consent should allow for the performance of a laparotomy.

Preparation in the Operating Room

Patients undergoing laparoscopic pelvic procedures should have both arms placed at their sides to allow the surgical team adequate room to maneuver around the operating table (Fig. 2-2). Additionally, a stretch-induced injury to the brachial plexus may result from overextension of the arms (>90 degrees). Shoulder braces have been used to keep the patient from falling off at the head of the table during extreme Trendelenburg. However, shoulder braces may push the clavicle into the retroclavicular space, causing compression of the brachial plexus.[8] Alternatively, the patient may be secured to the operating table by straps across the shoulders and legs. The straps must be carefully placed so as not to hinder ventilation or the circulation to any part of the body.

After the patient has been anesthetized, the bladder and stomach are respectively decompressed by a Foley catheter and nasogastric tube. Distention of the hollow viscera increases the likelihood of injury

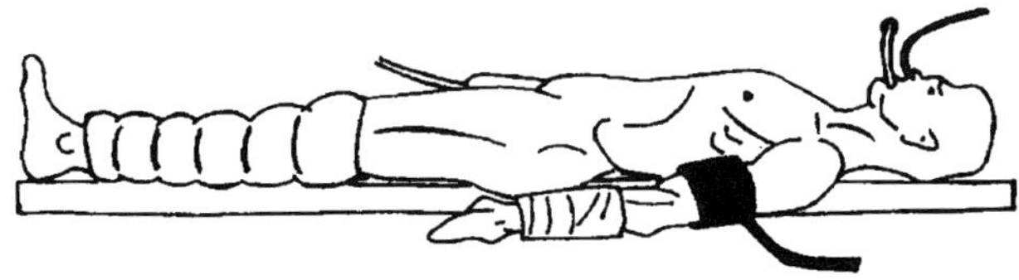

Figure 2-2 Standard patient position for routine laparoscopic surgery.

during pneumoperitoneum needle placement and trocar insertion.[9–13] Intermittent venous compression stockings are used to minimize venous stasis in the lower extremities during the operation. The patient is positioned on the table and padded in a manner that protects all areas prone to pressure injury to avoid neuropathies and soft tissue trauma. Finally, the patient is secured to the operating table so that rotation and tilting can be carried out to obtain exposure of the operative site.[14,15]

One dose of an intravenous broad spectrum antibiotic (usually a cephalosporin) is given 1 h before surgery. The abdomen is scrubbed with iodophor solution from the groin to the nipple line. The umbilical area is given a thorough cleansing. A sterile drape is placed to adequately expose the abdomen from the xiphoid process to the pubic bone and from one anterior superior iliac crest to the other. Wide exposure of the abdomen also allows the surgeon to percuss adequately all four quadrants to ascertain that total abdominal insufflation is being established. Additionally, the wide exposure is necessary for unimpeded trocar placement and to facilitate a quick, sterile conversion to an open laparotomy, if necessary. We have found it useful to include the genitalia in the surgical field in cases where manipulation of the vaginal vault or simultaneous endoscopy facilitates the proposed procedure (bladder surgery and laparoscopic assisted orchiopexy).

It cannot be stressed strongly enough that the availability and good working order of all laparoscopic equipment must be assured before the pneumoperitoneum needle is introduced. The laparoscope-video unit must be white balanced and ready for use. The insufflator must be operable, with a full tank of CO_2. Preparing the equipment after the initial trocar insertion will contribute to a long delay in the recognition and correction of an injury. A sterile laparotomy set should be readily available in the operating room so that if a major vessel or organ is injured, access to and control of the injury can be obtained without delay.

References

1. Sosa RE, Weingram J, Poppas D, Lyons J: Physiologic considerations in laparoscopic surgery in urology. *J Endourol* 6:85–87, 1992.
2. Wittgen CM, Andrus CH, Fitzgerald SD, et al: Analysis of the hemodynamic and ventilatory effects of laparoscopic cholecystectomy. *Arch Surg* 126:997–1000, 1991.
3. Johannsen G, Andersen M, Juhl B: The effect of general anesthesia on the hemodynamic events during laparoscopy with CO_2 insufflation. *Acta Anaesthesiol Scand* 33:132–136, 1989.
4. Liu S, Leighton T, Davis I, et al: Prospective analysis of cardiopulmonary responses to laparoscopic cholecystectomy. *J Laparoendosc Surg* 5:241–246, 1991.
5. Motew M, Ivankovich A, Bieniarz J, et al: Cardiovascular effects and acid-base and blood gas changes during laparoscopy. *Am J Obstet Gynecol* 115:1002–1012, 1973.
6. Marshall RL, Jebson PJR, Davie IT, Scott DB: Circulatory effects of carbon dioxide insufflation of the peritoneal cavity for laparoscopy. *Br J Anaesth* 44:680–684, 1972.
7. Ivankovich AD, Miletich DJ, Albrecht RF, et al: Cardiovascular effects of intraperitoneal insufflation with carbon dioxide and nitrous oxide in the dog. *Anesthesiology* 42:281–287, 1975.
8. Wilcox S, Vandon D: Alas, poor Trendelenburg and his position! *Anesth Analg* 67:574–578, 1988.
9. Thompson AG, Wheeless CR: Gastrointestinal complications of laparoscopy sterilization. *Obstet Gynecol* 41:669–676, 1973.
10. Milliken RA, Milliken GM: Gastric perforation during laparoscopic examination: Report of a case. *Anesth Analg* 53:239–240, 1974.
11. Reynolds RC, Pauca AL: Gastric perforation, an anesthesia- induced hazard in laparoscopy. *Anesthesiology* 38:84–85, 1973.
12. Yuzpe AA: Pneumoperitoneum needle and trocar injuries in laparoscopy. *J Reprod Med* 35:485–490, 1990.
13. Penfield AJ: Trocar and needle injuries, in *Laparoscopy*. Baltimore, Williams & Wilkins, pp 236–241, 1977.
14. Hershlag A, Loy RA, Lavy G, DeCherney AH: Femoral neuropathy after laparoscopy. *J Reprod Med* 35:575–576, 1990.
15. Prentice JA, Martin JT: The Trendelenburg position: Anesthesiologic considerations, in *Positioning in Anesthesia and Surgery*. Philadelphia, WB Saunders, pp 127–145, 1987.

3

Setup of the Operating Suite and Instrumentation for Laparoscopy

Charles H. Andrus

Introduction

Although minimal laparoscopic procedures have been performed in an outpatient clinic setting under intravenous sedation, most laparoscopic urologic interventions are performed in an operating room environment. Employment of electrocautery, which requires the presence of a carbon dioxide pneumoperitoneum, the use of general anesthesia, and the need for sophisticated monitoring dictate the surgical suite with anesthesiology assistance as the most appropriate setting for laparoscopic urologic surgery.

The Operating Room Setting

As with any procedure performed in an operating room, there should be a formalized localization of the patient and the operating and anesthesia personnel, as well as the video and laparoscopic equipment (Fig. 3-1).[1] The operating table should be centered in the room. The anesthetic equipment, monitoring devices, and anesthesia personnel are best located at the "head" of the table. The operating surgeon should be on the side of the patient opposite the surgeon's handedness (i.e., a right-handed surgeon should stand on the patient's left side). The assistant surgeon should be located directly across from the

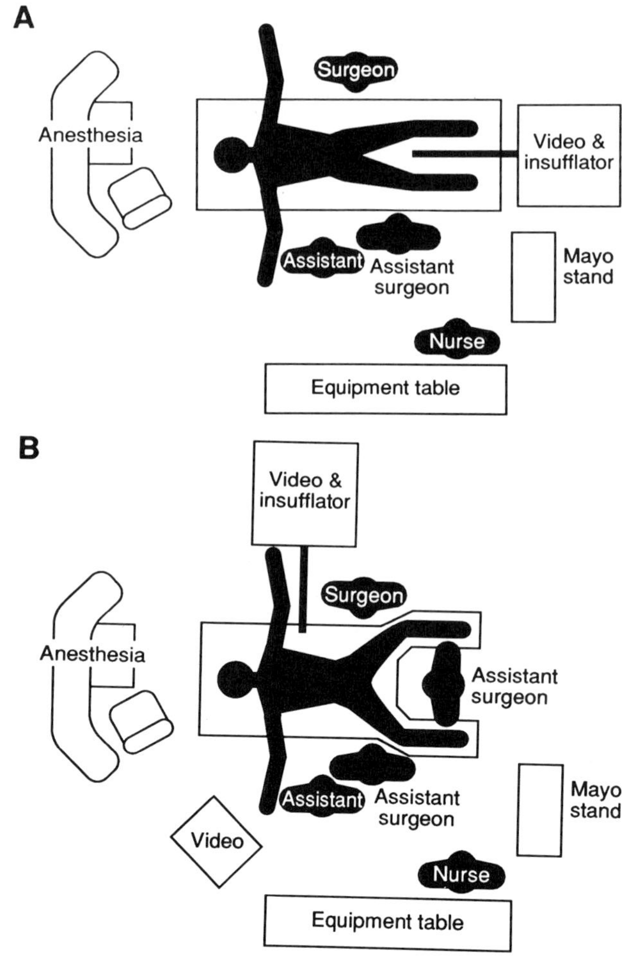

Figure 3-1 Possible OR suite arrangements for laparoscopic urologic procedures (a) when the patient is in a simple supine position and (b) when the patient is in a lithotomy position.

primary surgeon. The manipulation of the laparoscope with the video attachment can be performed by either surgeon, the scrub nurse, or an additional "video" technician.

If the patient is placed in the traditional supine position and the laparoscopic operation is to be performed in the pelvis and lower abdomen, the video monitor is best placed at the foot of the operating table to maximize the operating team's ability to coordinate their movements with what is visualized on the monitor (Fig. 3-1a). If the patient is placed in a lithotomy position to provide intraoperative access to the perineum, the video monitors should be placed lateral to the patient, preferably on both sides (Fig. 3-lb). If the patient is undergoing a mid- or upper-abdominal laparoscopic urologic operation (nephrectomy or adrenalectomy), the video monitors can be placed either at the foot of the table or laterally. All instrumentation cables (fiberoptic, video camera, gas insufflation, and cautery) and suction tubing are directed toward their respective equipment so as to allow maximum mobility of the instruments without hindering movement around the operating table.

Patient Preparation

Once the patient is placed on the operating table, routine preanesthetic preparation and general anesthetic induction is performed. Controversy remains as to the most appropriate route of anesthetic administration (inhalation versus intravenous),[2] tube or mask anesthetic techniques employed,[3] and variation of types of neuromuscular blocking agents utilized.[4,5]

Although placement of an NG tube and foley catheter can be disputed,[6] these techniques do allow for decompression of the respective hollow *visci* they catheterize, and a foley catheter will permit better identification of the bladder at time of laparoscopy. In those laparoscopic urologic procedures where manipulation of the ureters is anticipated (i.e., nephrectomy), preoperative catheterization of the ureters might be useful and helpful in both ureteral identification and prevention of inadvertent injury to the uninvolved ureter.[7] Although probably inconsequential during relatively brief diagnostic laparoscopies, the development of hypercarbia secondary to the carbon dioxide pneumoperitoneum during lengthy laparoscopic procedures performed on patients with poor cardiac and pulmonary status is real and necessitates capnography and in some cases intermittent arterial blood analysis.[8] A more detailed discussion of these issues may be found in Chapters 4 and 5.

Instrumentation

Table 3-1 includes a list of all the laparoscopic instruments recommended for a standard procedure.

Peritoneal Trocars

To establish a pneumoperitoneum, a "closed" technique utilizing a spring-loaded sheathed Veress needle[9] or an "open" method with direct peritoneal visualization and trocar placement in a Hasson-type fashion is employed (Fig. 3-2).[10,11] The abdominal cavity is then distended by gaseous insufflation utilizing a high-flow electronic insufflator (Chap. 5). Through the subumbilical skin incision site, a 10- to 12-mm standard trocar is placed "blindly" after adequate insufflation (12 to 16 mm Hg of pneumoperitoneum pressure) with a Veress needle, or a 10- to12-mm Hasson-type trocar is placed by the direct vision technique prior to insufflation. Additional trocars of varying sizes may be placed under direct laparoscopic visualization to provide ports through which one can retract intraabdominal tissues and operate (Table 3-1). Larger trocars (10, 12, or 15 mm in diameter) can be functionally reduced or "downsized" by add-on spacers (Chap. 6).

Laparoscopic Telescopes, Cameras, and Video Equipment

Excellent visualization of the placement of all subsequent trocars, peritoneal contents, and operative procedures depends directly on the magnification, clarity, and resolution provided by the laparoscopic telescope and video camera, and the intensity of the illumination source employed (Tables 3-1 and 3-2, Figs. 3-2 to 3-4). The standard, rigid laparoscopic telescope is a combination of fiberoptic bundles that deliver illumination from a light source to the intraperitoneal cavity and transmit an image to the extracorporeal eyepiece. Laparoscopic telescopes can be end-viewing (zero-degree scope) or provide angled viewing (25°, 30°, or 45° with regard to the

TABLE 3-1 Standard Operative Laparoscopic Instrumentation

Instrumentation	Variations	
Veress Needles:	(100 mm, 120 mm, 150 mm)	
Trochars:	5 mm	
	10–12 mm	
	10–12 mm Hasson	
	10- or 12-mm to 5-mm reducers (down sizers)	
Laparoscopic telescopes:	10 mm 0° (standard), 10 mm 30° or 45° (optional)	
	5 mm 0° (optional), 5 mm 30° or 45° (optional)	
Instrumentation that can be utilized through any 5-mm trocars		
Grasping forceps	Atraumatic	
	Atraumatic, locking	
	Traumatic	
	Traumatic, locking	
Needle holder and suture forceps		
Dissecting forceps	Atraumatic, straight	
	Atraumatic, curved	
Scissors	Straight	
	Curved	(optional)
	Hooked	(optional)
	Microscissors	(optional)
Semm endo-loop applicator		
Extracorporeal knot-pusher		
Palpation probes		
Suction / Irrigation tube		
Electrocauterization probes	Spatulated	
	Hooked	
Laser	CO_2 waveguide	(optional)
	YAG fiber and guide	(optional)
	KTP fiber and guide	(optional)
Disposable clip applicators (Multifire—usually 20 per applicator)		
Intracavitary multirow stapler (i.e., Endo-GIA)		
Pneumoperitoneum insufflation tubing		

long axis of the scope).[12] With these angled-tip scopes, one can better visualize intraabdominal structures whose surfaces parallel the long axis of the telescope. A video camera can be attached or permanently bonded (a laparocam) to the telescope.

TABLE 3-2 Standard Electronic Laparoscopic Instrumentation

Fiberoptic light cable
Xenon light source
Rapid flow automatic electronic insufflator
Color chip video camera with controller
Television monitor
VCR (optional)
Electro desiccator generator unit with cable
Lasers (CO_2, KTP, YAG, etc.) (optional)

Probably the single most important technologic advance in the development of laparoscopic urologic surgery was the development and refinement of the "chip" miniaturized color video camera (Fig. 3-3).[12–14] These miniaturized video cameras use the same CCD (charge-coupled device) technology employed in camcorders. The cameras are of a single- or triple-chip design, with the triple chip providing more lines of resolution (~450 horizontal lines of resolution for a single chip design compared to >700 horizontal lines of resolution for a triple chip design).[12] The camera is attached to a control box, which is connected to a high resolution color monitor. Through this technology, the entire operating team can view the laparoscopy and assist in much the same fashion as in the traditional "open" operation. Unlike traditional open urologic procedures, tactile sensation is quite limited during

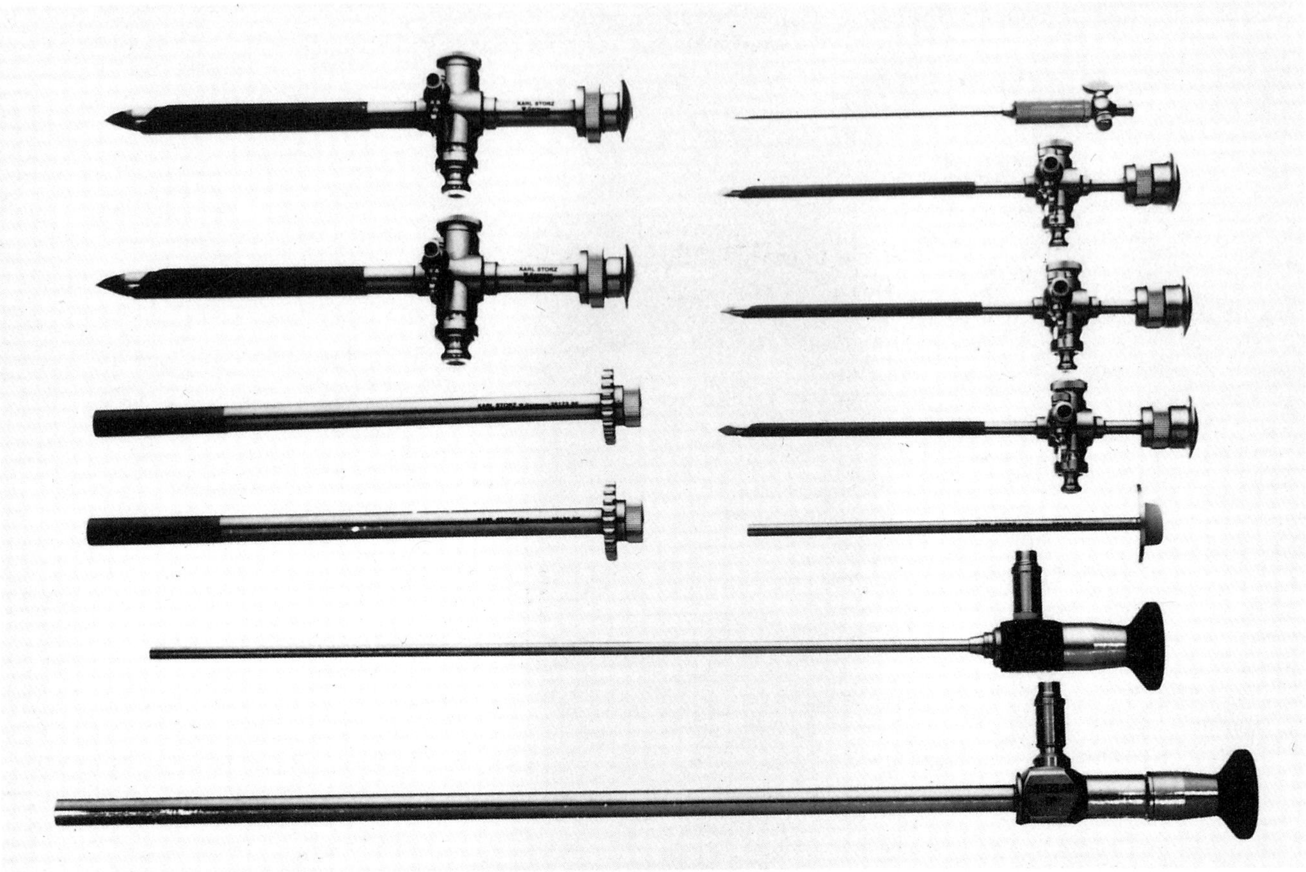

Figure 3-2 Laparoscopic trocars and telescopes. Left, 10-mm trocars (2), 10- to 5-mm downsizers (2), 5-mm straight laparoscopic telescope, 10-mm straight laparoscopic telescope. Right, Veress needle, 5-mm trocars (3), and SEMM endo-loop applicator. (Photograph provided by Karl Storz Endoscopy-America, Inc.)

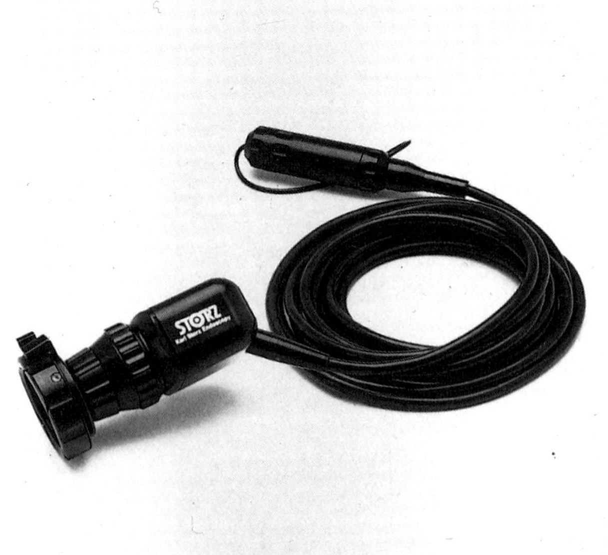

Figure 3-3 Color video chip-camera. (Photograph provided by Karl Storz Endoscopy-America, Inc.)

laparoscopy, and the ability to visualize structures clearly becomes paramount.

Laparoscopic Operative Instruments

General Instrumentation

A multitude of forceps, scissors, probes, staplers, cautery, and laser devices can be used during a laparoscopic urologic procedure (Fig. 3-5, Table 3-1).[13-15] To ensure a consistent pneumoperitoneum, the most critical issue regarding all hand instrumentation is the gas-tight seal formed between the shaft of the instrument and the trocar. The outer diameter of the instrumentation is critical and has become standardized. Most laparoscopic hand instruments are machined to appropriately fit either the 5-mm or 10-mm trocars. (A few 7-mm instruments were previously made for pelviscopy sets.) If an instrument is curved, the degree of curvature and the length of the "instrument jaws" are limited by the inner

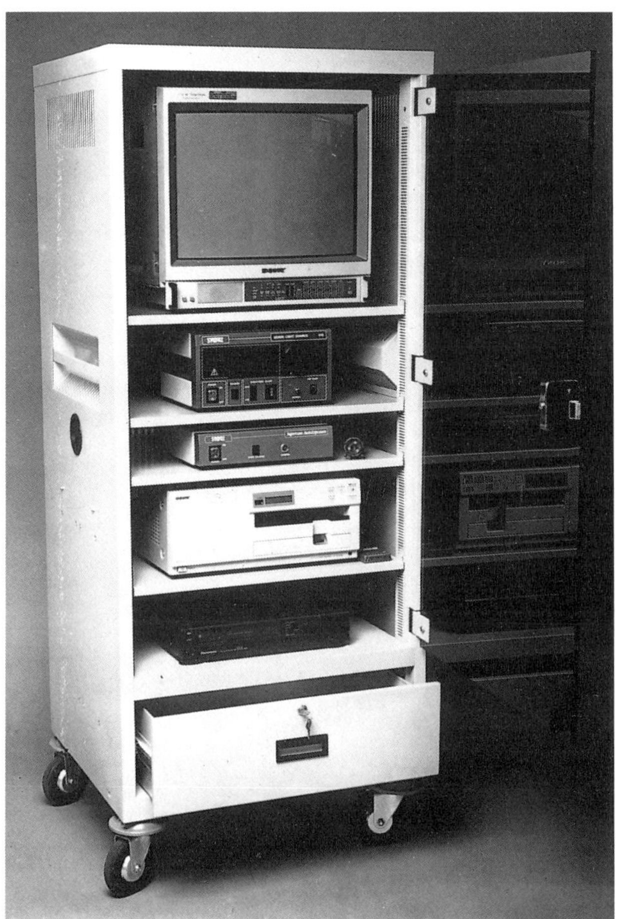

Figure 3-4 Laparoscopic cart containing a television monitor, high-intensity xenon light source, video camera modulator, Magnograph color print processor, and a VCR.

diameter of the trocar through which the instrument is designed to pass.

Most of the laparoscopic forceps are analogous to the instrumentation employed in a open intraabdominal operation. There are both straight and curved forceps that grasp atraumatically or traumatically (toothed forceps). These forceps can be nonlocking or locking. The locking forceps provide a constant grasping ability that is utilized in laparoscopic situations requiring continuous retraction. The curved, nonlocking forceps can be slightly pointed, and these are quite useful for dissection. (Eponyms: Maryland dissector, Petlin dissector, etc.)

Laparoscopic Clipping and Stapling Devices

Besides the recent development of video capabilities, the other major technologic enhancements that have made routine laparoscopic surgery feasible are the multifire, disposable clip applicators[16] (Fig. 3-6) and intracavitary stapling devices.[17–18] The ability to rapidly and repetitively apply clips or staples to tissue provides the surgeon with the capability to control vascular and lymphatic structures. Laparoscopic clipping and stapling techniques are found to be less awkward than suture ligation by most surgeons.

Instruments for Suturing During Laparoscopy

At times only ligature control is sufficient to control large or edematous structures. Thus, the capabilities to place preknotted suture ties on a structure (i.e., endo-loop)[19] or to perform intracavitary suturing become a necessity (Fig. 3-7). Although technically more demanding, these techniques should be developed and practiced by any laparoscopist.[20–22] As in any open operation, the size of the suture (absorbable or not) is totally dependent on the tissue being sutured or ligated, the amount of tension required, and the degree of permanency anticipated. A standard round, half-circle laparotomy needle (like an "sh" needle), a laparoscopic straight (Keith) needle, and a laparoscopic "ski" needle (a straight needle with a half-circle pointed end) have all been employed (Fig. 3-8). With the laparoscopic needle driver grasping the suture 1 to 4 cm from the swedged-on needle–suture junction, one of these needles can be introduced into the abdomen by dragging the needle through the trocar. As with other curved instrumentation, the ability to utilize a "half-circle" needle is limited by the needle's curvature diameter and by the inner diameter of the trochar through which the needle and suture are pulled.

Once the "stitch or stitches" have been placed in the tissues, the suture can be tied within the peritoneum (intracavity knot-tying) by instrument-tying techniques[19,22] or outside the abdomen (extracorporeal suturing).[20] With extracorporeal suturing, after the "stitch" has been placed, the laparoscopic needle driver again is used to grasp the suture 1 to 4 cm from the swedged-on needle–suture junction, and the needle with the suture withdrawn from the peritoneum through the trocar. A Roeder[19] or fisherman's knot (slipknots that are self-locking much like a hangman's noose) can be tied extracorporeally and advanced with a knot-pusher (Table 3-1) down through the trocar to approximate the tissues. Extracorporeal "square knots" can also be advanced one half hitch at a time using the knot-pusher.

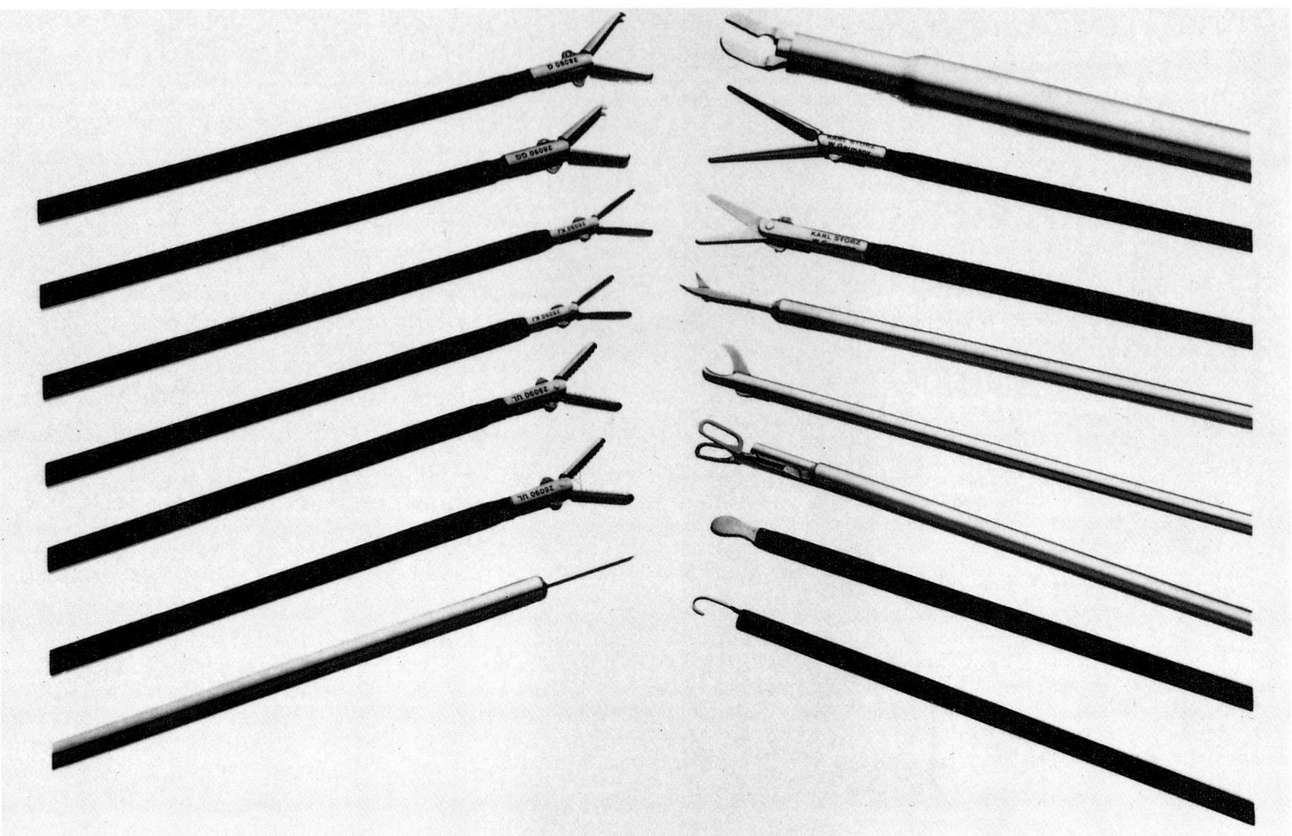

Figure 3-5 Laparoscopic instrument tips. Left, traumatic, grasping forceps (2), atraumatic grasping forceps (4), aspiration needle. Right, single-load clip applicator, needle holder, straight scissors, microscissors, hooked scissors, Olsen cholangiography clamp, spatulated monopolar cautery, and hook cautery. (Photograph provided by Karl Storz Endoscopy-America, Inc.)

Instrumentation for Dividing and Cauterizing Tissues Laparoscopically

Laparoscopic scissors have been developed for division of tissues and suture (Table 3-1, Fig. 3-5). With attachment to a standard electrosurgery cable and generator, many of the scissors can be employed with monopolar cauterization during tissue dissection. For similar purposes, monopolar electrosurgical cautery instruments with a multitude of tips have been developed, the spatulated and hooked types being the most frequently used. Previously, bipolar cauterizing instruments were developed specifically for the cauterization of tubular structures like blood vessels and the fallopian tubes. YAG lasers with contact tips, KTP lasers with bare fibers, and CO_2 lasers with waveguides (Table 3-2) have all been employed to coagulate and divide tissues laparoscopically.

Each of these electrosurgical and laser methods can be employed for dissection, tissue division, and coagulation (Table 3-2). All these methods are contraindicated in any pneumoperitoneum atmosphere (O_2, N_2O, air) that can support combustion and are thus limited to utilization with inert gases (CO_2 and the noble gases).[23] Much debate has arisen as to the relative efficacy, safety, and cost of electrocautery versus laser methods during laparoscopy.[24–28] With monopolar electrosurgery there can be secondary burning due to tissue transmission of the energy distally,[27] and lasers can demonstrate passpoint burning due to laser light transmission past the dissection area if there is no fiber contact with the tissues. The initial laser investment is more costly than electrocautery, although some would debate the long-term cost/benefit ratio.[25] The amount of thermal damage of adjacent tissues

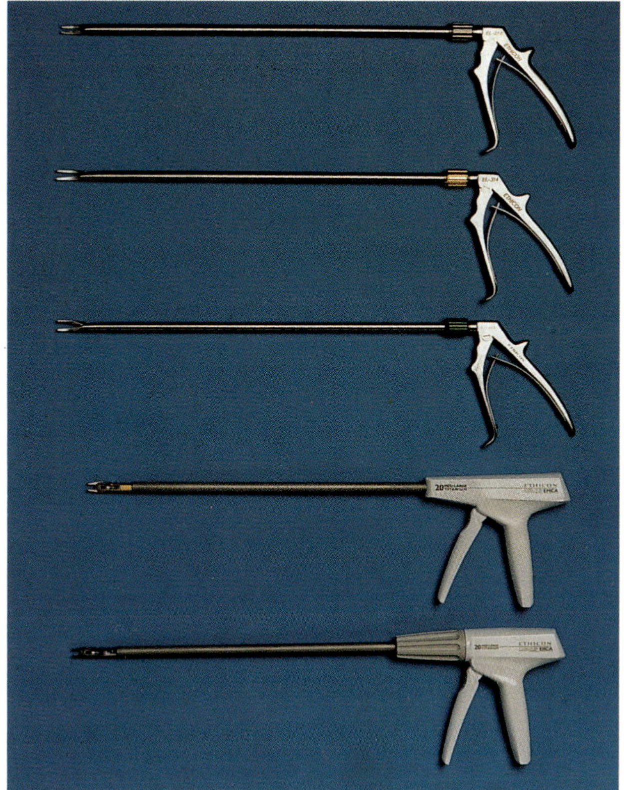

Figure 3-6 Laparoscopic clip applicators: single-load clip applicators (3) and multifire disposable clip applicators. (Photograph provided by Ethicon, Johnson & Johnson)

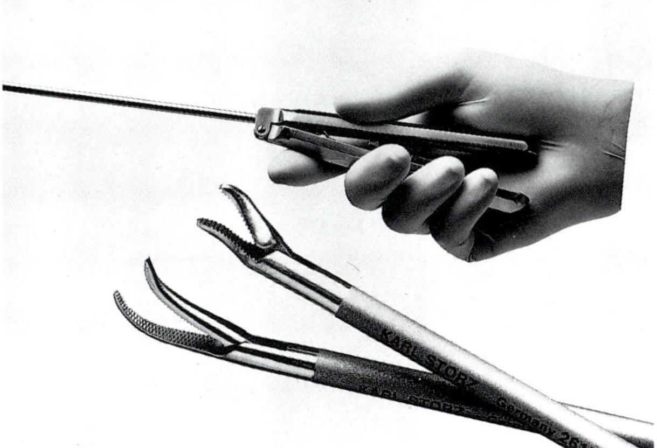

Figure 3-7 Laparoscopic needle holders. (Photograph provided by Karl Storz Endoscopy-America, Inc.)

varies with the type and settings of laser or cautery utilized.[26,27]

Preparation of the Instrumentation

Like traditional surgical instrumentation, laparoscopic instruments are placed in the abdominal cavity through surgical incisions and should therefore be sterilized prior to use.[13,29–35] Most nondisposable laparoscopic instrumentation is metal and can be sterilized by steam. Most of the optical laparoscopic equipment (telescopes, fiberoptic light cables, and video cameras) cannot be subjected to steam sterilization. Although ethylene oxide sterilization and aeration may take 4 to 8 h, optical instrumentation can most appropriately be sterilized in this manner.

Sterilization should be the ideal, but due to operating room scheduling and the limitation of available equipment it is still common practice for many institutions to practice high-grade disinfection by soaking the instruments in 2% glutaraldehyde for 15 to 20 min.[29–32,35] Large laparoscopic and arthroscopic series have failed to demonstrate any increase in peritoneal or wound contamination by the use of high-grade disinfection methods.[33–34] Unlike steam or ethylene oxide, increased sterilizer pressure is not a component of the process when high-grade disinfection is employed. However, adequate disinfection by wet techniques requires direct contact of the disinfecting agent with the instruments.

The FDA has classified one wet technique, peroxyacetic acid (Steris Corp., Painesville, OH), as a sterilizing method.[31] The method is fast (~30 min) and automated, which obviates the prolonged delays experienced with the use of ethylene oxide sterilization. Although some would still consider this a high-grade disinfecting technique due to the direct instrument contact constraints, peroxyacetic acid is an extremely effective agent against all bacteria and spores, and should be considered a "sterilizing method."

One often employed alternative to the exposure of the video and electronic equipment to ethylene oxide or high-grade disinfectants, is the intraoperative covering of the instrumentation with a presterilized, disposable plastic drape. The previously sterilized or high-grade disinfected laparoscopic telescopes can be attached to the video camera through a rubberized seal in the plastic drape; obviating the need for sterilization of sensitive electronic equipment.

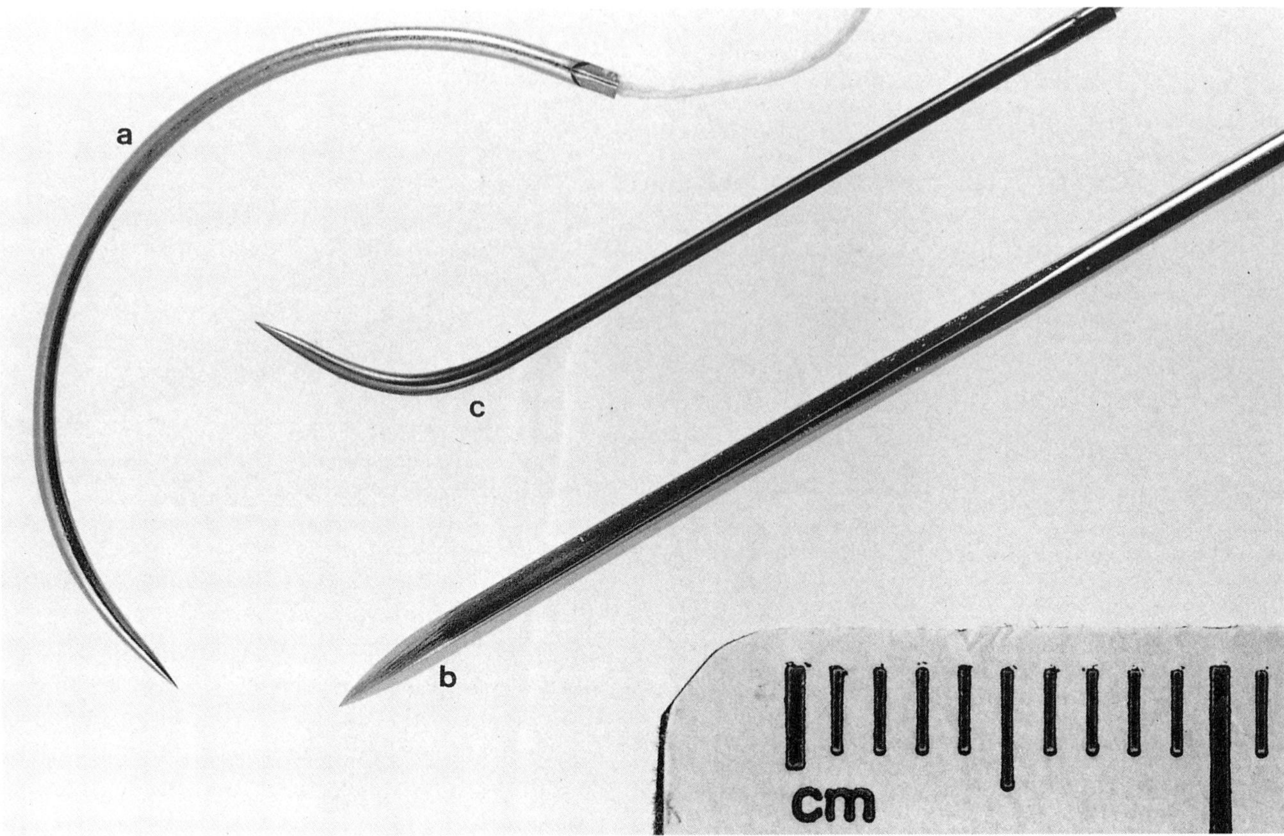

Figure 3-8 The three most commonly utilized needles for laparoscopic suturing: (a) sh, (b) Keith, and (c) "ski" needles.

References

1. Boyers SP: Operating room setup and instrumentation. *Clin Obstet Gynecol* 34:373–386, 1991.
2. DeGrood PMRM, Harbers JBM, van Egmond J, Crul JF: Anaesthesia for laparoscopy. A comparison of five techniques including propofol, etomidate, thiopentone, and isoflurane. *Anaesthesia* 42:815–823, 1987.
3. Kenefick JP, Leader A, Maltby JR, Taylor PJ: Laparoscopy. Blood-gas values and minor sequelae associated with three techniques base on isoflurane. *Br J Anaesth* 59:189–194, 1987.
4. Dodgson MS, Heier T, Steen PA: Atracurium compared with suxamethonium for outpatient laparoscopy. *Br J Anaesth* 58:40S–43S, 1986.
5. Sengupta P, Skagel M, Plantevin OM: Post-operative morbidity associated with the use of atracurium and vecuronium in day-case laparoscopy. *Eur J Anaesthesiol* 4:93–99, 1987.
6. Mowschenson PM, Weinstein ME: Why catheterize the bladder for laparoscopic cholecystectomy? *J Laparoendosc Surg* 2:215–217, 1992.
7. Winslow PH, Kreger R, Ebbesson B, Oster E: Conservative management of electrical burn injury of ureter secondary to laparoscopy. *Urol* 27:60–62, 1986.
8. Wittgen CM, Andrus CH, Fitzgerald SD, Baudendistel LJ, Dahms TE, Kaminski DL: Analysis of the hemodynamic and ventilatory effects of laparoscopic cholecystectomy. *Arch Surg* 126:997–1001, 1991.
9. Veress J: Neues Instrument zur Ausfuhrung von Bauchpunktionen. *Dtsch med Wochenschr* 64:1480–1484, 1938.
10. Hasson HM: Open laparoscopy: a modified instrument and method for laparoscopy. *Am J Obstet Gynecol* 110:880–884, 1971.
11. Colver RM: Laparoscopy: Basic technique, instrumentation, and complications. *Surg Laparosc Endosc* 2:35–40, 1992.
12. Phillips E, Daykhovsky L, Carroll B, Gershman A, Grundfest WS: Laparoscopic cholecystectomy: Instrumentation and technique. *J Laparoendosc Surg* 1:3–15, 1990.
13. Duppler DW: Laparoscopic instrumentation, videoimaging, and equipment disinfection and sterilization. *Surg Clin North Am* 72:1021–1032, 1992.

14. Eden CG, Ison KT, Popert RJ, Carter PG, Coptcoat MJ: A consumer's guide to laparoscopic equipment for urology. *Br J Urol* 72:1–5, 1993.

15. Reichert M: Laparoscopic instruments. *AORN Journal* 57:637–655, 1993.

16. Blatner ME, Wittgen CM, Andrus CH, Kaminski DL: Cystic duct cholangiography during laparoscopic cholecystectomy. *Arch Surg* 126:646–649, 1991.

17. Daniell JF, Gurley LD, Kurtz BR, Chambers JF: Instruments & Methods: The use of an automatic stapling device for laparoscopic appendectomy. *Obstet Gynecol* 78:721–723, 1991.

18. Parra RO, Andrus CH, Jones P, Boullier JA: Laparoscopic cystectomy: Initial report on a new treatment for the retained bladder. *J Urol* 148:1140–1144, 1992.

19. Semm K: Endoscopic appendectomy. *Endoscopy* 15:59–64, 1983.

20. Kennedy JS: A technique for extracorporeal suturing. *J Laparoendosc Surg* 2:269–272, 1992.

21. Meilahn JE: The need for improving laparoscopic suturing and knot-tying. *J Laparoendosc Surg* 2:267, 1992.

22. Pietrafitta JJ: A technique of laparoscopic knot tying. *J Laparoendosc Surg* 2:273–275, 1992.

23. Gunatilake DE: Case report: Fatal intraperitoneal explosion during electrocoagulation via laparoscopy. *Int J Gynaecol Obstet* 15:353–357, 1978.

24. Corbitt JD: Laparoscopic cholecystectomy: Laser versus electrosurgery. *Surg Laparosc Endosc* 1:85–88, 1991.

25. Lane GE, Lathrop JC: Comparison of results of KTP/532 laser versus monopolar electrosurgical dissection in laparoscopic cholecystectomy. *J Laparoendosc Surg* 3:209–214, 1993.

26. Luciano AA, Frishman GN, Maier DB: A comparative analysis of adhesion reduction, tissue effects, and incising characteristics of electrosurgery, CO_2 laser, and Nd:YAG laser at operative laparoscopy: An animal study. *J Laparoendosc Surg* 2:287–292, 1992.

27. Saye WB, Miller W, Hertzmann P: Electrosurgery thermal injury: Myth or misconception? *Surg Laparosc Endosc* 1:223–228, 1991.

28. Soper NJ, Barteau JA, Clayman RV, Becich MJ: Safety and efficacy of laparoscopic cholecystectomy using monopolar electrocautery in the porcine model. *Surg Laparosc Endosc* 1:17–22, 1991.

29. Corson SL, Block S, Mintz C, Dole M, Wainwright A: Sterilization of laparoscopes: Is soaking sufficient? *J Reprod Med* 23:49–56, 1979.

30. Corson SL, Dole M, Kraus R, Richards L, Logan B: Studies in sterilization of laparoscopes: II. *J Reprod Med* 23:57–59,1979.

31. Favero MS, Bond WW: Sterilization, disinfection, and antisepsis in the hospital. *Manual of Clinical Microbiology*, Washington: American Society for Microbiology, Chap. 24, pp. 183–200, 1991.

32. Gregory E, Simmons D, Weinberg JJ: Care and sterilization of Endourologic instruments. *Urol Clin North Am* 15:541–546, 1988.

33. Huezo CM, DeStefano F, Rubin GL, Ory HW: Risk of wound and pelvic infection after laparoscopic tubal sterilization: Instrument disinfection versus sterilization. *Obstet Gynecol* 61:598–602, 1983.

34. Johnson LL, Shneider DA, Austin MD, Goodman FG, Bullock JM, DeBruin JA: Two per cent glutaraldehyde: A disinfectant in arthroscopy and arthroscopic surgery. *J Bone Joint Surg Br* 64A:237–239, 1982.

35. Rutala WA, Clontz EP, Weber DJ, Hoffmann KK: Disinfection practices for endoscopes and other semicritical items. *Infect Control Hosp Epidemiol* 12:282–288, 1991.

4

Physiologic and Anesthetic Principles of Laparoscopy

Charles H. Andrus
Catherine M. Wittgen
Raul O. Parra

Introduction

The anesthetic care of the patient during laparoscopy is largely determined by the alterations in physiology observed during the pneumoperitoneum. These changes can be considered as secondary to abdominal distension or to the pharmacologic effects of the gas employed for insufflation. Abdominal wall distension or retraction by external elevators maintain exposure at the same pressure (normal atmospheric) that a patient would experience during laparotomy.[1] With these devices, physiologic responses to anesthesia should be no different than those observed during laparotomy. With peritoneal insufflation, however, significant alterations in hemodynamics, pulmonary function, acid-base balance, and hormonal secretion can occur in response to the anesthesia administered.

Physiology During Urologic Laparoscopy

Hemodynamic Effects

During most laparoscopies, the insufflation pressures used to establish and maintain abdominal distension for adequate intraperitoneal visualization range from 12 to 20 mm Hg (average 15 mm Hg). At these pressures, inferior vena cava and portal vein pressures increase, and flow is decreased in the superior mesenteric artery and portal vein.[2,3] This results in a measurable decrease in venous return to the heart. These effects can be minimized as demonstrated in an experimental canine model where insufflation pressures were decreased to 8 to 12 mm Hg.[4] Numerous studies in humans have documented that cardiac output and stroke volume decrease or remain unchanged, while heart rate is increased or unchanged.[2,5–14] These effects appear to be independent of the gas utilized, since they are reproducible with many different insufflation agents. Two studies, however, have reported an increase in cardiac output with insufflation.[15,16] One study suggests that this increase may be the true cardiac response to the pneumoperitoneum and is observed only in the absence of myocardial depressant anesthetic agents like halothane.[15]

With rapid systemic absorption, the peritoneal insufflation of carbon dioxide produces additional hemodynamic changes not observed with other, more inert gases. This may result in hypercapnia and acidemia, and has been shown to initiate pulmonary hypertension and systemic vasodilation.[13] These effects are masked by the hypercapnia also stimulating a sympathomimetic response with hyperventilation and systemic vasoconstriction.[5,17] Clinically these effects may be difficult to observe, since they are overshadowed by the baroeffects of the pneumoperitoneum or the myocardial depressant effects of the anesthetics.

Acid-Base and Pulmonary Effects

No matter what the insufflation agent for the pneumoperitoneum, the positive intraperitoneal pressure employed causes a linear increase in peak airway pressure during artificial ventilation.[6,11] This effect is purely mechanical and is a result of the increased intraabdominal pressure, which causes an upward displacement and distension of the diaphragm, reducing the space in the thoracic cavity. In order to maintain an adequate minute ventilation, the anesthesiologist must compensate for these decreased tidal volumes by hyperventilating the patient with increased airway pressures. This appears to be a pure alteration in ventilatory capacity without an associated defect in oxygenation, since hypoxia has not been a complication detected with the use of any of the insufflation agents studied.

While the need for increased minute ventilation has been observed during pneumoperitoneum with any gas, the development of a persistent respiratory acidosis is a complication unique to the utilization of CO_2 for insufflation. This hypercapnia and acidosis first concerned gynecologists, who found these effects to be reproducible. They concluded that nitrous oxide was superior to CO_2 due to the elimination of these complications.[18–20] As an alternative agent, N_2O is not without potential hazard either. While it is not flammable, it does support combustion as an oxidizer. Consequently, for most urologic procedures requiring the use of electrocautery or laser, the most commonly used and frequently available gas is CO_2.

With laparoscopic procedures of increased complexity and prolonged insufflation, the development of hypercapnia and subsequent acidosis has been documented in patients with underlying pulmonary pathology.[8] Subsequent reports in both animal and human subjects have repeatedly documented the consistent development of hypercapnia and acidosis during prolonged periods of CO_2 pneumoperitoneum.[6,9–13,16] No increase in ventilatory dead space has been observed with the insufflation of any gas, including CO_2, which eliminates this commonly observed phenomenon as a major cause of the observed acidosis.[21] A chronic obstructive pulmonary disease (COPD) canine model has demonstrated that the severity of the hypercarbia is a function of the pulmonary excretory ability of the individual dog's diseased lungs.[16]

Prospective studies are now underway employing alternate inert gases during laparoscopy. Currently, helium seems most promising as shown in both human and animal studies.[12,13,16] No adverse outcomes have been reported, but the diminished solubility of helium versus carbon dioxide in the serum remains a concern, since gas emboli can be a potentially life-threatening complication. Another alternative would be to perform laparoscopy using an external abdominal lift device without a pneumoperitoneum.[1]

Avoidance of CO_2 insufflation in clinical practice is impractical and not indicated for all patients. Preoperative evaluation of patients can help identify those individuals at risk to develop severe CO_2 retention, marked hypercapnia, and subsequent significant acidosis. Patients with abnormal preoperative pulmonary function tests (especially in those with a decreased diffusing capacity of the lung for carbon monoxide) and those individuals with cardiac atherosclerosis, diabetes, and renal failure have been demonstrated to be at higher risk for the development of intraoperative hypercapnia and acidosis.[22] Since capnography (end-tidal carbon dioxide measurement by mass spectrometer) may underestimate the severity of hypercapnia secondary to the defect in the diffusing capacity of the lung, intermittent arterial blood gas monitoring is recommended in these patients during laparoscopy.[8,23] To minimize severe hypercapnia, modifications in the choice of anesthetic (intravenous versus inhaled), better ventilatory support (increase in the minute ventilation), and less insufflation pressure (8 to 12 mm Hg vs. 15 to 20 mm Hg) may be beneficial.

Although carbon dioxide retention has been observed, most laparoscopic surgeries can be completed successfully without undue risk to the patient.[24,25] In fact, when "high-risk" patients undergoing laparoscopic cholecystectomy were compared with similar individuals undergoing the equivalent open procedure, the overall morbidity and mortality was less.[26,27] Consistent with the minimally invasive nature of these procedures, pulmonary function testing has also demonstrated significantly fewer changes in the immediate postoperative period in individuals undergoing laparoscopic cholecystectomies.[28,29] In short, during any laparoscopic procedure requiring over 1 h of carbon dioxide insufflation time, intraoperative capnography and intermittent arterial blood gas sampling should be utilized in those patients at potential risk for pneumoperitoneum-induced hypercarbia and acidosis.

Hormonal Effects

As with any intraabdominal operation, stimulation of hormone release during laparoscopic procedures is in part due to the manipulation of the abdominal contents and subsequent postoperative pain. Some serum metabolites and hormones that are influenced by operative stress that have been studied in relation to laparoscopy are glucose, b-endorphin, cortisol, prolactin, epinephrine, norepinephrine, dopamine, and interleukin-6 (IL-6).[30,31] All have been observed to increase during laparoscopic procedures. The increase in b-endorphin secretion is notably less during laparoscopy, however, when compared to laparotomy.[32] The observed increase in serum cortisol levels during laparoscopic colectomy was similar to that observed during traditional open colectomy, while the IL-6 response was muted.[33] In addition, immune function, as measured by T-cell proliferation, is observed to be less inhibited.[34]

Patients undergoing pneumoperitoneum-assisted laparoscopy have demonstrated a rapid rise in serum arginine vasopressin levels upon abdominal insufflation that is independent of hypotension or amount of blood lost. These levels are comparable to the increased antidiuretic hormone (ADH) levels of severely cirrhotic patients.[35,36] The actual physiologic mechanism causing this increased ADH secretion with elevated intraabdominal pressure due to ascites is unknown, but appears to be in response to peritoneal distension and not mediated through baroreceptors in the aortic or carotid bodies. The response to the pneumoperitoneum during laparoscopy may be by a similar mechanism.

Although "surgical stress" pre- and postoperatively is not completely eliminated, the diminished hormonal responses observed when compared to open laparotomy demonstrates laparoscopy to be a physiologically minimally invasive procedure.

Anesthesia During Urologic Laparoscopy

Although brief gynecologic procedures have been performed laparoscopically with the aid of intravenous sedation and local anesthesia, most urologic laparoscopic procedures are performed under general anesthesia. This allows for better overall airway control, muscle relaxation, and an adequate pneumoperitoneum with less pain. In the conscious, nonintubated patient, the utilization of local anesthetic is limited by the peritoneal irritation induced by a carbon dioxide pneumoperitoneum and the very real potential of hypercarbia, hypoxia, and emesis with subsequent aspiration.[37]

General Anesthesia During Laparoscopy

With laparoscopy under a general anesthesia, the anesthetic technique employed can vary with regard to the different types of inhalation versus intravenous agents,[38] tube versus mask anesthetic techniques,[39] and neuromuscular blocking agents,[40,41] to allow for both inpatient and outpatient procedures.[42–44] Laparoscopy requiring longer than an hour of pneumoperitoneum is usually performed under controlled conditions with a general anesthesia. Endotracheal intubation with a cuffed-type tube helps insure an adequate airway, allows adequate ventilation, and prevents aspiration during the period of pneumoperitoneum.[45] In order to minimize reflux of gastric contents intraoperatively, nasogastric decompression is also recommended. With increased intraabdominal pressure (pneumoperitoneum of usually 12 to 20 mm Hg), increased ventilation pressures are required to ventilate the patient adequately throughout the procedure.[46] Patient positioning, with the employment of a steep Trendelenburg position for lower abdominal and pelvic urologic laparoscopy, may also increase ventilatory pressures.[47]

Patient monitoring during laparoscopic urologic procedures should include continuous electrocardiographic monitoring, intermittent noninvasive blood pressure monitoring, precordial or esophageal stethoscope monitoring, and pulse oximetry.[47] When carbon dioxide is employed as the insufflating agent, the procedure is longer than one hour, or the patient has COPD, capnography (measured exhaled end-tidal CO_2) should also be employed.[45] One should note, however, that the end-tidal CO_2 monitoring may severely underestimate serum arterial CO_2 levels in patients with impaired carbon dioxide exchange (as seen in COPD patients). Serial arterial blood gas analyses are, therefore, often indicated to provide more precise representation of the patient's acid-base balance.[8]

During laparoscopic procedures the anesthetic agents and methods utilized may vary greatly. Standard inhalation anesthesia with halogenated hydrocarbons such as halothane, isoflurane, and enflurane with or without nitrous oxide (N_2O) are routinely employed.[45] Although there may be increased bowel distension when N_2O is utilized as the anesthetic method, the occurrence of N_2O bowel distension during laparoscopy is neither absolute nor predictable.[45,48] With N_2O, though, postlaparoscopic emesis seems to be increased, which may be due to a direct effect on intestinal motility.[49]

Propofol, etomidate, and ketamine with midazolam have been employed for total intravenous anesthesia.[38,50] A more rapid recovery and diminished postoperative nausea and vomiting have been observed with this technique (specifically with propofol).[38] During laparoscopy, a balanced general anesthesia technique utilizing fentanyl or butorphanol with N_2O has failed to demonstrate a similar advantage over inhalational anesthesia.[51,52] Total intravenous anesthesia, therefore, may be the most appropriate method of general anesthesia.

Some form of abdominal distension, either positive pressure pneumoperitoneum or mechanical retraction, must be employed for adequate visualization during laparoscopy.[1] Neuromuscular blockade during general endotracheal anesthesia greatly augments the distensibility of the abdomen and aids visualization. Neuromuscular blocking agents such as atracurium, vecuronium, pancuronium, and alcuronium have demonstrated equivalent usefulness with only minor differences.[53–57] The reversal of all such agents is readily accomplished by standard techniques[58] although some prolongation of postoperative muscle weakness has been observed with pancuronium[54] and alcuronium.[55]

Regional and Local Anesthesia During Laparoscopy

Although general anesthesia may provide better airway control, ventilation, and muscular relaxation, regional and local anesthesia continue to be utilized in shorter pelvic laparoscopic procedures such as tubal ligation.[59,60] Due to the rapid systemic absorption and diaphragmatic and peritoneal irritation with CO_2, N_2O is frequently utilized as the insufflation agent during laparoscopy under local anesthesia.[61] Unfortunately, N_2O, although not flammable, is an oxidizer and thus precludes the extensive use of electro- or laser cauterization. Epidural anesthesia has also been employed during brief pelvic laparoscopic procedures for regional abdominal anesthesia. Comparable levels of circulating stress hormones can be measured during epidural anesthesia when compared to general anesthesia, leaving the advantage of epidural anesthesia during laparoscopy debatable.[30]

Although it has been implied that a general anesthesia during laparoscopy is "safer" than local or regional anesthesia, this has yet to be proven. With conscious anesthesia, the patient's airway is not controlled, but there is no documented increase in the frequency of gastroesophageal reflux. This may be in part explained by the concomitant increase in lower esophageal sphincter pressure observed with the pneumoperitoneum.[62] While laparoscopy for pelvic and limited diagnostic procedures can be readily accomplished with local or regional anesthesia, there has been no definite physiologic advantage demonstrated for the utilization of local anesthesia except in those cases where a genetic defect or previous adverse reaction precludes the utilization of a general anesthetic or neuromuscular blocking agents.[60,63–65]

Postanesthesia Recovery and Perioperative Complications

The patient's perception of diminished postoperative pain, discomfort, length of hospital stay, and the early return to routine activities of life have made laparoscopic surgery extremely popular. Laparoscopy does demonstrate real postanesthetic and postoperative morbidity, however, including incisional pain, nausea, vomiting, anorexia, constipation, and urinary retention. Although these complications are less severe in intensity and duration when compared to standard laparotomy, postoperative analgesia and antiemetics are sometimes required.

Although postoperative discomfort seems to be diminished during laparoscopy when compared to the comparable laparotomy, postlaparoscopic incisional pain and abdominal discomfort are still experienced by some of the patients. Attempts to further decrease postlaparoscopic pain with the use of preoperative analgesia have been unsuccessful.[66,67] The incidence of both postoperative dysphagia and abdominal muscle pain are significantly decreased by the utilization of neuromuscular blocking agents during laparoscopy.[68] At the completion of the laparoscopy, local abdominal rectus muscular blockade with 0.25% bupivacaine also seems to diminish the need for postoperative analgesia.[69]

Nausea and emesis in the postlaparoscopic period occur in approximately one half of the patients studied.[49] Nitrous oxide, etomidate, and fentanyl have all been implicated as potential causes.[38] Droperidol seems to diminish postlaparoscopic nausea and emesis, but metaclopramide's efficacy has been equivocal in comparative trials.[70,71] As with any general anesthesia, it has been documented that patients without supplemental oxygen will become relatively hypoxemic in the immediate postlaparoscopic period.[72] A small supplementation of O_2 (21 oxygen/min nasal prongs) will usually prevent this transient effect.

Most of the complications unique to laparoscopy that influence anesthetic care are attributable to the pneumoperitoneum. Subcutaneous emphysema, pneumothorax, pneumopericardium, pneumomediastinum, or gas embolism are dependent on the gaseous properties of the insufflation agent employed. During prolonged laparoscopy the insufflation gas may escape into the subcutaneous tissues around the trocars, and with higher-than-normal insufflation pressures, subcutaneous emphysema is frequently seen.[73] Scrotal subcutaneous emphysema is commonly seen in laparoscopic varicocelectomy patients after the retroperitoneal dissection. Regardless of the extent, the subcutaneous emphysema generally resolves over a 24-hour period when CO_2 is used. More inert, insoluble gases such as helium may require many weeks for the subcutaneous emphysema to subside.

Pneumothorax, pneumomediastinum, or pneumopericardium are rare but life-threatening complications of the pneumoperitoneum.[74–76] When one of these is recognized, immediate deflation of the pneumoperitoneum is indicated, with additional corrective actions such as tube thoracostomy or pericardiocentesis if symptoms persist.

Venous gas embolism (incidence of 0.0016% to 0.013%)[77,78] is the most dreaded of the laparoscopic complications directly attributable to the insufflation agent. During any laparoscopy performed with a positive pressure pneumoperitoneum, gas emboli can gain entry to the heart through many major venous structures: uterine veins, hepatic veins, the portal vein, or the inferior vena cava.[77–81] With significant embolization, sudden cardiovascular collapse with an acute loss of pulse and blood pressure will be observed, and a "mill wheel" cardiac murmur may be auscultated. The patient should then be placed in a left lateral decubitus (left-side-down) Trendelenburg (head-down) position to help alleviate the pulmonary outflow obstruction created by the gas embolus in the right ventricle.[78] CO_2 and N_2O are highly soluble in blood, and the ventricular embolus will rapidly dissolve, but if a relatively insoluble gas such as helium has been used as the insufflation agent, this dissolution process may require a considerable length of time.

With positive abdominal pressure from the pneumoperitoneum, there is loss of venous pulsation, diminution in venous blood velocities and a decrease in venous flow, which may result in a diminished venous return to the heart.[2–4,82] Deep venous prophylaxis with pneumatic compression stockings is therefore warranted during any laparoscopy in which a positive pressure pneumoperitoneum is utilized.

Hypothermia and cardiac arrhythmias are complications indirectly related to the pneumoperitoneum. As with any operative procedure, the patient's core temperature decreases with time due to patient exposure in a cool environment. In addition, there has been reported a 0.3°C decrease in core temperature per 50 l volume flow of carbon dioxide pneumoperitoneum.[83] Warming the insufflation gas may avoid this added temperature decrease.[84]

During laparoscopy, cardiac arrhythmias occur more frequently during CO_2 pneumoperitoneum than during N_2O (17% vs. 4.4%).[85] Acid-base disturbances are felt to be the major causative factors for this observation during CO_2 pneumoperitoneum. Although arrhythmias are relatively common, cardiac arrest and cardiovascular collapse are fortunately extremely rare (0.04% incidence). The causes of these severe cardiac complications are most likely multifactorial in origin and may include a combination of increased ventricular irritability, decreased venous return, decreased cardiac output, hypoventilation, gas embolization, and/or profound vagal response due to peritoneal insufflation.[86,87]

Conclusions

The pneumoperitoneum is the major cause of the physiologic changes observed during anesthesia for urologic laparoscopic procedures. Although laparoscopy can be performed under local or regional anesthesia, general anesthesia allows for a potentially safer and technically superior procedure due to better abdominal distension, visualization, and patient cooperation. With infrequent and usually minimal complications, the administration of anesthesia is extremely safe during the vast majority of laparoscopic urologic procedures.

References

1. Smith RS: Gasless laparoscopy systems. In: *Gasless laparoscopy with conventional instruments: The next phase in minimally invasive surgery*. Edited by Smith RS, Organ Ch Jr. San Francisco: Norman Publishing, ch 2, pp 11–32, 1993.
2. Ishizaki Y, Bandai Y, Shimomura K, Abe H, Ohtomo Y, Idezuki Y: Changes in splanchnic blood flow and cardiovascular effects following peritoneal insufflation of carbon dioxide. *Surg Endosc* 7:420–423, 1993.
3. Pricolo VE, Demaria EJ, Burchard KW: Venous return: Physiology, monitoring, and manipulation: Part I. *Surg Rounds* Sept:703–707, 1993.
4. Ishizaki Y, Bandai Y, Shimomura K, Abe H, Ohtomo Y, Idezuki Y: Safe intraabdominal pressure of carbon dioxide pneumoperitoneum during laparoscopic surgery. *Surgery* 114:549–554, 1993.
5. Marshall RL, Jebson PJR, Davie T, Scott DB: Circulatory effects of carbon dioxide insufflation of the peritoneal cavity for laparoscopy. *Br J Anaesth* 44:680–684, 1972.
6. Motew M, Ivankovich AD, Bieniarz J, et al: Cardiovascular effects and acid-base and blood gas changes during laparoscopy. *Am J Obstet Gynecol* 115:1002–1012, 1973.
7. McKenzie R, Wadhwa RK, Bedger RC: Noninvasive measurements of cardiac output during laparoscopy. *J Reprod Med* 24:247–250, 1980.
8. Wittgen CM, Andrus CH, Fitzgerald SD, Baudendistel LJ, Dahms TE, Kaminski DL: Analysis of the hemodynamic and ventilatory effects of laparoscopic cholecystectomy. *Arch Surg* 126:997–1001, 1991.
9. Liu SY, Leighton T, Davis I, Klein S, Lippmann M, Bongard F: Prospective analysis of cardiopulmonary responses to laparoscopic cholecystectomy. *J Laparoendosc Surg* 1:241–246, 1991.
10. Ho HS, Gunther RA, Wolfe BM: Intraperitoneal carbon dioxide insufflation and cardiopulmonary function. *Arch Surg*127:928–933, 1992.
11. Williams MD, Murr PC: Laparoscopic insufflation of the abdomen depresses cardiopulmonary function. *Surg Endosc* 7:12–16, 1993.
12. Leighton TA, Liu SY. Bongard FS: Comparative cardiopulmonary effects of carbon dioxide versus helium pneumoperitoneum. *Surgery* 113:527–531, 1993.
13. Bongard FS, Pianim NA, Leighton TA, et al: Helium insufflation for laparoscopic operation. *Surg Gynecol Obstet* 177:140–146, 1993.
14. Eisenhauer DM, Saunders CJ, Ho HS, Wolfe BM: Hemodynamic effects of argon pneumoperitoneum. *Surg Endosc* 8:315–321, 1994.
15. Smith I, Benzie RJ, Gordon NLM, Kelman GR, Swapp GH: Cardiovascular effects of peritoneal insufflation of carbon dioxide for laparoscopy. *Br Med J* 14:410–411, 1971.
16. Fitzgerald SD, Andrus CH, Baudendistel LJ, Dahms TE, Kaminski DL: Hypercarbia during carbon dioxide pneumoperitoneum. *Am J Surg* 163:186–190, 1992.
17. van de Bos GC, Drake AJ, Noble MI: The effect of carbon dioxide upon myocardial contractile performance, blood flow and oxygen consumption. *J Physiol* 287:149–161, 1979.
18. Alexander GD, Brown EM: Physiologic alterations during pelvic laparoscopy. *Am J Obstet Gynecol* 105:1078–1081, 1969.
19. Mango R, Medegard A, Bengtsson R, Tronstad SE: Acid-base balance during laparoscopy. *Acta Obstet Gynecol Scand* 58:81–85, 1979.
20. El-Minawi MF, Wahbi O, El-Bagouri IS, Sharawi M, El-Mallah SY: Physiologic changes during CO_2 and N_2O pneumoperitoneum in diagnostic laparoscopy—A comparative study. *J Reprod Med* 26:338–346, 1981.
21. Leighton T, Pianim N, Liu SY, Kono M, Klein S, Bongard F: Effectors of hypercarbia during experimental pneumoperitoneum. *Am Surg* 52:717–721, 1992.
22. Wittgen CM, Naunheim KS, Andrus CH, Kaminski DL: Preoperative pulmonary function evaluation for laparoscopic cholecystectomy. *Arch Surg* 128:880–886, 1993.
23. Brampton WJ, Watson RJ: Arterial to end-tidal carbon dioxide tension differences during laparoscopy. Magnitude and effect of anaesthetic technique. *Anaesthesia* 45:210–214, 1990.

24. Holzman M, Sharp K, Richards W: Hypercarbia during carbon dioxide gas insufflation for therapeutic laparoscopy: A note of caution. *Surg Laparosc Endosc* 2:11–14, 1992.
25. Safran D, Sgambati S. Orlando R: Laparoscopy in high-risk cardiac patients. *Surg Gynecol Obstet* 176:548–554, 1993.
26. Massie MT, Massie LB, Marrangoni AG, D'Amico FJ, Sell HW: Advantages of laparoscopic cholecystectomy in the elderly and in patients with high ASA classifications. *J Laparoendosc Surg* 3:467–476, 1993.
27. Wittgen CM, Andrus JP, Andrus CH, Kaminski DL: Cholecystectomy: Which procedure is best for the high-risk patient? *Surg Endosc* 7:395–399, 1993.
28. Barnett RB, Clement GS, Drizin GS, Josselson AS, Prince DS: Pulmonary changes after laparoscopic cholecystectomy. *Surg Laparosc Endosc* 2:125–127, 1992.
29. Johnson D, Litwin D, Osachoff J, et al: Postoperative respiratory function after laparoscopic cholecystectomy. *Surg Laparosc Endosc* 2:221–226, 1992.
30. Lehtinen AM, Laatikainen T, Koskimies AI, Hovorka J: Modifying effects of epidural analgesia or general anesthesia on the stress hormone response to laparoscopy for in vitro fertilization. *J in Vitro Fert Embryo Trans* 4:23–29, 1987.
31. Cooper GM, Scoggins AM, Ward ID, Murphy D: Laparoscopy—A stressful procedure. *Anaesthesia* 37:266–269, 1982.
32. Lefebvre G, Thirion AV, Vauthier-Brouzes D, et al: Laparoscopic surgery versus laparotomy. Comparative analysis of stress markers. *J Gynecol Obstet Biol Reprod* (Paris) 21:507–511, 1992.
33. Senagore A, Kilbride M, Luchtefeld M, MacKeigan J, Warzynski M: Cortisol and IL-6 response attenuated following laparoscopic colectomy. *Surg Endosc* 7:121 (abstract), 1993.
34. Griffith J, Everitt N, Curley P, McMahon M: Laparoscopic versus "open" cholecystectomy—Reduced influence upon immune function and the acute phase response. *Surg Endosc* 7:123 (abstract), 1993.
35. Melville RJ, Frizis HI, Forsling ML, LeQuesne LP: The stimulus for vasopressin release during laparoscopy. *Surg Gynecol Obstet* 161:253–256, 1985.
36. Solis Herruzo JA, Castellano G, Larrodera L, et al: Plasma arginine vasopressin concentration during laparoscopy. *Hepato-gastroenterology* 36:499–503, 1989.
37. Gomar C, Fernandez C, Villalonga A, Nalda MA: Carbon dioxide embolism during laparoscopy and hysteroscopy. *Ann Fr Anesth Reanim* 4:380–382, 1985.
38. De Grood PMRM, Harbers JBM, Egmond J, Crul JF: Anaesthesia for laparoscopy: A comparison of five techniques including propofol, etomidate, thiopentone, and isoflurane. *Anaesthesia* 42:815–823, 1987.
39. Kenefick JP, Leader A, Maltby JR, Taylor PJ: Laparoscopy: Blood-gas values and minor sequelae associated with three techniques based on isoflurane. *Br J Anaesth* 59:189–194, 1987.
40. Dodgson MS, Heier T, Steen PA: Atracurium compared with suxamethonium for outpatient laparoscopy. *Br J Anaesth* 58:40S–43S, 1986.
41. Sengupta P, Skagel M, Plantevin OM: Postoperative morbidity associated with the use of atracurium and vecuronium in day-case laparoscopy. *Eur J Anaesth* 4:93–99, 1987.
42. Millard PR: Laparoscopy in a small community free-standing surgicenter. *Am J Obstet Gynecol* 156:1480–1485, 1987.
43. Myatt JK, Smith M, Plantevin OM, Crowther A: Anaesthesia for day-stay laparoscopy. *Br J Anaesth* 58:1200–1201, 1986.
44. Harvey DC, Charloton AJ, Findley IL: Comparison of morbidity between inpatients and outpatients following gynaecological laparoscopy. *Ann R Coll Surg Engl* 67:103–104, 1985.
45. Monk TG, Weldon BC: Anesthetic considerations for laparoscopic surgery. In: *Laparoscopic Urology*. Edited by Clayman RV, Ellspeth EM. St. Louis: Quality Medical Publishing, ch 3, pp 19–27, 1993.
46. Alexander GD, Noe FE, Brown EM: Anesthesia for pelvic laparoscopy. *Anesth Analg* 48:14–18, 1969.
47. Marco AP, Yeo CJ, Rock P: Anesthesia for a patient undergoing laparoscopic cholecystectomy. *Anesthesiology* 73:1268–1270, 1990.
48. Taylor E, Feinstein R, Soper N, White PF: Effect of nitrous oxide on surgical conditions during laparoscopic cholecystectomy. *Anesthesiology* 75:541–543, 1991.
49. Lonie DS, Harper NJN: Nitrous oxide anaesthesia and vomiting: The effect of nitrous oxide anaesthesia on the incidence of vomiting following gynaecological laparoscopy. *Anaesthesia* 41:703–707, 1986.
50. Bailie R, Craig G, Restall J: Total intravenous anaesthesia for laparoscopy. *Anaesthesia* 44:60–63, 1989.

51. Rising S, Dodgson MS, Steen PA: Isofluarane v fentanyl for outpatient laparoscopy. *Acta Anaesthesiol Scand* 29:251–255, 1985.
52. Pandit SK, Kothary SP, Pandit UA, Mathai MK: Comparison of fentanyl and butorphanol for outpatient anaesthesia. *Can J Anaesth* 34:130–134, 1987.
53. Collins KM, Plantevin MB, Docherty PW: Comparison of atracurium and alcuronium in day-case gynaecological surgery. *Anaesthesia* 39:1130–1134, 1984.
54. Fragen RJ, Shanks CA: Neuromuscular recovery after laparoscopy. *Anesth Analg* 63:51–54, 1984.
55. Kong KL, Cooper GM: Recovery of neuromuscular function and postoperative morbidity following blockade by atracurium, alcuronium, and vecuronium. *Anaesthesia* 43:450–453, 1988.
56. Raynes MA, Chisholm R, Woolner DF, Gibbs JM: A clinical comparison of atracurium and vecuronium in women undergoing laparoscopy. *Anaesth Intensive Care* 15:310–316, 1987.
57. Sleigh JW, Matheson KH: The use of atracurium besylate for laparoscopy. *Anaesthesia* 39:277–279, 1984.
58. Engbaek J, Ording H, Ostergaard D, Viby-Mogensen J: Edrophonium and neostigmine for reversal of the neuromuscular blocking effect of vecuronium. *Acta Anaesthesiol Scand* 29:544–546, 1985.
59. Hegarty JH, Brennan TG: Laparoscopy under local anesthesia: Our experience in 400 non-gynaecological patients. *Ir J Med Sci* 152:276–278, 1983.
60. Poindexter AN, Abdul-Malak M, Fast JE: Laparoscopic tubal sterilization under local anesthesia. *Obstet Gynecol* 75:5–8, 1990.
61. Phillips RS, Goldberg RI, Watson PW, Marshall JR, Barkin JS: Mechanism of improved patient tolerance to nitrous oxide in diagnostic laparoscopy. *Am J Gastroenterol* 82:143–144, 1987.
62. Jones MJ, Mitchell RW, Hindocha N: Effect of increased intra-abdominal pressure during laparoscopy on the lower esophageal sphincter. *Anesth Analg* 68:63–65, 1989.
63. Wheeler AS, James FM: Local anesthesia for laparoscopy in a case of myotonia dystrophia. *Anesthesiology* 50:169, 1979.
64. Peterson HB, Hulka JF, Speilman FJ, Lee S, Marchbanks PA: Local versus general anesthesia for laparoscopic sterilization: A randomized study. *Obstet Gynecol* 70:903–908, 1987.
65. Spielman FJ, Hulka JF, Ostheimer GW, Mueller RA: Pharmacokinetics and pharmacodynamics of local analgesia for laparoscopic tubal ligations. *Am J Obstet Gynecol* 146:821–824, 1983.
66. Dunn GL, Morison DH, Fargas-Babjak AM, Goldsmith CH: A comparison of zomepirac and codeine as analgesic premedicants in short-stay surgery. *Anesthesiology* 58:265–269, 1983.
67. Edwards ND, Barclay K, Catling SJ, Martin DG, Morgan RH: Day case laparoscopy: a survey of postoperative pain. *Anaesthesia* 46:1077–1080, 1991.
68. Skacel M, Sengupta P: Morbidity after day case laparoscopy. A comparison of two techniques of tracheal anaesthesia. *Anaesthesia* 41:537–541, 1986.
69. Smith BE, Suchak M, Siggins D, Challands J: Rectus sheath block for diagnostic laparoscopy. *Anaesthesia* 43:947–948, 1988.
70. Ho RT, Jawan B, Fung ST, Cheung HK, Lee JH: Electro-acupuncture and postoperative emesis. *Anaesthesia* 45:327–329, 1989.
71. Parris WCV, Lee EM: Anaesthesia for laparoscopic cholecystectomy. *Anaesthesia* 46:997, 1991.
72. Vegfors M, Cederholm I, Lennmarken C, Lofstrom JB: Should oxygen be administered after laparoscopy in healthy patients? *Acta Anaesthesiol Scand* 32:350–352, 1988.
73. Kent RB: Subcutaneous emphysema and hypercarbia following laparoscopic cholecystectomy. *Arch Surg* 126:1154–1156, 1991.
74. Doctor NH, Hussain Z: Bilateral pneumothorax associated with laparoscopy—A case report of a rare hazard and review of literature. *Anaesthesia* 28:75–81, 1973.
75. Batra MS, Driscoll JJ, Cobum WA, Marks WM: Evanescent nitrous oxide pneumothorax after laparoscopy. *Anesth Analg* 62:1121–1123, 1983.
76. Murray DP, Rankin RA, Lackey C: Bilateral pneumothoraces complicating peritoneoscopy. *Gastrointest Endosc* 30:45–46, 1984.
77. Wadhwa RK, McKenzie R, Wadhwa SR, Katz DL, Byers JF: Gas embolism during laparoscopy. *Anesthesiology* 48:74–76, 1978.
78. Yacoub OF, Cardona I, Coveler LA, Dodson MG: Carbon dioxide embolism during laparoscopy. *Anesthesiology* 57:533–535, 1982.
79. Root B, Levy MN, Pollack S, Lubert M, Pathak K: Gas embolism death after laparoscopy delayed by "trapping" in portal circulation. *Anesth Analg* 57:232–237, 1978.

80. Gomar C, Fernandez C, Villalonga A, Nalda MA: Carbon dioxide embolism during laparoscopy and hysteroscopy. *Ann Fr Anesth Reanim* 4:380–382, 1985.

81. DePlater RMH, Jones ISC: Non-fatal carbon dioxide embolism during laparoscopy. *Anaesth Intensive Care* 17:359–361, 1989.

82. Beebe DS, McNevin MP, Crain JM, et al: Evidence of venous stasis after abdominal insufflation for laparoscopic cholecystectomy. *Anesthesiology* 77:A147, 1992.

83. Ott DE: Laparoscopic hypothermia. *J Laparoendosc Surg* 1:127–131, 1991.

84. Ott DE: Correction of laparoscopic insufflation hypothermia. *J Laparoendosc Surg* 1:183–186, 1991.

85. Scott DB, Julian DG: Observations on cardiac arrhythmias during laparoscopy. *Br Med J* 1:411–413, 1972.

86. Brantley JC, Riley PM: Cardiovascular collapse during laparoscopy: A report of two cases. *Am J Obstet Gynecol* 159:735–737, 1988.

87. Shifren JL, Adlestein L, Finkler NJ: Asystolic cardiac arrest: A rare complication of laparoscopy. *Obstet Gynecol* 79:840–841, 1992.

5

Pneumoperitoneum During Urologic Laparoscopy

Charles H. Andrus

Introduction

During laparoscopic urologic procedures, the surgeon is almost totally dependent on the image transmitted through the laparoscopic telescope, the video camera, and the television. Adequate visualization of the structures to be examined and operated upon is paramount. In order to create an operating environment in which visualization has been optimized, continuous abdominal distension is obtained by establishing and maintaining a pneumoperitoneum. Positive pressure pneumoperitoneum has been and can be instituted with a variety of gases: air, oxygen, carbon dioxide (CO_2), nitrous oxide (N_2O), and mixtures of CO_2, O_2, and nitrogen (N_2).[1] With the employment of electrocautery and other forms of thermal or electromagnetic energy transmission, any of the gases that are oxidizers (air, O_2, and the gaseous mixtures) should be avoided due to potential combustion during the procedure. Traditionally, nitrous oxide (N_2O) has been utilized during short diagnostic laparoscopic interventions. This is an ideal pneumoperitoneum when used in association with intravenous sedation and local subcutaneous anesthesia because of its slow peritoneal absorption, nonirritating nature to the peritoneum and diaphragm, and lack of changes in acid-base and metabolic balance.[2] Unfortunately, it does have the potential to support combustion in the presence of hydrogen or methane gas and thus should not be utilized in conjunction with electrocautery.[1,3] Consequently, the gas routinely employed today to create the pneumoperitoneum is carbon dioxide (CO_2). Although CO_2 has the disadvantages of being readily absorbable, being irritating to the peritoneum and diaphragm, and having the potential to produce hypercarbia and acidosis, it is inert, noncombustible, and relatively safe with regard to embolization.[4] During most urologic laparoscopic procedures, the potential need to utilize electrocautery is always present. Thus, for the present, CO_2 seems to be the gas of choice during laparoscopic urologic operations.

Investigators are at present attempting to find an alternate gas or technique that might prove to be the "ideal" way to promote abdominal distension and guarantee adequate visualization in all laparoscopic procedures. At present, research is being conducted both in animal models and in man utilizing several of the noble gases (helium[5-7] and argon[8]) as alternate pneumoperitoneum media. Another alternative being explored is the development of non-pneumoperitoneum systems employing mechanical abdominal distension devices.[9,10] An example of this is the Origin Laparolift System (Origin Medsystems Inc., 135 Constitution Dr., Menlo Park, CA 94025)[11] (Fig. 5-1).

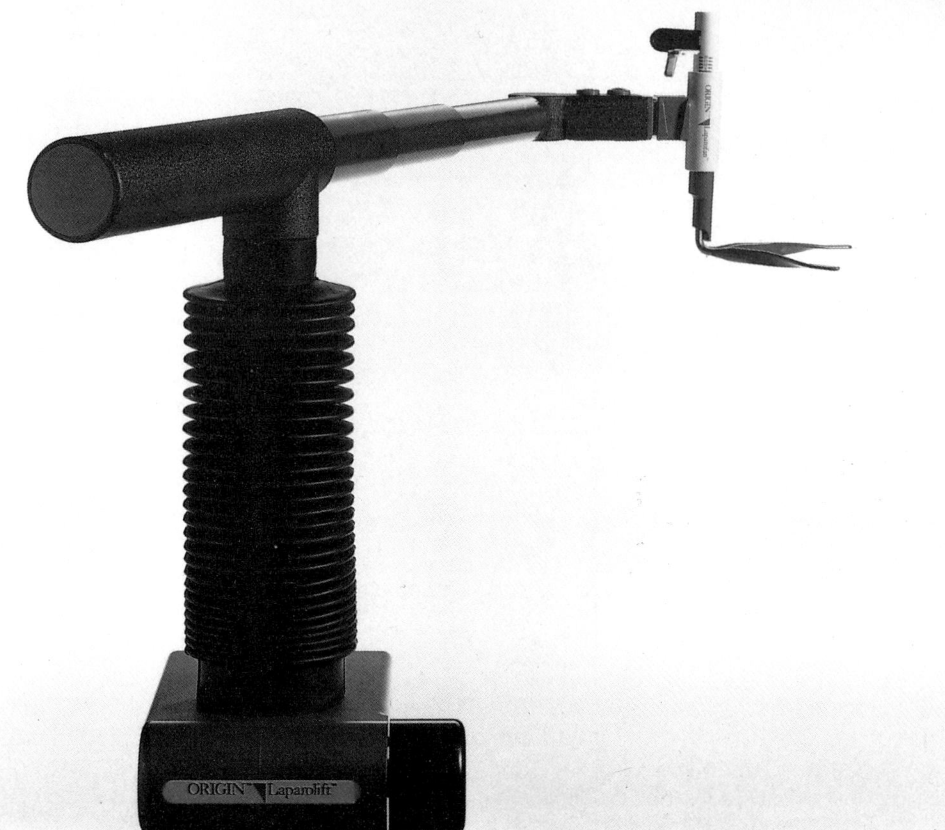

Figure 5-1 The Origin Laparolift System.

Establishing the Pneumoperitoneum

The Closed Technique

Problems associated with insufflation and trocar placement can be minimized by identifying individuals at risk for intraperitoneal adhesions. After the patient has been induced with a general anesthetic, endotracheally intubated, and the Foley catheter placed, the abdominal wall is prepared in a standard fashion and the operative field draped. The initial laparoscopic procedure is the establishment of the pneumoperitoneum. The patient is placed in the Trendelenburg position in preparation for insufflation. With the head down the bowel moves out of the pelvis and enters the upper abdomen. Potential morbidity exists from this posture. Augmented venous return to the heart increases myocardial oxygen demands. In patients with compromised ejection fractions (less than 54%), subendocardial ischemia may readily occur.[12] Elevations of left atrial blood pressures in relation to alveolar pressures can lead to atelectasis and pulmonary edema.[13] In the Trendelenburg position jugular venous pressures can rise to four times normal levels. The resultant cerebral venous stasis and pressure elevation is compounded by vasodilation of the cerebral vessels secondary to hypercarbia. Cerebral edema may be produced.[13]

The traditional method of inducing a pneumoperitoneum is to insufflate the abdominal cavity with CO_2 or N_2O through a spring-loaded, guarded needle (Veress needle) that has been placed through a small skin incision[14] (Fig. 5-2). The subumbilical area is the most common location for the placement of the Veress needle and the first trocar due to the

(a)

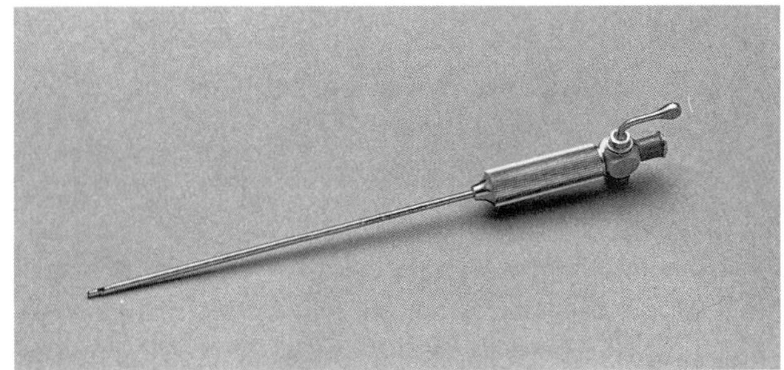

Figure 5-2 (a) Reusable spring-loaded Veress cannula.

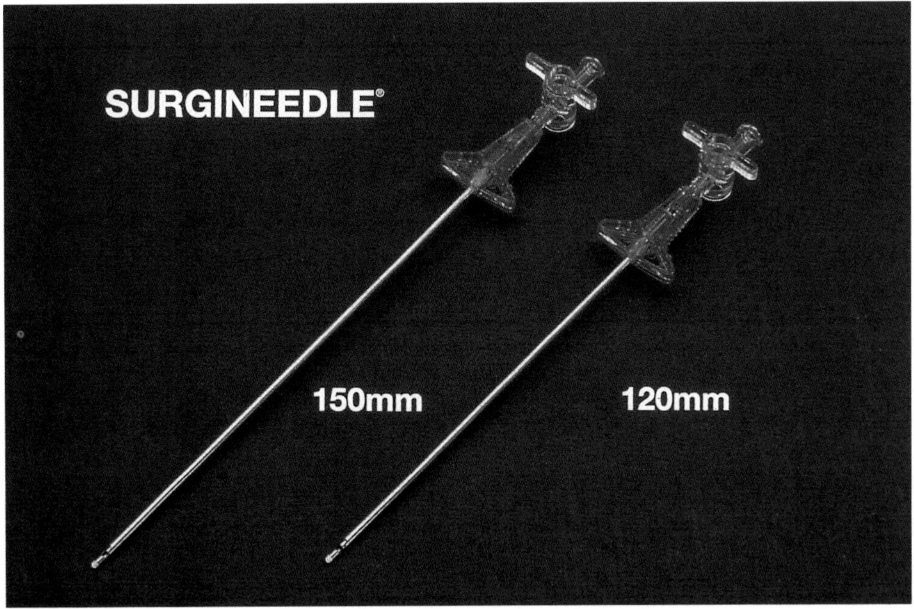

Figure 5-2 (b) Examples of a commonly used disposable Veress needle.

fusion of the fascial layers in the abdominal midline and the proximity of the peritoneal lining to the fascia. To insert the Veress needle, the skin incision is performed in the inferior edge of the umbilicus. We have found the technique described by Mitchell and colleagues[15] to be an extremely useful aid in safely introducing the insufflating needle (Fig. 5-3). The needle is then directed through this skin incision and the subcutaneous tissues angled down toward the sacrum but in a midline vertical orientation (Fig. 5-4). The needle should be held like a pencil at midshaft so as to limit its excursion into the abdomen. The entrance through the linea alba and peritoneum will be felt as two distinct "pops." Correct placement of the cannula can be evaluated by several methods. When a syringe of sterile saline is injected through a correctly placed Veress needle, there will be a loss of resistance to the injection. If a drop of

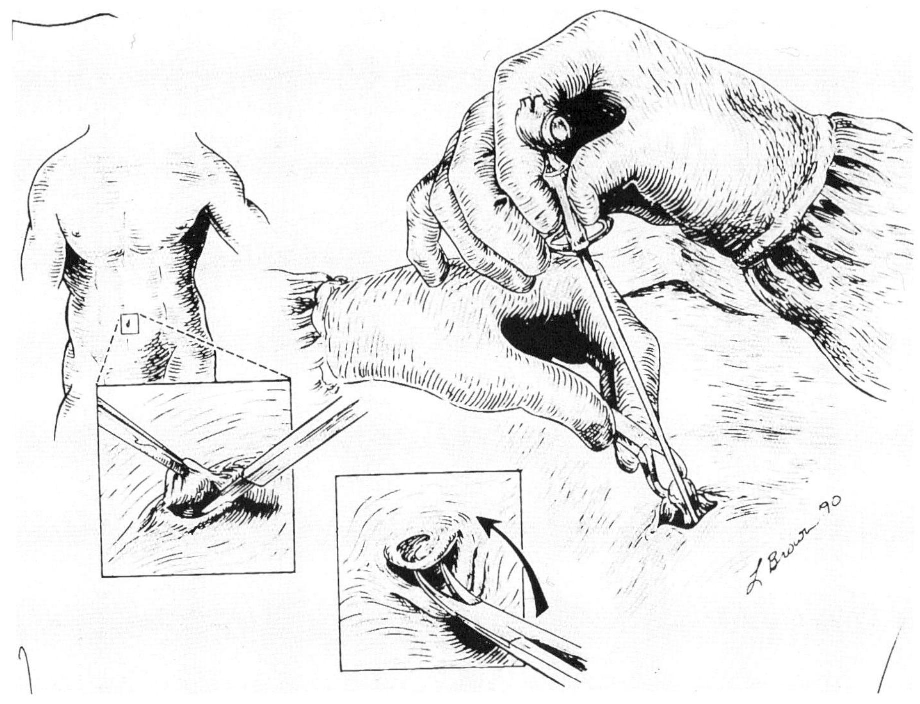

Figure 5-3 *Left*, A 1-cm curilinear incision is made in the inferior aspect of the umbilicus. *Center bottom*, A penetrating towel clamp is used to grasp the umbilical ring. *Right*, Elevation of the clamp away from the abdominal wall draws the umbilical ring and linea alba (with which the ring is fused) away from underlying peritoneal cavity contents.

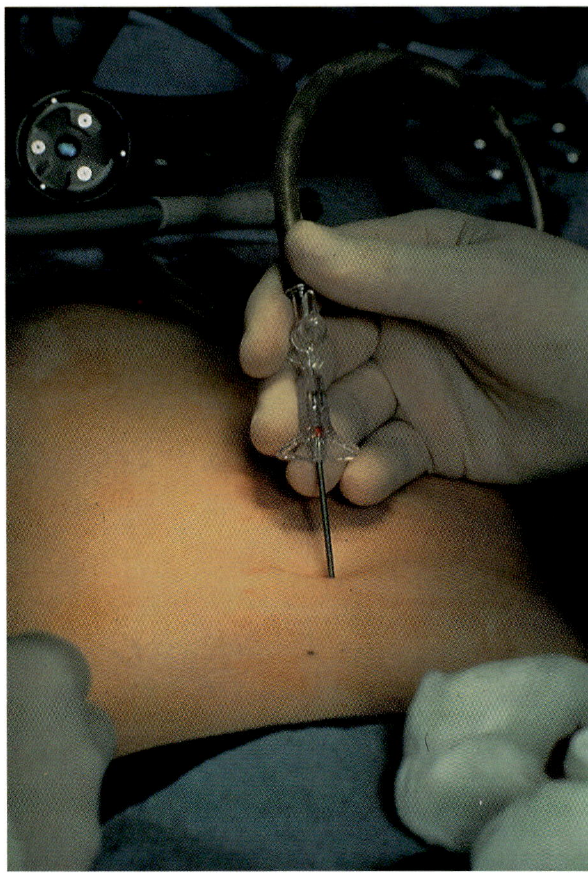

Figure 5-4 A Veress needle in place.

sterile saline is placed on the open end of the stopcock of the Veress needle and the abdominal wall is manually elevated by grasping the abdominal skin with a towel clamp, a negative abdominal pressure is induced that will draw the drop into the needle if the cannula has been placed in the peritoneal cavity. Finally, when the insufflation tubing is attached to the Veress needle's stopcock, the measured abdominal pressure on the initiation of insufflation gas flow should be less than 6 mm Hg.[16]

The umbilical area should be avoided as the entry site if (1) it was the site for a prior laparotomy, as there is risk of encountering adherent omentum or bowel underneath, (2) there is an umbilical hernia, or (3) there is portal hypertension, as the paraumbilical veins are likely to be greatly distended. If an alternative site is selected for Veress needle placement, careful evaluation should assure that the bowel, bladder, and stomach are not distended and that the liver and spleen are not enlarged. Despite the safety spring mechanism that is present in the needle, penetration into bowel is possible if there is intestinal distension, bowel adhesions, or forceful needle introduction. An alternative location that has been used safely and repeatedly is a position 2 cm to the left of the patient's umbilicus and 2 cm cephalad.[16] This area is relatively avascular and is infrequently involved with adhesions in the "virgin" abdomen. If this site is utilized, the Veress needle will pass through the anterior and posterior rectus

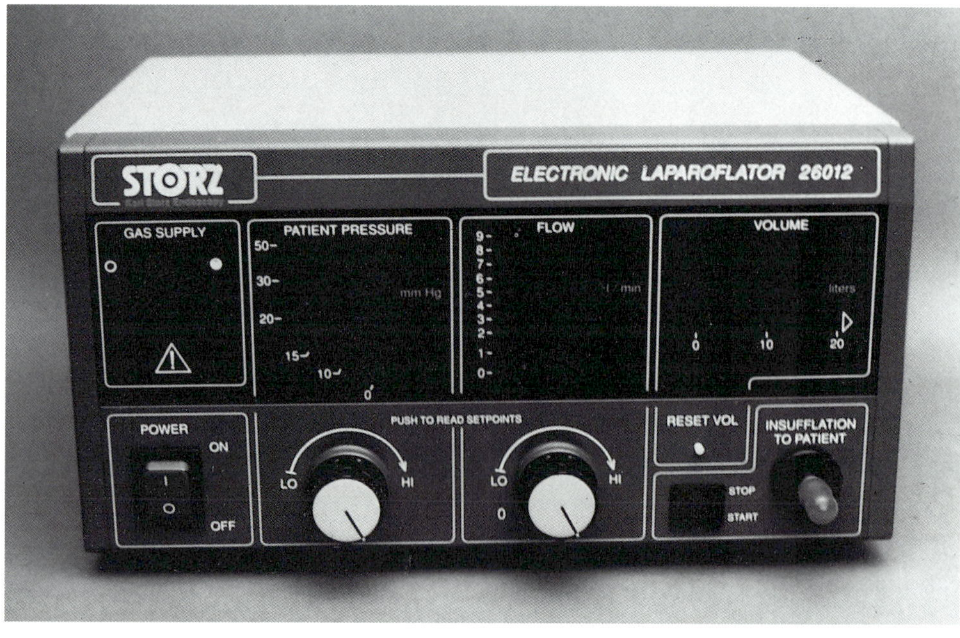

Figure 5-5 High-flow electronic automatic insufflator.

fascias and the peritoneal lining. Thus, the operator introducing the needle at this point will feel the sensation of "pops" as the resistance of each of the layers in succession is overcome. As with the subumbilical site, confirmation of the peritoneal cavity position of the Veress needle is confirmed by the injection of saline with loss of resistance, the "hanging drop" technique, and the initial low pressure (< 6 mm Hg) when insufflator gas flow is initiated.

The abdomen should initially be insufflated at a low-flow rate of about 1 L/min until the maximum pressure is reached (approximately 15 mm Hg in adults and 12 mm Hg in children). This slow insufflation rate is performed to minimize the rapid change in abdominal pressure, which can stimulate adrenal release of sympathomimetic amines and subsequent transient hypertension and tachycardia. Once the maximum pressure is reached, the rate setting of insufflator flow can be increased to 5 to 10 liters per minute (Fig. 5-5). Adequate peritoneal insufflation can be indirectly assessed by percussion of the abdominal wall and the resultant tympany noted. When satisfied that no problems exist, the initial trocar is placed (Chap. 6).

The Open Technique

The previously described "closed" method is felt by many to be unnecessarily risky when open techniques of trocar placement prior to peritoneal insufflation are probably safer.[17] As in the previous technique, a subumbilical placement is utilized as the site of initial trocar introduction. A subumbilical incision is made in the skin in a vertical or horizontal fashion (~ 1.5 to 2 cm in length). Placement of a Kocher clamp at the base of the umbilicus with subsequent cephalad traction exposes the linea alba caudal to the clamp even in an obese patient. A vertical incision (~ 1 cm) is made in the linea alba, and a blunt hemostat is spread cephalad under the umbilicus to produce an entry into the peritoneum. Placement of a gloved finger through this peritoneal defect with a sweeping motion against the inferior side of the anterior abdominal wall will help insure the absence of adhesions to this area.[18] Once free entry into the peritoneal cavity is confirmed by the finger palpation method, a trocar with a blunt obturator (Hasson trocar) is introduced into the peritoneal cavity[19] (Chap. 6). The gas-tight seal around this trochar can be secured by means of a purse-string ligature placed in the surrounding fascia or by

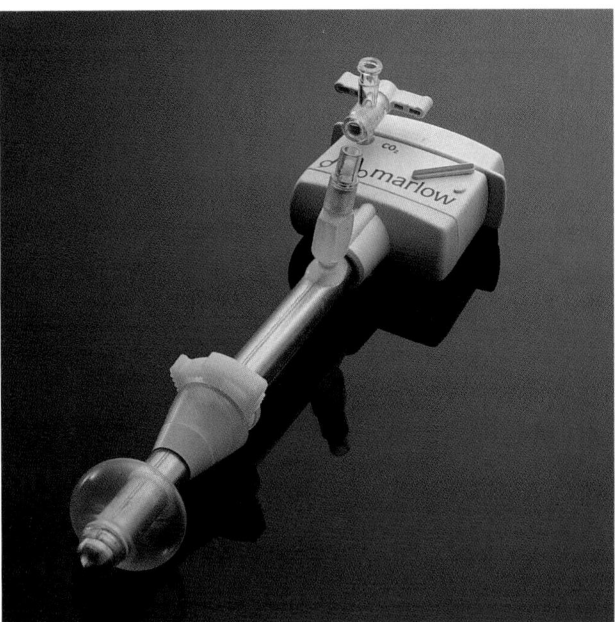

Figure 5-6 Balloon-tipped "Hasson"-type blunt trochar for open trochar introduction without prior establishment of a pneumoperitoneum.

the utilization of a balloon-type trocar [20,21] (Fig. 5-6). Although this technique seems to be safer than the "closed" method, complications of wound infections and lacerations of adherent bowel have been reported.[22]

As in the "closed" technique, the abdomen should initially be insufflated at a low-flow rate of about 1 L/min until the maximum pressure is reached. Confirmation of appropriate trocar placement in the peritoneum can be performed by direct visualization through the laparoscopic telescope prior to reaching the maximum insufflation pressure.

Potential Complications of a Pneumoperitoneum

Laparoscopic urologic surgery may be "minimally invasive," but like any other operation these procedures have complications common to operative therapy in general and unique to laparoscopic techniques. Many of the major and minor complications specific to laparoscopy can be attributed to the establishment or maintenance of the pneumoperitoneum. Injury of vascular structures, hemorrhage in the abdominal wall, pelvic vessel injury, and mesenteric injury with hemorrhage have all been attributable to mechanical injury during Veress needle or trocar placement.[1] Mechanical injury to the bowel and peritonitis are similarly attributable to trochar and Veress needle injury.[23] Hernia formation in one of the trochar sites is a documented postoperative mechanical complication of trocar placement.[24]

The utilization of a positive pressure pneumoperitoneum has been associated with many unique complications. The inherent acid-base changes seen with the utilization of CO_2 gas as the pneumoperitoneum agent have already been mentioned. Cardiac arrhythmias and cardiac arrest attributable to carbon dioxide pneumoperitoneum have been reported.[25,26] Neck and shoulder pain attributable to residual CO_2 irritation of the diaphragm has been reported to occur in as many as 80 percent of patients.[27] Hypothermia due to the continued and prolonged high flow of room-temperature gas into the patient has been estimated to occur at a rate of decrease of 0.3°C in core temperature per 50 L of carbon dioxide delivered.[28,29] Pressure complications secondary to the pneumoperitoneum range from minor emphysema in the subcutaneous tissues, omentum, and mediastinum to major life-threatening pneumothoraces and pneumopericardium, and even venous gas embolization.[1,30-37] However, by following well established techniques induction of a pneumoperitoneum may be safely achieved.

References

1. Ohlgisser M, Sorokin Y, Heifetz M: Gynecologic laparoscopy. A review article. *Obstet Gynecol Surg* 40:385–396, 1985.
2. Phillips RS, Goldberg RI, Watson PW, Marshall JR, Barkin JS: Mechanism of improved patient tolerance to nitrous oxide in diagnostic laparoscopy. *Am J Gastroenterol* 82:143–144, 1987.
3. Gunatilake DE: Case report: Fatal intraperitoneal explosion during electrocoagulation via laparoscopy. *Int J Gynecol Obstet* 15:353–357, 1978.
4. Gomar C, Fernandez C, Villalonga A, Nalda MA: Carbon dioxide embolism during laparoscopy and hysteroscopy. *Ann Fr Anesth Reanim* 4:380–382, 1985.
5. Fitzgerald SD, Andrus CH, Baudendistel LJ, Dahms TE, Kaminski DL: Hypercarbia during carbon dioxide pneumoperitoneum. *Am J Surg* 163:186–190, 1992.
6. Leighton TA, Bongard FS, Liu SY, Lee TS, Klein-SR: Comparative cardiopulmonary effects of helium and carbon dioxide pneumoperitoneum. *Surg Forum* 42:485–487, 1991.
7. Leighton TA, Se-Yuan L, Bongard FS: Comparative cardiopulmonary effects of carbon dioxide versus helium pneumoperitoneum. *Surgery* 113:527–531, 1993.
8. Eisenhauer DM, Saunders CJ, Ho HS, Wolfe BM: Hemodynamic effects of argon pneumoperitoneum. *Surg Endosc* 8:315–320, 1994.
9. Hashimoto D, Nayeem SA, Kajiwara S, Hoshino T: Laparoscopic cholecystectomy: an approach without pneumoperitoneum. *Surg Endosc* 7:54–56, 1993.
10. Akimaru K, Michiya I, Saitoh M, et al: Subcutaneous wire traction technique with CO_2 insufflation for laparoscopic cholecystectomy. *J Laparoendosc Surg* 3:59–62, 1993.
11. Tsoi EKM, Smith RS, Fry WR, Henderson VJ, Organ CH: Laparoscopic surgery without pneumoperitoneum: A preliminary report. *Surg Endosc* 7:139, 1993.
12. Prentice JA, Martin JT: The Trendelenberg position: Anesthesiologic considerations. In: *Positioning in Anesthesia and Surgery*. Edited by Martin JT: Philadelphia: WB Saunders, pp 127–145, 1987.
13. Rasmussenk JP, Dauchot PJ, Depalma RG, et al: Cardiac Function and Hypercarbia. *Arch Surg* 113:1196–1200, 1978.
14. Veress J: Neues Instrument zur Ausfuhrung von Bauchpunktionen. *Dtsch med Wochenschr* 64:1480–1484, 1938.
15. Mitchell MB, Stiegmann GV, Mansour A: Improved technique for establishing pneumoperitoneum for laparoscopy. *Surg Laparosc Endosc* 1:198–199, 1992.
16. Colver RM: Laparoscopy: Basic technique, instrumentation, and complications. *Surg Laparosc Endosc* 2:35–40, 1992.
17. Fitzgibbons RJ, Schmid S, Santoscoy R, et al: Open laparoscopy for laparoscopic cholecystectomy. *Surg Laparosc Endosc* 1:216–222, 1991.
18. Grundsell H, Larsson G: A modified laparoscopic entry technique using a finger. *Obstet Gynecol* 59:509–510, 1982.
19. Hasson HM: Open laparoscopy: a modified instrument and method for laparoscopy. *Am J Obstet Gynecol* 110:880–884, 1971.

20. Oshinsky GS, Smith AD: Laparoscopic needles and trocars: An overview of designs and complications. *J Laparoendosc Surg* 2:117–125, 1992.
21. Brooks DC, Becker JM: A simplified technique for open laparoscopy using disposable trocars. *J Laparoendosc Surg* 2:357–359, 1992.
22. Penfield AJ: How to prevent complications of open laparoscopy. *J Reprod Med* 30:660–663, 1985.
23. Kane M, Krejs GJ: Complications of diagnostic laparoscopy in Dallas: A 7-year prospective study. *Gastrointest Endosc* 30:237–240, 1984.
24. Hogdall C, Roosen JU: Incarcerated hernia following laparoscopy. *Acta Obstet Gynecol Scand* 66:735–736, 1987.
25. Scott DB, Julian DG: Observations on cardiac arrhythmias during laparoscopy. *Br Med J* 1:411–413, 1972.
26. Shifren JL, Adlestein L, Finkler NJ: Asystolic cardiac arrest: A rare complication of laparoscopy. *Obstet Gynecol* 79:840–841, 1992.
27. Collins KM, Docherty PW, Plantevin OM: Postoperative morbidity following gynecological outpatient laparoscopy. A reappraisal of the service. *Anaesthesia* 39:819–822, 1984.
28. Ott DE: Laparoscopic hypothermia. *J Laparoendosc Surg* 1:127–131, 1991.
29. Ott DE: Correction of laparoscopic insufflation hypothermia. *J Laparoendosc Surg* 1:183–186, 1991.
30. Orlando R, Lirussi F, Nassuato G, Okolicsanyi L: Complication of laparoscopy in the elderly: A report on 345 consecutive cases and comparison with a younger population. *Endoscopy* 19:145–146,1987.
31. Doctor NH, Hussain Z: Bilateral pneumothorax associated with laparoscopy. *Anaesthesia* 28:75–81, 1973.
32. Batra MS, Driscol JJ, Coburn WA, Marks WM: Evanescent nitrous oxide pneumothorax after laparoscopy. *Anesth Analg* 62:1121–1123, 1983.
33. Murray DP, Rankin RA, Lackey C: Bilateral pneumothoraces complicating peritoneoscopy. *Gastrointest Endosc* 30:45–46, 1984.
34. Nicholson RD, Berman ND: Pneumopericardium following laparoscopy. *Chest* 76:605–607, 1979.
35. Root B, Levy MN, Pollack S, Lubert M, Pathak K: Gas embolism death after laparoscopy delayed by "trapping" in portal circulation. *Anesth Analg* 57:232–237, 1978.
36. Gomar C, Fernandez C, Villalonga A, Nalda MA: Carbon dioxide embolism during laparoscopy and hysteroscopy. *Ann Fr Anesth Reanim* 4:380–382, 1985.
37. de Plater RMH, Jones ISC: Non-fatal carbon dioxide embolism during laparoscopy. *Anesthesia Intensive Care* 17:359–360, 1989.

6

Types and Techniques of Trocar Insertion

Jose M. Hernandez-Graulau
Nicholas Stroumbakis

Introduction

One of the key elements in both percutaneous and laparoscopic surgery is developing methods that achieve correct accessibility time after time. Therefore, before any discussion of the various laparoscopic procedures, it is vital that techniques of trocar placement be thoroughly analyzed for the beginning urologist interested in laparoscopic surgery. As will be discussed, initial correct placement of needles and trocars is perhaps the most important part of successful laparoscopic surgery, as it will prevent delays and reduce the risk of complications. This chapter will deal primarily with the different types of trocars and techniques of insertion as well as the potential complications of trocar placement.

Cannula/Trocar Design

The principal surgical assistant for the laparoscopic surgeon is the cannula trocar unit. The trocar is an extension of the urologist's hand. The cannula is the sleeve in which the trocar is fitted. The main purpose of the cannula is to permit instrument passage and to prevent gas leakage when an instrument is removed from the abdominal cavity.

Cannula Design

There are many types of cannulas sold, with diameters ranging from 3 to 20 mm for the standard models. Some new trocars even have a 30-mm diameter.[1] The most commonly used are the 5 mm and 12 mm. The 5-mm trocar allows passage of most working elements such as forceps and scissors. The larger ports permit the placement of the 10-mm laparoscope and staple applicators. The length of the cannulas range from 6 cm to 15.8 cm.

Both reusable and disposable cannulas are available with metal, fiberglass, or plastic as the main constituent. The plastic cannulas are preferable because of their relatively safer usage with no chance of electrical injury. Metal sheaths are durable but may act as capacitors and cause an electrical discharge. Fiberglass cannulas are insulated but may be less durable.

Gas Containment Mechanism

Cannulas prevent CO_2 leakage by either a trumpet or a flapper valve. The trumpet valve permits manual opening and closing necessitating the use of two hands to exchange instruments. The flapper or automatic valve allows instrument exchanges with one hand and works automatically (self-occluding valve). In addition "reducers" are supplied that allow downsizing of the larger trocars to accomodate the passage of smaller instruments without escape of CO_2

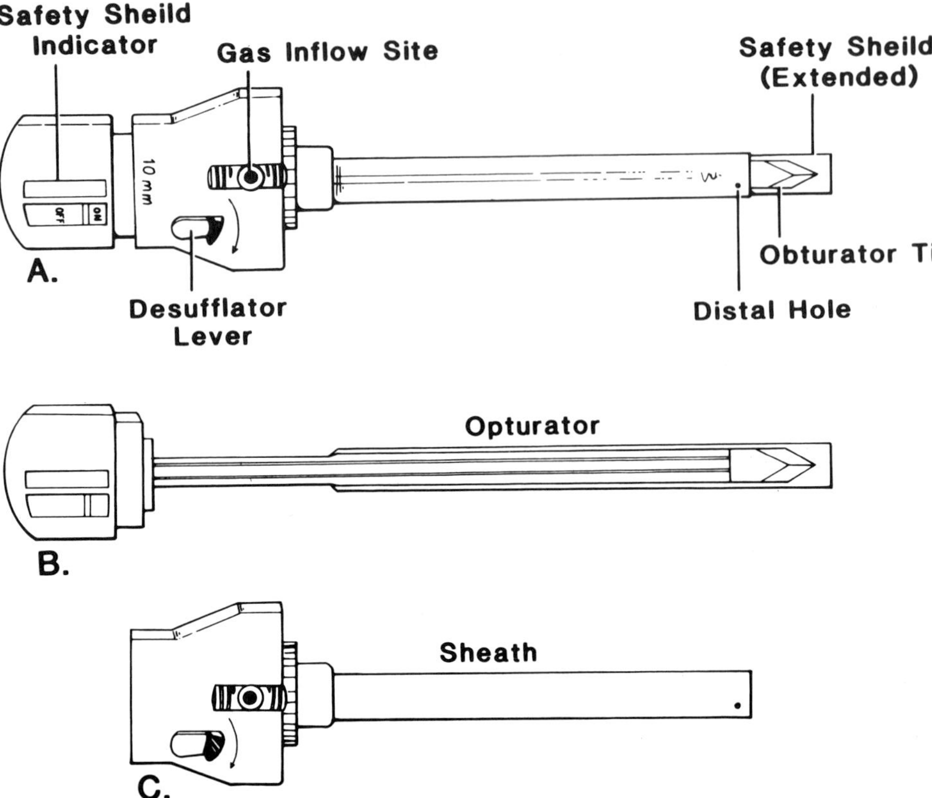

Figure 6-1 (a) Diagrammatic illustration of a disposable cannula/trocar unit. (b) & (c) Diagrammatic illustration of the cannula/trocar unit disasembled.

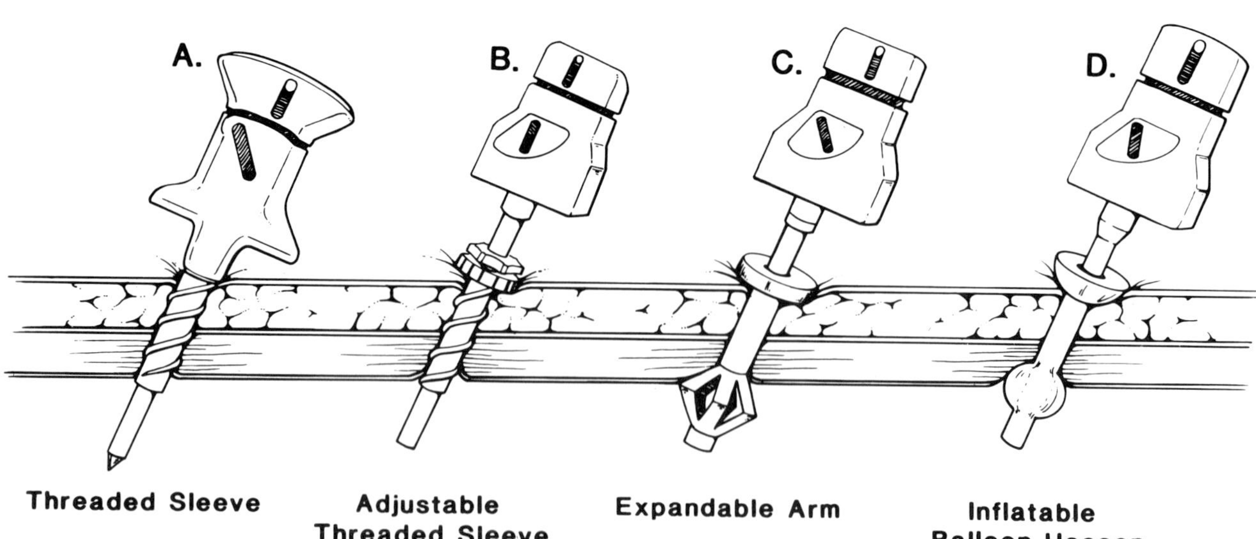

Figure 6-2 Diagrammatic representation of disposable cannulas with different retention mechanisms. (a) Threaded sleeve. (b) Adjustable threaded sleeve. (c) Expandable arm. (d) Inflatable balloon Hasson.

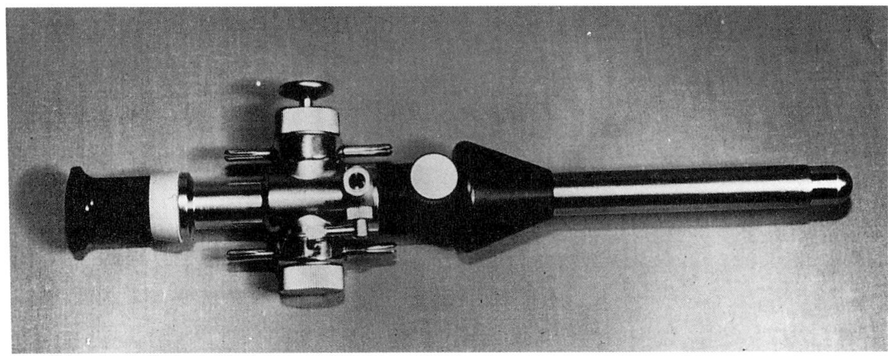

Figure 6-3 The Hasson-Eder cannula.

Vacuum Prevention Mechanism

Another important feature common to all cannulas is a small distal hole to prevent the formation of a vacuum that may pull the viscera into the cannula during removal of the particular trocar. Fig. 6-1 illustrates a typical disposable trocar with its cannula and obturator, showing the distal hole mechanism. Additionally, as seen in the Veress needle, this hole may permit insufflation if the distal cannula is occluded with mesentery or any other tissue.

Retention Mechanism

During laparoscopy, it is desirable to secure sheaths to the abdominal wall to avoid their inadvertent dislodgment. Early cannulas were secured with stay sutures. At present, however, there are disposable trocars that have a retention mechanism to prevent inadvertent removal and allow trocar adjustment. Both threaded sleeve (Ethicon) (Fig. 6-2a) and adjustable threaded sleeve (U.S. Surgical) (Fig. 6-2b) designs are available. These cannulas are threaded into the fascia, which results in secure placement and also provides an element of hemostasis. There are others with a different retention mechanism that uses the peritoneum as a tent (Fig. 6-2c). The expandable arm trocar with a locking screw (Dexide Inc.) also furnishes excellent stability and exposure. A cannula with a retention balloon at the end is also available (Marlow Inc.) (Fig. 6-2d).

For high-risk patients who have had previous abdominal surgery or when an adequate pneumoperitoneum cannot be achieved, a mini-laparotomy may be required. In the case where direct trocar insertion is contraindicated, one of the special blunt cannulas should be considered.

Special Cannulas

Hasson-Eder Design

The Hasson-Eder design (Fig. 6-3) is one of the early cannulas used to obtain direct access into the abdominal cavity. It has a 10-mm port and uses stay sutures as the retention mechanism.

Surgiport Blunt Design

Recently produced by U.S. Surgical, the Surgiport Blunt cannula (Fig. 6-4) requires no stay suture and is leakproof because of its adjustable collar. It has a 12-mm trocar diameter. This cannula is more mobile than the Hasson.

Trocar Design

Trocars are available in various widths and lengths. These instruments are constructed of stainless steel or plastic and are available with a blunt, pyramidal, or conical tip (Fig. 6-5).

Although no definitive study has demonstrated which tip is the best, each particular type has its own advantage. The pyramidal trocar may require less force of entry and therefore lessens the risk of injury to abdominal organs.[2] Conical tips create less trauma to surrounding tissue. A blunt-tip trocar, passed through a small initial incision, may reduce the incidence of complications.

The biggest controversy in trocar usage is between disposable and reusable units. The controversy involves concerns about patient safety, ease of function, maintenance, and possibly environmental implications. For each type of trocar, there are potential benefits and risks.

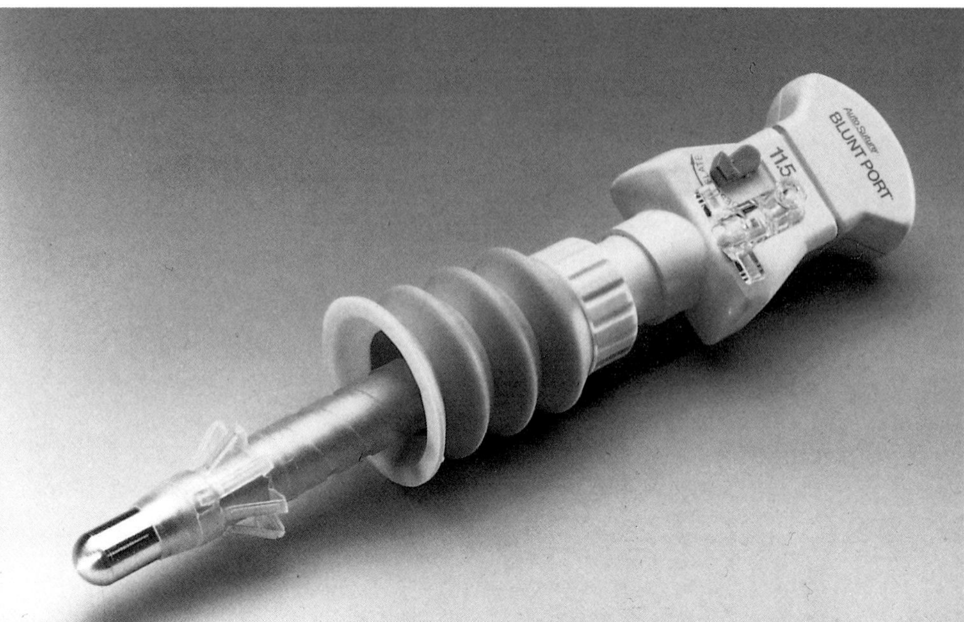

Figure 6-4 The Surgiport Blunt cannula (U.S. Surgical).

Disposable

Several sizes of disposable trocars are available. The tip may be conical or pyramidal The 5-mm and 10-mm sizes are popular, with trocars 5.5 mm to 11 mm in outer diameter also being available (Fig. 6-6). The disposable trocars are made of plastic and have three standard features: (1) a safety indicator, (2) a gas inflow site, and (3) a desufflation lever (Fig. 6-1).

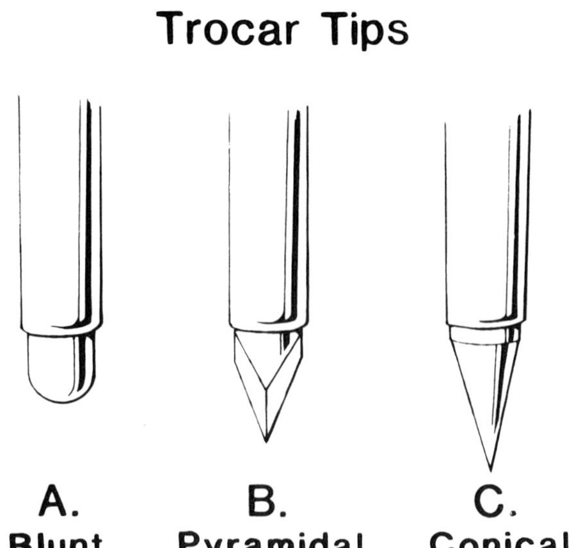

Figure 6-5 Trocar tip configurations. (a) Blunt tip. (b) Pyramid tip. (c) Conical tip.

Disposable trocars have many advantages over the reusable units. The disposable trocars are relatively lighter in weight and always sharp. They have a control handle for easier access into the peritoneal cavity, are available commercially in different arrangements, require less force to enter the abdominal cavity,[3] and contain a protective shield. The trocar's sharpness is maintained because it is not subject to repeated use.

The key advantage of the disposable trocar is the protective shield, which protrudes automatically on entry into the abdominal cavity to cover the sharp obturator tip and therefore protect the intraabdominal organs (Fig. 6-7). It is important to note however, that an adequate pneumoperitoneum should be established in order to maximize the safety of the disposable trocar. Because there is a time interval between the entry of the trocar and the release of the protective shield, an inadequate pneumoperitoneum and excessive force of placement may not allow the shield time to act appropriately. In addition, the disposable trocars offer no advantage to high-risk patients with previous surgery and adhesions.

Reusable

Reusable trocars were the first ones used in laparoscopy (Fig. 6-8). These trocars are made of metal and hence are radiopaque. They have either a conical or pyramidal obturator. The valve is usually

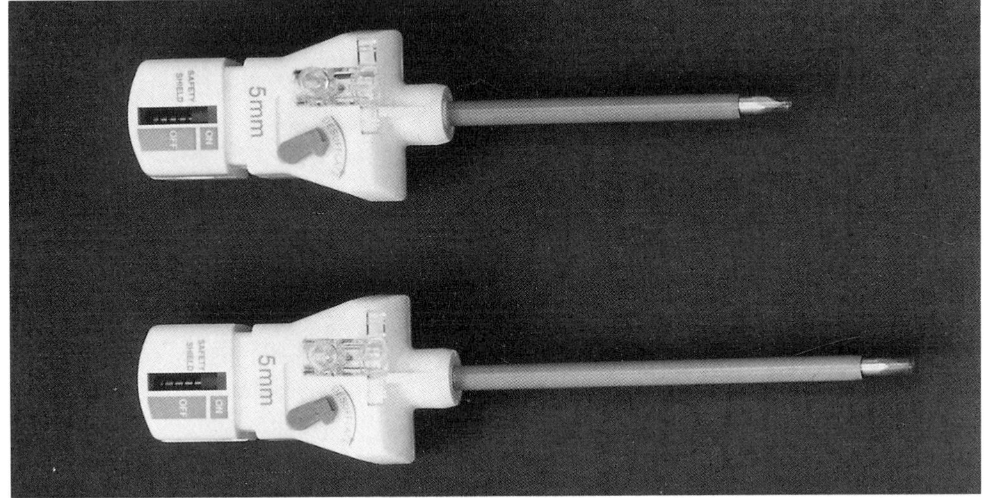

(a)

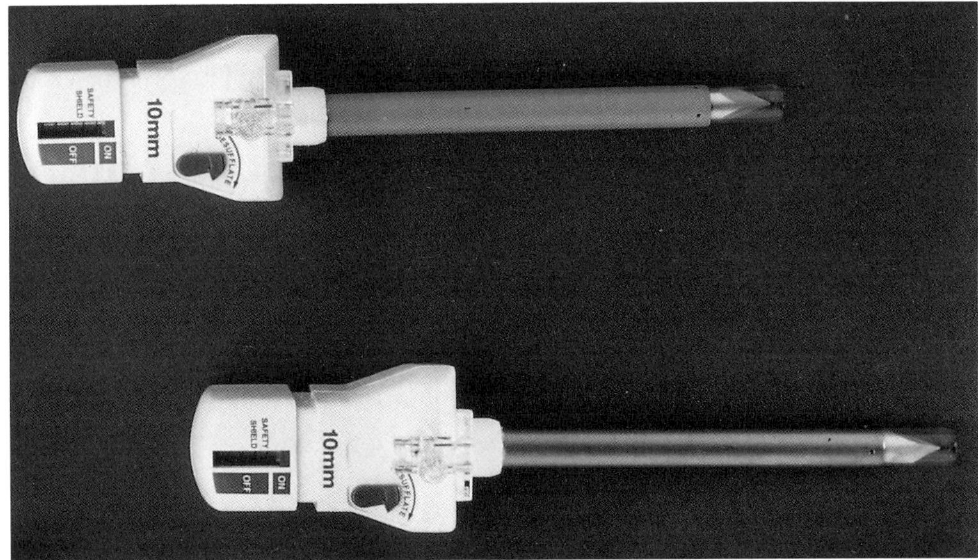

(b)

Figure 6-6 (a) Five-mm cannula/trocar unit. (b) Ten-mm cannula/trocar unit.

of a trumpet type and therefore requires two hands to exchange instruments through the ports. The only retention mechanism is a rough outer ridge along the sheath. This limits maneuverability and overall performance. Most reusable cannula/trocar units were imported and not readily available. As a result, disposable trocars were used in some centers by default.

Because the reusable trocar lacks many of the attributes of its disposable counterpart, it seems theoretically that it may be associated with more complications, require more insertions and result in more failures. However, literature from gynecologists and general surgeons demonstrate that in *experienced* hands,[4,5] these conjectural disadvantages do not affect the overall performance of the reusable trocars. Moreover, the criticism that reusable tips are not always sharp may not be warranted, as they are usually inserted through an incision made in the fascia.[6] Similarly, the metal component of these trocars may seem initially to be a disadvantage, a possible cause of electrical injury. However, according to various authors, the metal cannula may actually be advantageous if an electrosurgical accident occurs, because the heat generated by the current will disperse at the abdominal wall, whereas the plastic cannulas can concentrate heat at the bowel surface.[7]

Perhaps the most important issue in these days of cost containment is that reusable trocars are less costly than disposable ones. In general surgery, it has been estimated that the employment of reusable trocars in laparoscopic cholecystectomies yielded a savings in excess of $250 million.[8] The argument for

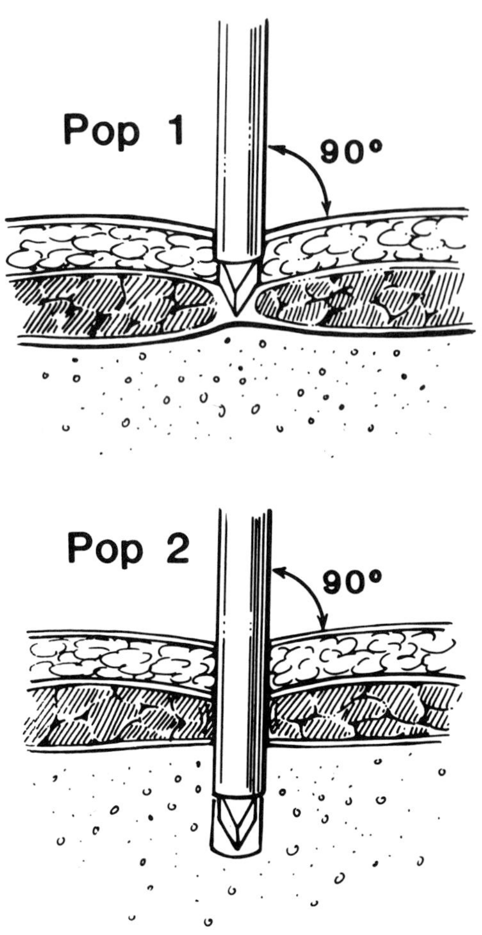

Figure 6-7 Typical "pop" sound heard when trocar tip enters the abdominal wall. Note the protusion of the protective shield over the obturator tip ("pop" 2).

disposable vs. reusable trocars will undoubtedly continue as more urologic procedures are performed.

Whichever trocar is used, two issues are important. First, the surgeon should always check the trocars for malfunction. Second, the particular trocar used should carry the greatest benefit to the patient. For the beginning urologist, the disposable trocar may be the preferred instrument, because (at least theoretically) it offers a safer, lighter, and sharper tool and a greater variety of designs.

Trocar Placement

At the present moment creation of a pneumoperitoneum is considered necessary for the initial trocar insertion. In the gynecologic literature, direct trocar insertion without pneumoperitoneum has been reported with excellent results. However, for the

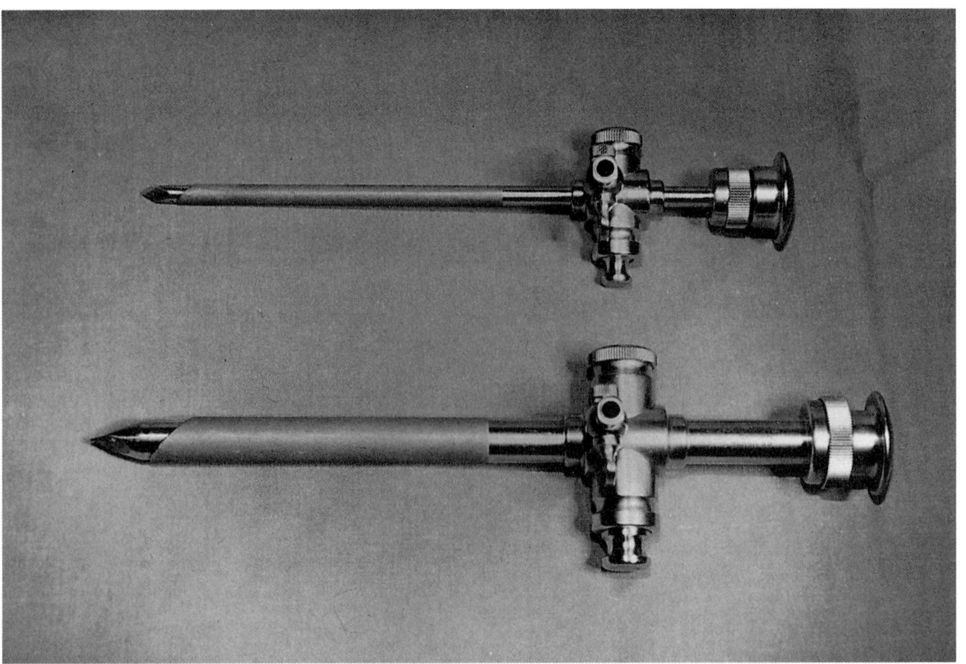

Figure 6-8 Reusable cannula (Hasson).

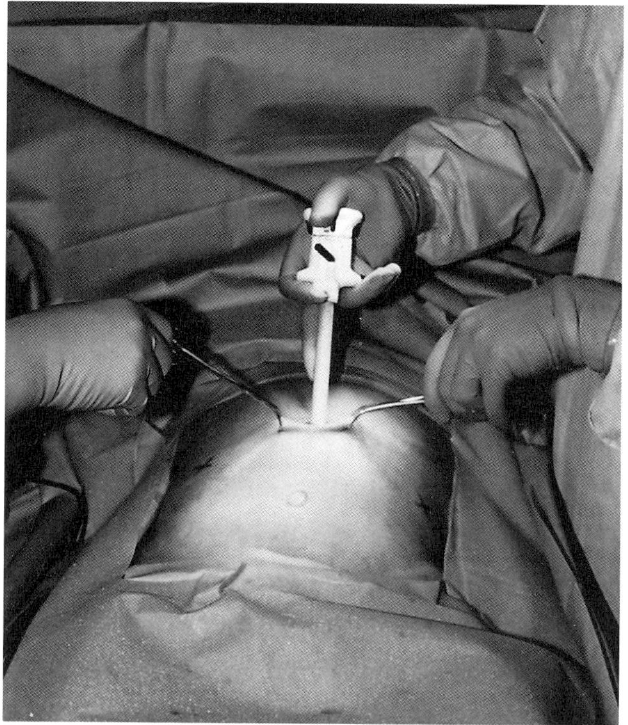

Figure 6-9 Intraoperative demonstration of primary trocar placement.

beginning laparoscopist, creating a pneumoperitoneum may provide a cushion against potentially more catastrophic complications such as viscus and vasculature injuries. The classic method of creating a pneumoperitoneum is the insertion of a Veress needle in the umbilical area. The saline-drop test can be used to confirm its proper placement. Carbon dioxide is then insufflated at the rate of 1 to 6 L/min, usually to an initial pressure of 14 to 20 mm Hg, with higher pressures being used during the insertion of the primary trocar. Malpositioning of the needle can lead to subcutaneous emphysema, preperitoneal insufflation, or insufflation of a hollow organ.

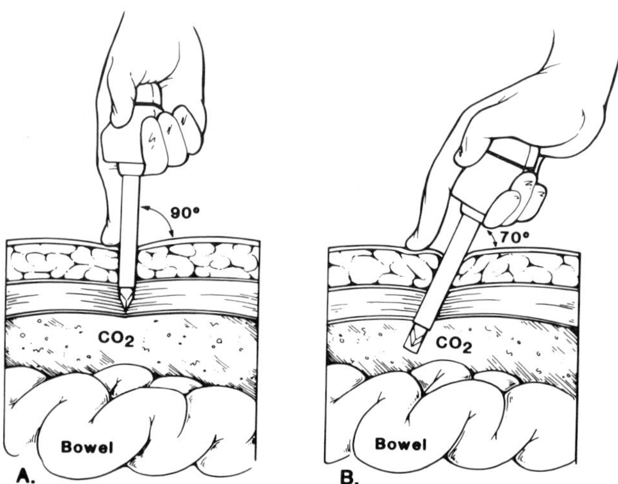

Figure 6-10 Diagrammatic illustration of proper positioning and insertion of the cannula/trocar unit.

Standard Technique

Primary Trocar

Once the pneumoperitoneum has been achieved, we enlarge the initial supraumbilical or infraumbilical incision to accept the 10- or 11-mm trocar. This is the final blind procedure. The incision is carried down to and including the rectus fascia. Usually, a hemostat is all that is required for the dissection. To diminish the chance of intraperitoneal injury, the abdominal wall is elevated with towel clips or hands. The trocar is grasped with the palm of the dominant hand, with either the index or the middle finger used to buffer it against advancement too posteriorly into the abdominal wall (Fig. 6-9). The trocar handle is aimed at the sacrum, with careful attention to avoid underlying large vessels. The initial angle of entrance to the abdominal cavity is 90 degrees. As the trocar penetrates the abdominal wall, the angle is decreased to 70 degrees (Fig. 6-10). Gentle continuous pressure is used to advance the trocar through the abdominal layers. Recognition of the two "pops" of penetration of the anterior rectus fascia and the peritoneum should provide the surgeon assurance that the trocar is in the peritoneal cavity. Once the trocar is in an intraperitoneal location, a gush of air will be heard, indicating correct placement. The obturator is removed, the retention mechanism is secured, and the 10-mm laparoscope introduced into the sheath. The sheath is secured into the abdominal wall either by stay sutures or by the threaded sleeve. The CO_2 insufflator is connected to the cannula, and insufflation is restarted.

The remaining operation is done under visual assistance of the high resolution cameras. The initial trocar site is examined, including bowel and other structures. The remaining intraperitoneal structures —the liver, spleen, stomach and pelvic organs—are systematically examined. This sequence of trocar insertion is illustrated in Fig. 6-11.

Secondary Trocar Placement

The positions of the remaining (secondary) trocars will depend on the procedure and the preference of

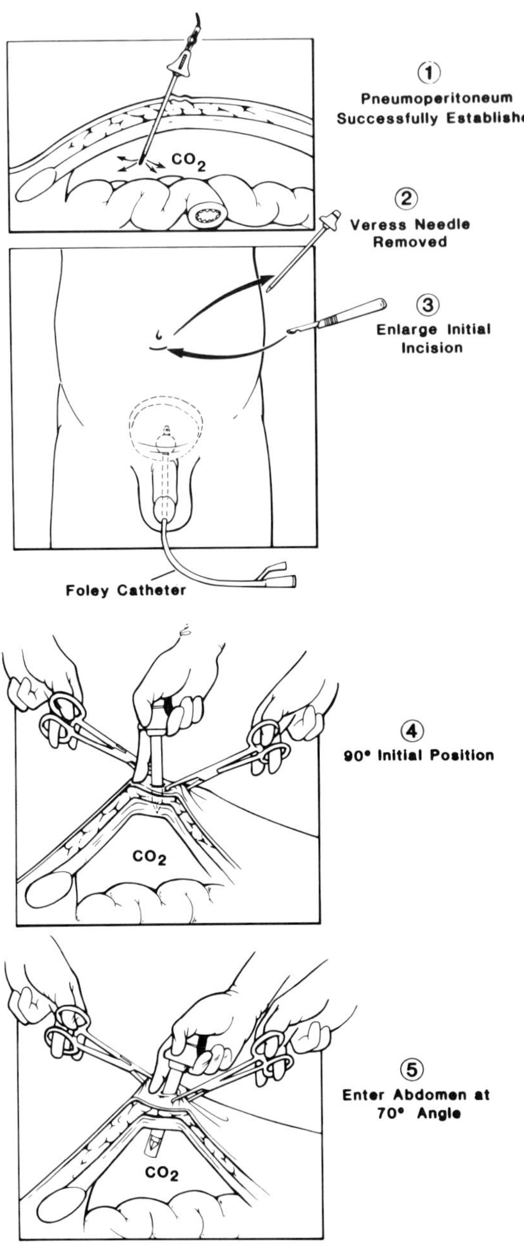

Figure 6-11 Step by step diagrammatic representation of the trocar unit insertion.

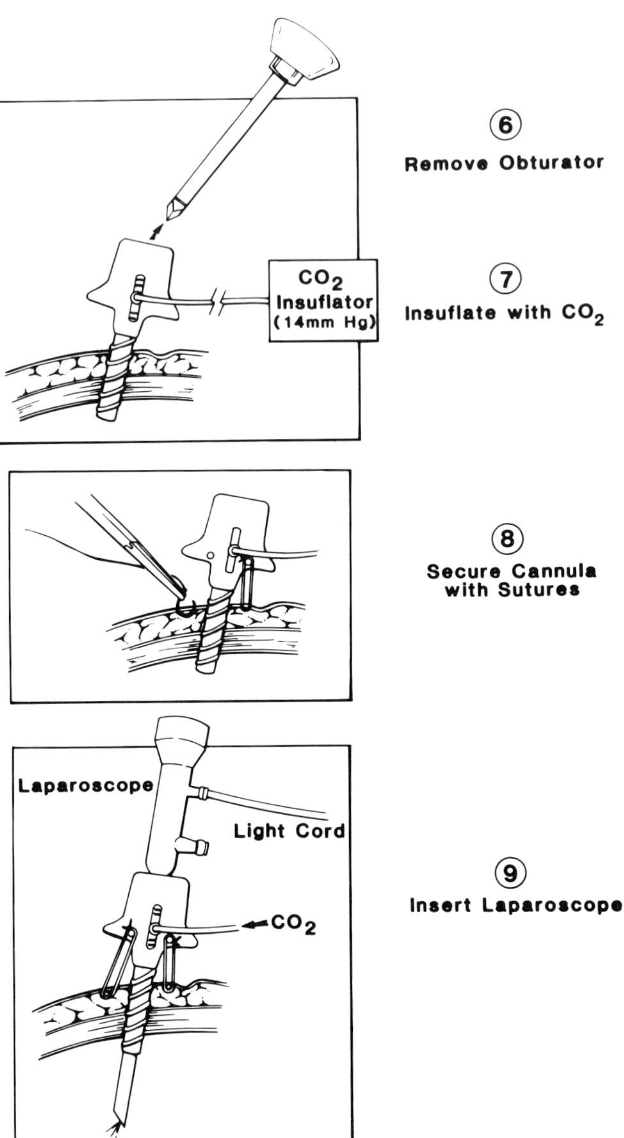

the surgeons. However, as in any trocar placement, it is important that each potential site be inspected for hernias, masses, or superficial vascular anomalies (caput medusa). Once the initial trocar is in the peritoneum, the lights of the operating room are dimmed so that the light of the laparoscope transilluminates the anterior abdominal wall to identify the branches of the superior and inferior epigastric vessels (Fig. 6-12). Placement of trocars lateral to the rectus muscle also will help avoid injury to the epigastrics. The secondary site is incised, and the subcutaneous tissue is spread with the tips of a hemostat to expose the underlying fascia. Once the pyramidal tip impression is seen in the peritoneum laparoscopically, the trocar is introduced with the same technique as the first trocar.

Closed (Seldinger) Technique

Alternatively, one may use a "closed" trocar placement, which is well known to urologists who are familiar with percutaneous surgery. This technique involves using a needle and a curved-tipped wire that is placed into the abdominal cavity. The needle is removed, and fascial dilators are introduced over

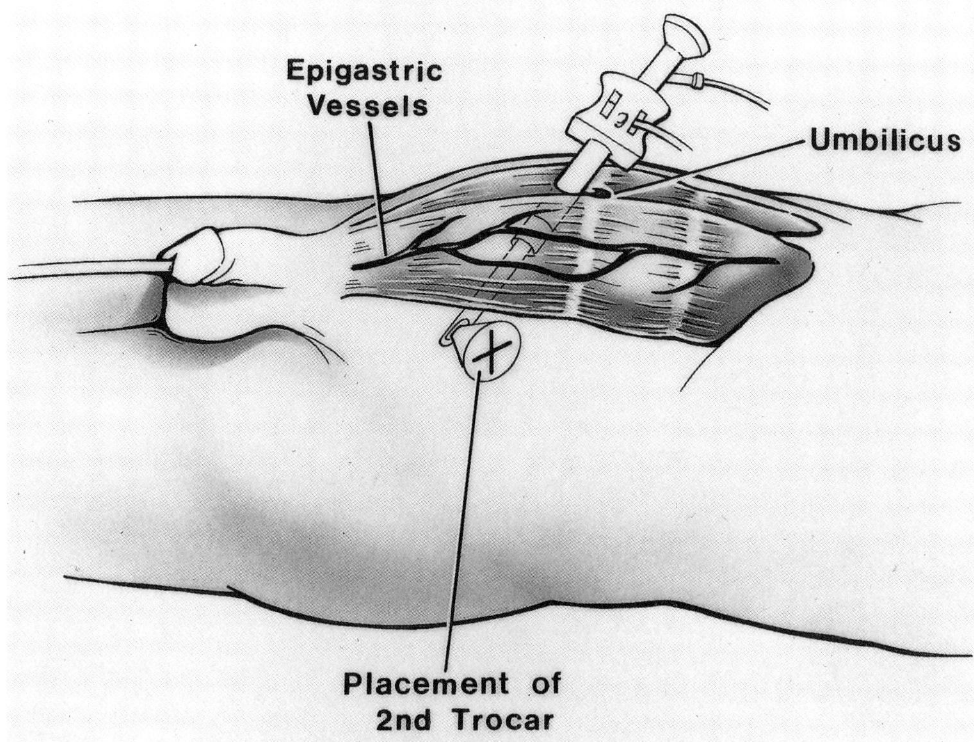

Figure 6-12 Placement of secondary trocar. Notice the avoidance of the epigastric vessels.

the guidewire to dilate the tract. The trocar is introduced after the desired size of the tract has been established. This method rarely is used but may be valuable in children and adults with an enormous amount of superficial epigastric vessels, such as those with portal hypertension. This technique may also be used to exchange trocars of different sizes to prevent escape of CO_2 from the peritoneal cavity (Fig. 6-13).

Hasson Open Technique

In 1971, Hasson first described a technique to enter the abdominal cavity safely through a mini-laparotomy with subsequent placement of a laparoscope. He developed a cone-shaped stainless steel sleeve trocar that was mounted on a laparoscope cannula to avoid gas leakage. The trocar consists of a blunt-tipped obturator and a cone-shaped sleeve with a standard trumpet valve design. This technique involves making a 2-cm supraumbilical incision away from any abdominal scar. The incision is carried down to the anterior fascia. The fascia is incised, and heavy silk sutures are placed through each fascial edge for retraction. The peritoneum is lifted and the abdominal cavity may then be entered under direct vision (Fig. 6-14). A small incision is made in the peritoneum, and the Hasson trocar with the laparoscope is introduced into the peritoneal cavity. When the obturator is in the peritoneal cavity, the collar slides down the sheath to secure the entire unit. The fascial sutures can be secured to the cannula. Petrolatum gauze can be wrapped around the bottom of the cannula to prevent air leakage. Insufflation ensues, and the remaining trocars are placed in the usual fashion. The indications for this technique are patients who are considered high-risk for laparoscopic surgery, primarily those with previous abdominal surgery and abdominal adhesions. We also recommend its use in very thin patients. Finally, this method may be used when initial Veress needle placement is unsuccessful.

Modified Laparoscopic Entry Technique

A similar method of "open" trocar placement, proposed by Grundsell and Larsson,[9] uses blunt finger dissection to penetrate the peritoneum (Fig. 6-15). A No. 11 scalpel is used to make a 1-cm incision on the skin. The fascia is similarly incised, and the peritoneum is penetrated by the physician's finger. A 20F red rubber catheter or a pediatric feeding tube is then introduced into the peritoneal cavity.

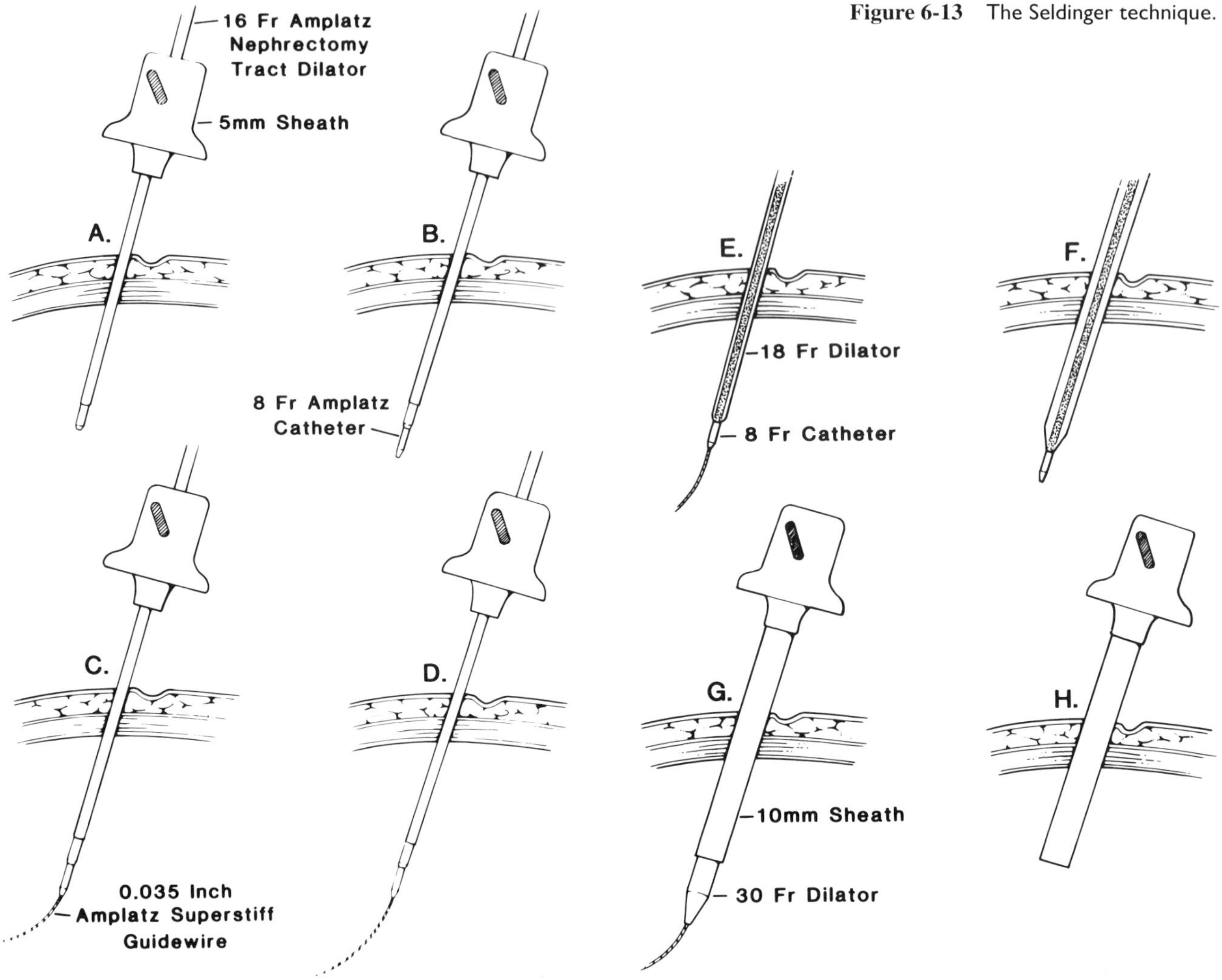

16 Fr Amplatz
Nephrectomy
Tract Dilator
5mm Sheath
A.
B.
8 Fr Amplatz
Catheter
E.
F.
18 Fr Dilator
8 Fr Catheter
C.
D.
G.
H.
10mm Sheath
30 Fr Dilator
0.035 Inch
Amplatz Superstiff
Guidewire

Figure 6-13 The Seldinger technique.

Incision
Umbilicus
Peritoneum

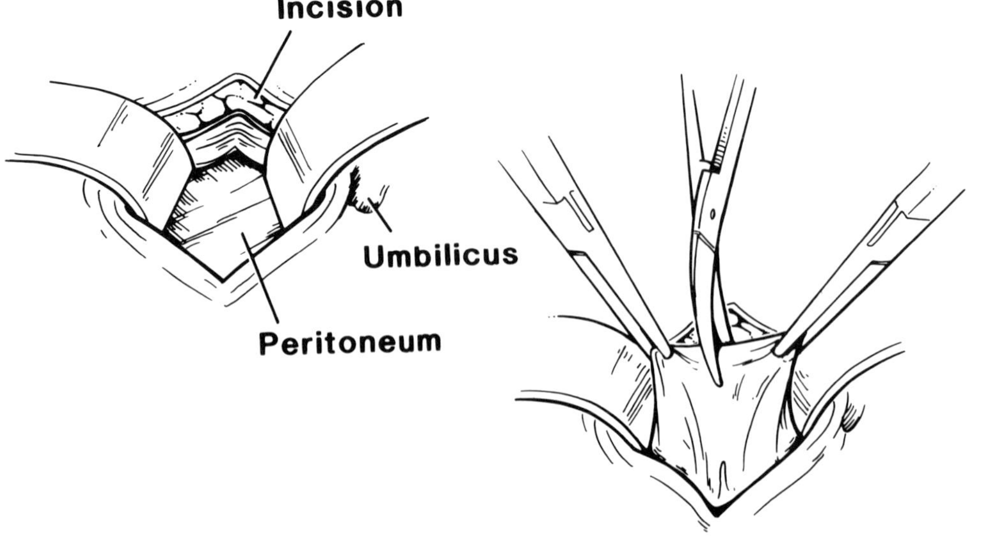

Figure 6-14 The Hasson open technique. Note that the peritoneum is lifted and the abdominal cavity entered under direct vision.

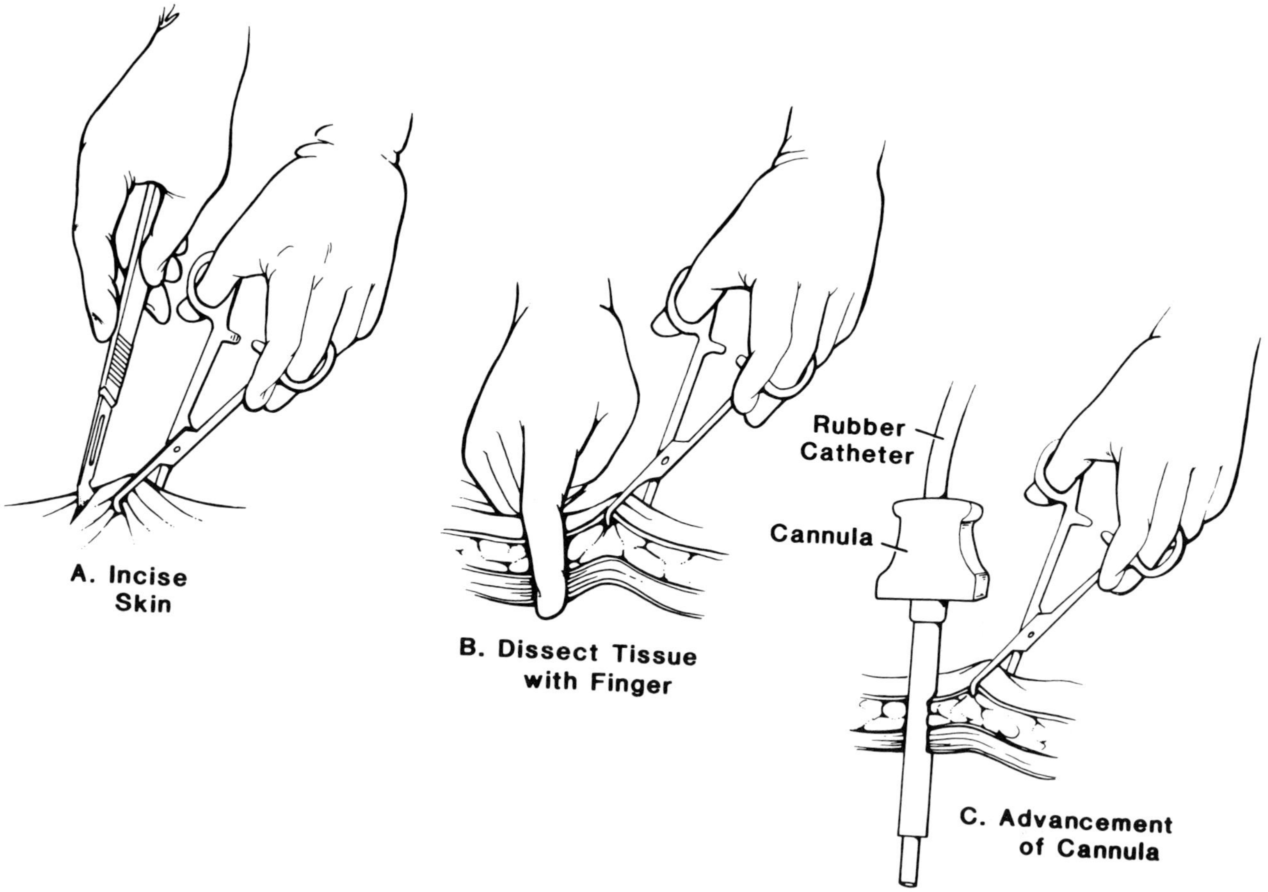

A. Incise Skin
B. Dissect Tissue with Finger
Rubber Catheter
Cannula
C. Advancement of Cannula

Different Trocar Arrangements

11mm
11mm
5mm
5mm
Diamond
Tent
House

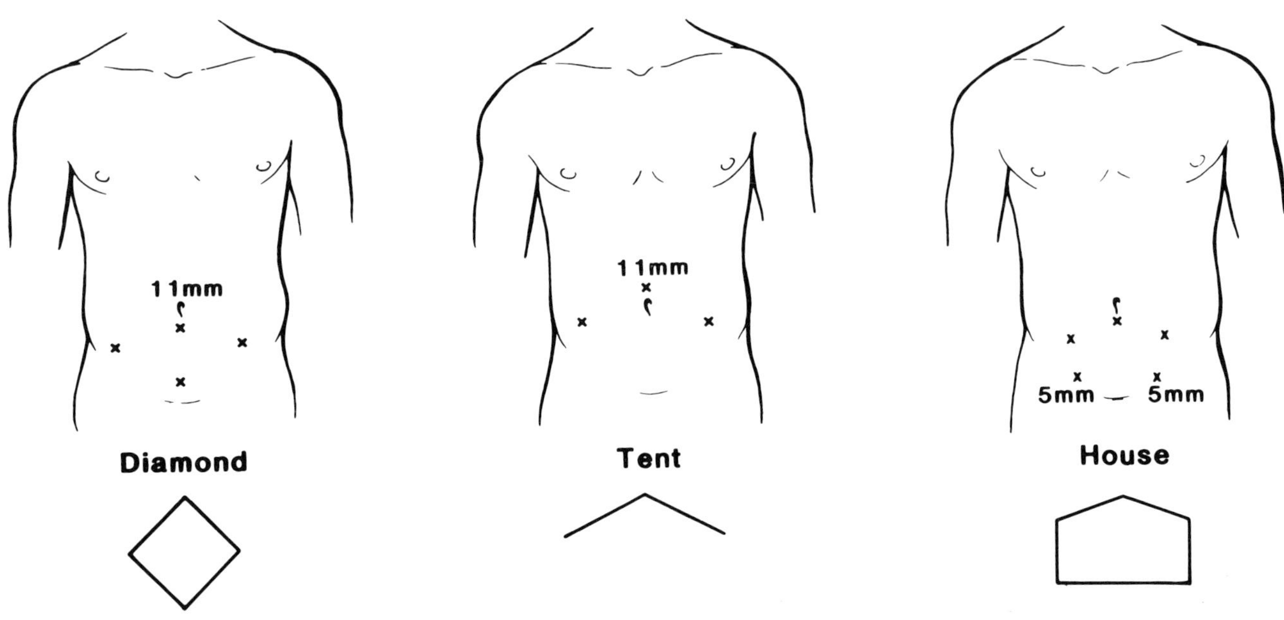

The cannula is inserted over the catheter, and confirmation of placement is made laparoscopically. The purpose of this technique is to achieve a tight seal with a percutaneous technique while avoiding viscus injury, which is possible with a blind insertion of a No. 10 trocar.

Different Trocar Arrangements

Although the ultimate placement of trocars and their size will depend on the surgeon's preference, the following arrangements are recommended (Fig. 6-16).

Potential Hazards of Trocar Placement

It is important to place trocars in a symmetrical and orderly fashion. They should not be close to one another, because this may cause the "chopstick" phenomenon and thus compromise visualization. In addition, trocars should be placed away from sites that will limit their mobility (i.e., ileum, rib cage, long surgical scars). No trocar should traverse the rectus muscle. All trocar/cannula units should be aligned in a parallel fashion along the surgical plane. This will prevent continuous movement of trocars to redirect them to the surgical field. Such movements produce larger holes in the peritoneum and allow the escape of intraabdominal gas.

For obese individuals, a common problem that one confronts when placing the supraumbilical trocar is abundant fatty tissue that hangs in the region of the obliterated umbilical ligaments. When pelvic laparoscopy is performed in an obese patient, it may be advisable to place a total of five trocars (Fig. 6-16).

Removal of Trocars

Removal of trocars is the final step of laparoscopy and should not be untidy: One should consider it similar to the closing of the abdominal wall in standard open operations. Trocars are removed and the peritoneum closed while a pneumoperitoneum is still present to prevent inadvertent trapping of intraperitoneal contents in the closure.

The entire abdominal cavity should be inspected for bleeding and other injuries. The laparoscope is then removed and reinserted in a secondary trocar site. This step is critical, as the primary trocar was placed blindly and the peritoneum at this site must be examined to identify potential bleeding points. Each subsequent trocar site is inspected in turn for bleeding and for bowel and omental herniation as the trocar is removed. If reusable trocars have been employed, the valve should be opened when removing them from the abdominal cavity. The laparoscope-video unit is removed last.

Although a 5-mm fascial site does not need to be closed, the 10-mm sites should be approximated with a 2-0 Vicryl suture. The skin is closed with Steri-Strips.

Trocar Complications and Pitfalls

Complications and problems may occur in either of the two phases of trocar insertion, namely penetration of the abdominal wall and passage into the peritoneal cavity.

First Phase

Proper handling of the instrument with the palm of the hand using the index finger as guide is a simple concept that is critical in obtaining the proper angle and force of entry past the abdominal wall. Occasionally, one is unable to advance the trocar. To avoid this problem, one must always check the tip's sharpness prior to usage. More commonly, the problem does not lie with the trocar. Rather, the initial skin incision needs to be enlarged to allow passage of the safety shield. In obese patients, we have found that a vertical infraumbilical incision makes insertion easier. Another maneuver to facilitate entrance is to hold the trocar perpendicular to the skin.

Another potential problem at the skin level is air leakage around the sheath. This problem can be prevented by refraining from excessive movement of the trocars, which creates larger holes in the peritoneum. Securing a 0-silk or 0-nylon purse-string suture often will eliminate this problem. Also, petrolatum gauze wrapped around the sheath and secured to the skin may help. If all these measures fail, exchanging the initial trocar for a larger one using the Seldinger technique may obliterate the gap causing the gas leakage.

Occasionally, when the trocar is placed the cannula will be in an extraperitoneal location. This usually is attributable to an incorrect angle of entrance, although rarely, in obese patients, the sheath is too short to enter the abdominal cavity. In this instance, the cannula can be guided into the peritoneal cavity under direct vision with the laparoscope. In some cases, the trocar cannot be inserted into the abdominal cavity because of the properitoneal fat or inadequate tension of the peritoneum. A simple maneuver is to displace the fat with a Kelly clamp. Otherwise, either lifting the abdominal wall or using an already placed sheath to exert upward pressure may allow penetration through the fat.

Second Phase

In placing the secondary trocars, it is important to avoid the underlying abdominal contents. If a loop of bowel appears to adhere to the underside of the peritoneum, one should move the trocar to one side and enter the peritoneum in a clear space. Another problem is the actual final position of the trocars. Portions of the sheaths may be too close to each other and crossing one another (chopstick phenomenon). The best way to deal with this problem is to pull the sheath of each trocar, which may allow better vision and maneuverability. Similarly, the trocar handles may strike each other and cause difficulties in the dissection. Keeping all trocars parallel and pointed toward the surgical field is the best way to avoid these problems.

Trocar injury to intraabdominal organs is one of the most serious complications of laparoscopy. Bowel injuries can include superficial (serosa) and deep lacerations. Such injury can be immediately recognized when the laparoscope is moved to a secondary trocar site and used to examine the primary site. Occasionally, however, a complete perforation may be missed if the cannula is not removed under direct vision. The treatment of a bowel injury will depend on its extent and on the skill of the operator. Superficial injuries (less than 0.5 cm) may be managed conservatively. However, deep lacerations mandate immediate repair. If the cannula is stuck in the bowel, it should not be removed, as this maneuver may cause more contamination. Most operators would deal with deep lacerations by open repair. Skilled laparoscopists may remedy this injury endoscopically with either sutures or GIA staplers. Formal colostomy is rarely required.

Trocar insertions also may cause urinary tract injuries. Bladder damage is more likely with inadequate emptying or secondary to faulty technique, the presence of adhesions, or congenital anomalies. Trocar injuries to the bladder are more severe than those created by the Veress needle and may be recognized by hematuria or pneumaturia. Additionally, bladder injuries may be missed intraoperatively and present with hematuria, fever, and peritoneal signs. All bladder injuries are considered intraperitoneal and should be assessed with a cystogram using indigo-carmine. Small lacerations may be repaired laparoscopically; otherwise, formal repair is mandatory. Ureteral injuries may be caused by off-center trocar insertion. Also, extensive dissection past the common iliac vessels may lead to injury from dissection or thermal effects. Often, these injuries are recognized postoperatively. The management options are immediate exploration, temporary bypass with a ureteral catheter, or delayed repair with interim percutaneous nephrostomy drainage.

Life-threatening injuries undoubtedly can result from trocar vascular damage, although to date only 15 major vessel injuries have been reported in the literature as a result of needle and trocar insertion. Major vessel injury is a true emergency and necessitates immediate laparotomy. If a vascular injury is identified, it is advantageous to leave the trocar in place and elevate the laparoscope against the abdominal wall for the emergency incision. Lesser vascular injuries caused by trocar insertion involve abdominal wall vessels. They may be recognized by excessive bleeding during the dissection without identifying the source. The primary trocar site should always be examined for bleeding at the peritoneal entrance. This bleeding can be controlled by simple coagulation or with a Keith needle.

References

1. Oshinsky SG, Smith AD: Choosing the proper trocar and cannula. *Contemp Urol* Oct:15–24, 1992.
2. Corson SL, Batzer FR, Gocial B, et al: Measurement of the force necessary for laparoscopic trocar entry. *J Reprod Med* 34:282–284, 1989.
3. Levinson CJ: Complications. In: *Laparoscopy*. Baltimore, Williams & Wilkins, chap 20, pp 220–230, 1977.
4. Dingerfelder JR: Direct laproscope trocar insertion without prior pneumoperitoneum. *J Reprod Med* 21:45–47, 1978.
5. Jarret CJ: Laparoscopy: Direct trocar insertion without pneumoperitoneum. *Obstet Gynecol* 75:725–727, 1990.
6. Tews G, Arzt W, Bohaumilitzky T, et al: Significant reduction of operational risk in laparoscopy through the use of a new blunt trocar. *Surg Gynecol Obstet* 173:67–68, 1991.
7. Tuker RD: The physics of electrosurgery. *Contin Educ Famil Phys* 20:574–589, 1985.
8. Voyles CR, Haick AJ, Koury AM, et al: Trocar/cannula systems in laparoscopic surgery. *Surg Rounds*:799–804, 1992.
9. Grundsell H, Larsson G: A modified laparoscopic entry technique using a finger. *Obstet Gynecol* 59:509–510, 1982.

7

Laparoscopic Suturing and Stapling Techniques

Michael E. Moran

Introduction

In this chapter we will address the pertinent technical problems of intracorporeal suturing and stapling. Theories of laparoscopic hemostasis and the techniques currently practiced for extracorporeal knotting and intracorporeal suturing, knotting, clipping, and stapling will also be addressed.

History of Laparoscopic Suturing and Stapling

The early history of laparoscopic surgery is dominated by diagnostic endeavors of those interested in hepatobiliary and gynecologic pathology. Instruments and procedures were limited. Increasing experience prompted an interest in reproducing open surgical interventions as laparoscopic procedures. In 1972, Clarke described a series of instruments and techniques applicable for suturing and ligation.[1] Extracorporeal knots and new suturing techniques followed.[2,3] The production of instruments designed both to gently reapproximate tissues and to firmly grasp laparoscopic needles has been a difficult manufacturing goal. Nevertheless, a number of devices specifically addressing the shortcomings of intracorporeal suturing are becoming available.

Surgical stapling has its foundations in the large, cumbersome prototypes investigated and utilized by the Russians during the 1950s.[4] In the United States the investigation and refinement of these instruments led to acceptance and widespread surgical applications in the 1970s.[5] Limitations imposed by the closed endocavitary environment favor a quick mechanical system to achieve hemostasis or reconstruct an organ. Laparoscopic implementation of a linear stapler was initially utilized for intracorporeal bowel resections and reconstruction.[6,7] Urologic adaptation of such an instrument in renal pedicle division and for the distal portion of a nephroureterectomy have been reported.[8–11] This device has also been used to aid in the formation of a laparoscopic ileal conduit.[12] Detractors of these techniques cite the fact that metallic staples within the urinary tract can provide a foreign body nidus with well-recognized risks of encrustation and stone formation. However, with the continued advancement in the development of absorbable clips and staples this problem may be overcome.[12,13]

Laparoscopic Hemostasis

Hemostasis in the closed environment imposed by minimal access surgery is one obstacle blocking progression to more complex intracorporeal techniques. There are five basic modalities presently available for the augmentation of local hemostasis (Table 7-1).

The performance of laparoscopic suture ligation is complicated by the fixed location of the portals, the "relative" position of the angle of view of the laparoscope, the two-dimensional nature and magnification of the electronic image, the length of the suturing instruments, and the mechanical difficulties of manipulating needle and thread. Such problems have led to the implementation of numerous extracorporeally applied pretied slipknots.[14] Nevertheless, concerns regarding slippage and speed of application have prompted preference for a stapled alternative for hemostasis.[9]

Vascular pedicles have been safely ligated and divided by autostaplers for two decades.[15] Although arteriovenous fistula development remains a concern, the vascular autostapling devices are theoretically designed to separate the artery and the vein prior to fixing into the staple delivery mode. Studies on the amount of load that these vascular staples can withstand indicate that they maintain hemostasis at superphysiologic pressures (1137 to 1551 mmHg).[9]

Titanium clips are the most commonly utilized automated devices for achieving hemostasis. One investigation of the two major manufacturers of laparoscopic clip appliers studied the pressures necessary to dislodge each type of clip in vitro and in vivo. Both types had an unusually high rate of distractibility during the in vivo studies.[16] The surgeon should be aware that these clips can become dislodged during the course of subsequent dissecting if either radial or horizontal traction is applied near or at the clip.

TABLE 7-1 Methods of Laparoscopic Hemostasis

- Mechanical
  - pressure
  - clamping
- Thermal
  - radiofrequency
  - electrocautery
    - monopolar
    - bipolar
  - endothermal
  - argon beam coagulator
  - lasers
  - cryoprobes
  - radiofrequency energy
  - microwave energy
- Chemical
  - fibrin glue
  - calcium impregnated swabs
  - Endo-Avitene
- Suture/ligation
- Stapling/clipping

Laparoscopic Extracorporeal Knotting

Extracorporeal knotting has had its most common application with loop ligation techniques. A variety of loop knots are utilized, and the laparoscopic surgeon can use pretied ligatures or nontied ones as desired. Several knot configurations are available, and the surgeon can choose from variants of the fly-fishing or sailor's knots for the same purpose.[2] The most commonly utilized loop ligature employs the Roeder knot.[17] This type of knot can be applied pretied as a loop ligature or can be tied after intracorporeal needle ligature placement and then cinched (Fig. 7-1).[3,18] Clarke described the basic tenets of the prepackaged, slipknot loop ligatures in 1972.[1] An endoscopic loop ligature is passed backward through a reducer sleeve (3 mm) and then into the appropriate trocar. The pushrod is then advanced until the loop is fully opened within the abdomen. A grasping instrument is passed through the loop, and the targeted tissue is grasped. The back end of the plastic pushrod is snapped and the rod advanced to tighten the slipknot. The same knots can be tied with any suture material and cinched with a pusher.

Other knot configurations recommended for endocavitary use include the Duncan (with or without a half hitch), Fisherman's clinch, jamming loop, and Weston's knots.[19-21] Loop ligatures by design incorporate any of these aforementioned slipknot modalities. Several manufacturers offer prepackaged, slipknot loop ligatures. Common features include a variable-length pusher (usually 80 cm) with a variety of commonly used sutures. Application of pretied slipknot loop ligatures has been simplified by disposable applicators.

Extracorporeal knotting can also be utilized with intracorporeal suturing when knot-pushers are available.[21] Any available suture material can be utilized for these extracorporeal techniques, providing that adequate length is available to traverse the trocar

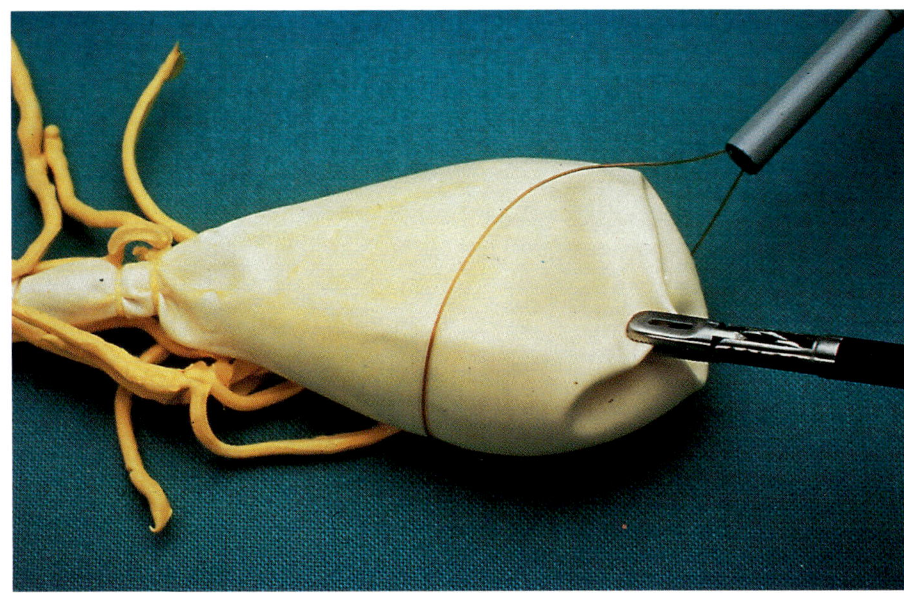

Figure 7-1 (a) Application of Roeder slipknot loops. Technique of applying pretied loop ligatures. (b) Completion of the extracorporeally tied Roeder knot.

(a)

(b)

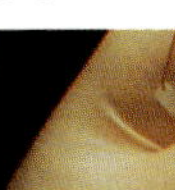

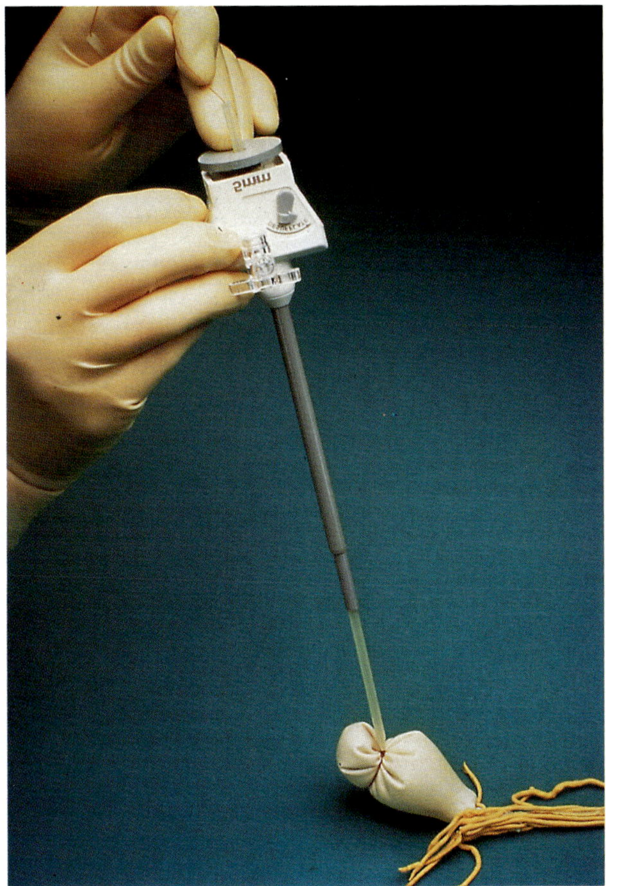

(usually 80 cm). Braided sutures do not slide as well as others if standard square knots are utilized and should be avoided. Prepackaged endoscopic ligatures with variable needle configurations are available for this purpose from most manufacturers.

Some surgeons advocate hemoclips or specially designed absorbable suture securement devices (Laparotie, Ethicon, Cincinnati, OH, or Surgitie, U.S. Surgical, Norwalk, CT) to secure the intracorporeal suture or suture line. Proponents of this method of suture anchoring cite advantages such as avoidance of the potential loosening of slipknot ties and the cumbersome multiple trocar passages required by extracorporeal knotting. Metallic and absorbable clips have been successfully used to secure intracorporeal sutures.[14]

Laparoscopic Intracorporeal Suturing and Knotting

Intracorporeal Suturing Difficulties

Laparoscopic urologic reconstruction is currently hampered by difficulties inherent in the acquisition

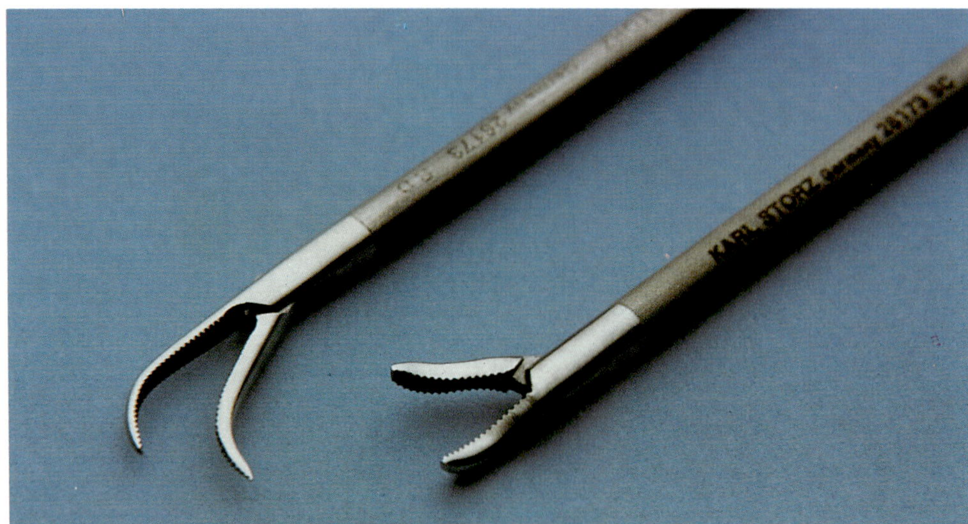

Figure 7-2 Top, flamingo-type assistant instrument for intracorporeal suturing. Below, parrot-jawed needle driver (Karl Storz, Culver City, CA).

of intracorporeal suturing skills. The reasons for the difficulty in performing intracorporeal suturing are multifactorial. The closed operating environment and fixed portals of entrance limit the "approach" to the targeted suture site. In addition, the intraabdominal viscera are rarely stationery, compounding the technical difficulties of immobile access portals. Special assisting instruments (Fig. 7-2) have been designed to manipulate nonfixed tissues for correct alignment.

Flexible trocar portals have been introduced (Fig. 7-3) that may permit some degree of the fine movement assistance currently lacking in endoscopic suturing. Some experienced laparoscopists advocate the utilization of curved needle graspers, which allows continuous visualization of the needle and driver's tip during all aspects of intracorporeal suturing.

Instrumentation and Skills

The limitation of general purpose endoscopic graspers as needle drivers is their inability to hold and maintain the torque needed for driving needles through tissue. To overcome this problem several

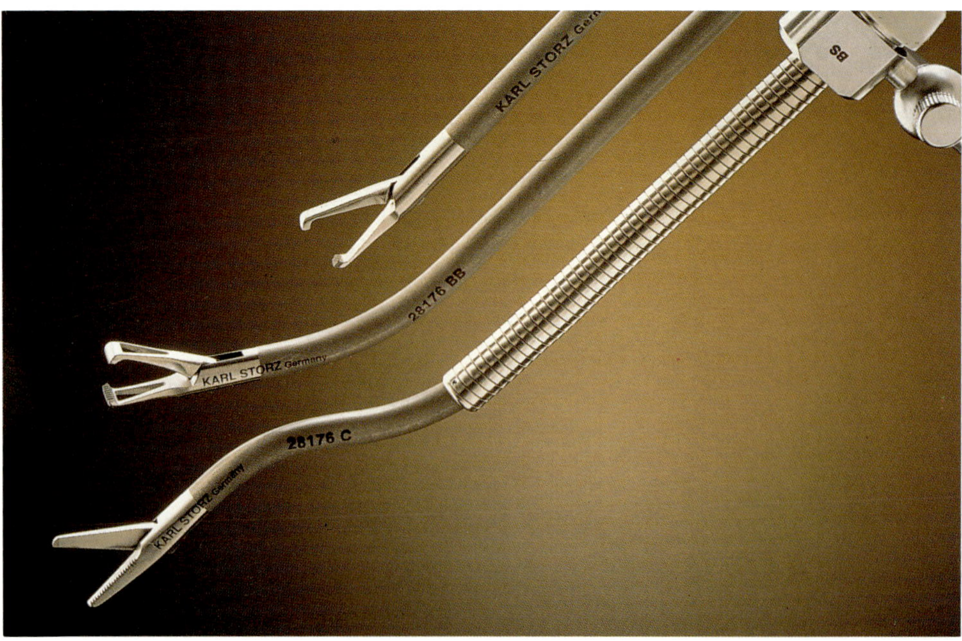

Figure 7-3 Flexible trocars that give the surgeon some suturing control at the wrist with long laparoscopic suturing instruments (Karl Storz, Culver City, CA).

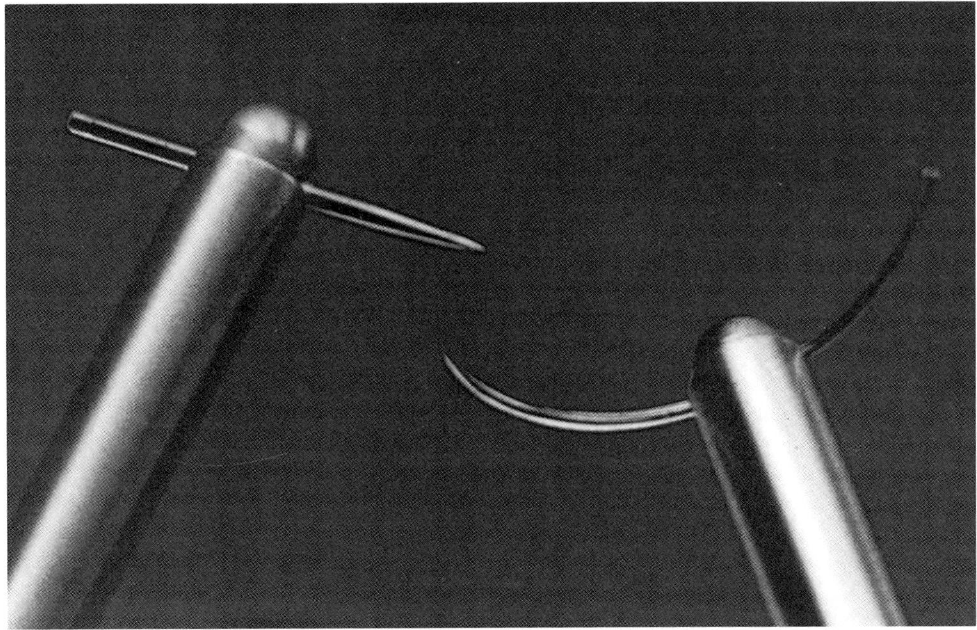

(a)

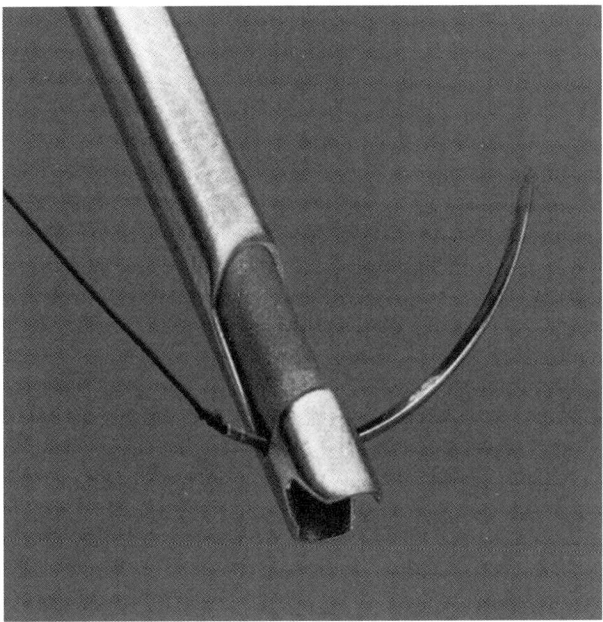

(b)

Figure 7-4 Pin-vise laparoscopic suturing instruments. The design limits utilization of these needle drivers for any other purpose. (a) WISAP U.S.A., Tomball, TX. (b) Cook Urologic, Cook OB/Gyn, Spencer, IN.

manufacturers developed pin-vise-like needle drivers, which facilitate needle passage (Fig. 7-4). The result is a perfectly good needle driver but not a specialized intracorporeal suturing instrument. Specifically designed intracorporeal suturing instruments have emerged. Shorter needle drivers to preclude magnification of small movements at the tip and instruments with the finger rings removed to free the surgeon's hands for performance of fine suturing movements are currently available. The needle driver's jaws are another essential feature affecting performance. Although most instruments rely upon the standard open diamond jaw configuration to firmly grasp the needle, other variations are emerging as effective alternatives (Fig. 7-5). An intracorporeal suturing set that provides an assistant tissue grasper and a dedicated needle driver is composed of the Szabo-Berci flamingo and parrotjawed instruments (Fig. 7-6).

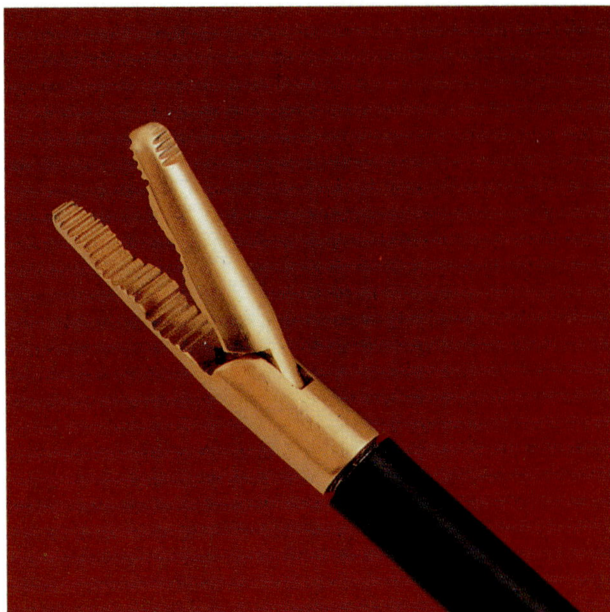

Figure 7-5 A unique laparoscopic needle driver's jaws (Endolap Inc., contour tip with rack and pinion power drive).

Intracorporeal suturing can be divided into three distinct tasks that can be practiced and mastered separately. These are needle driving, suturing, and knot-tying.

Needle Driving

Laparoscopic intracorporeal needle driving requires successful, safe introduction of the needle and suture material through a trocar or through the anterior abdominal wall. This requires knowing which needles will pass through a trocar of a specific size. The safest method to avoid inadvertent injury to the trocar's flapper valve mechanism and the patient's underlying viscera is to grasp the suture 2 to 3 mm behind the swage, open the valve, and begin passing the needle driver and suture simultaneously. Next, the needle and suture must be grasped by the needle driver and correctly aligned prior to beginning. Here, the assisting instrument grasps either the suture close to the needle or the needle itself, then the needle is turned by both instruments close to the

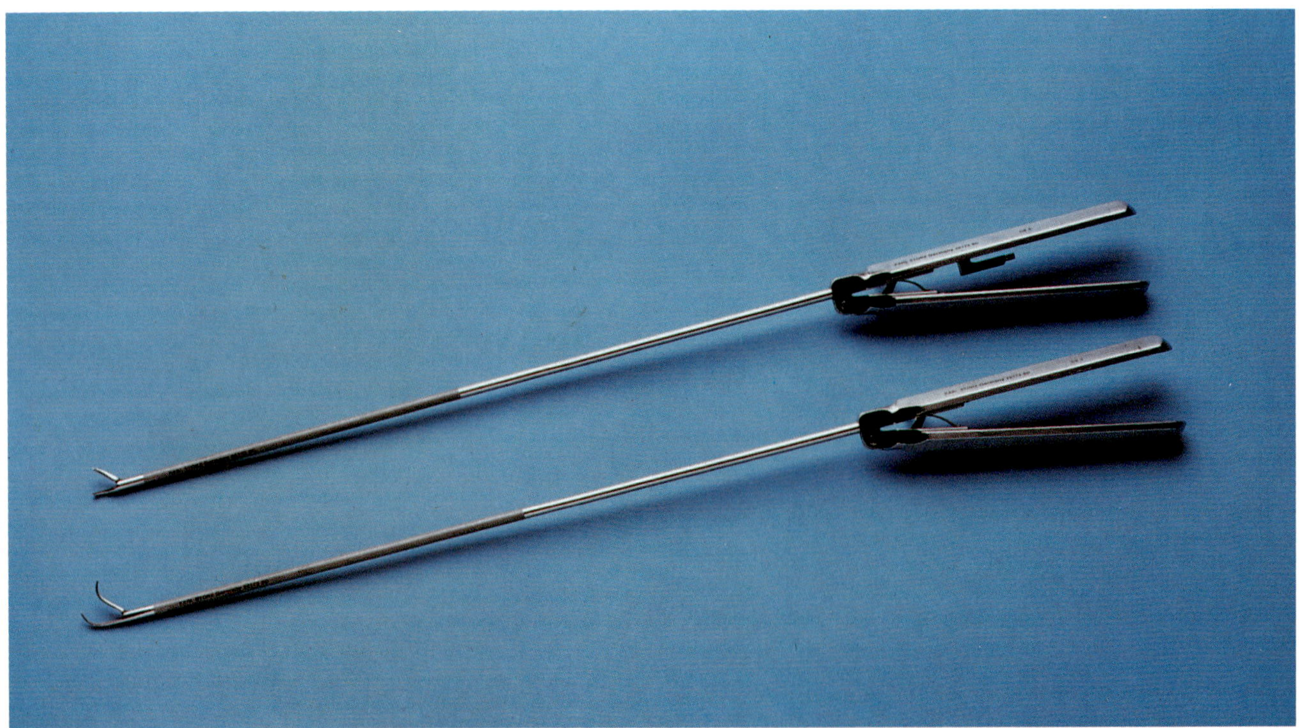

Figure 7-6 The Szabo-Berci laparoscopic intracorporeal suturing set (Karl Storz, Culver City, CA).

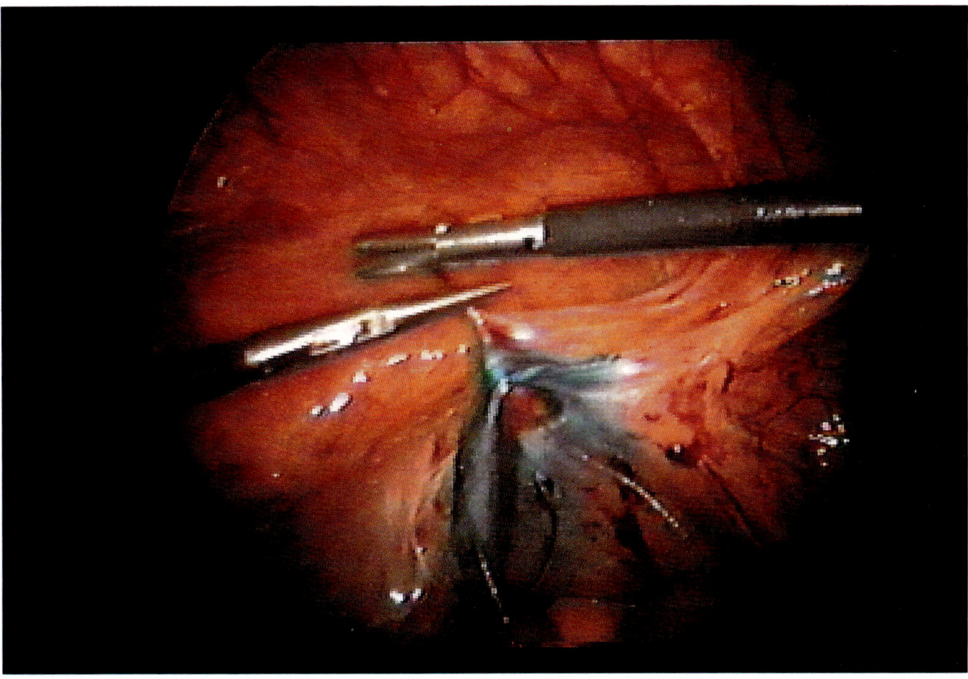

Figure 7-7 The principles of intracorporeal needle driving. Preventing frustrating needle deflections requires slow, careful alignment of tissues and countertraction by the assisting instrument.

laparoscope until proper alignment is achieved. Needles are best held perpendicular to the jaws of the driver and in line with the proposed suture line. A curved needle is best grasped halfway along its circumference, whereas the "ski" types can be grasped along the straight shaft. An assisting instrument is utilized for tissue alignment and countertraction. The most common problem encountered during initial experiences with intracorporeal suturing is frustrating deflections during the entrance bite, needle advancement, or exit bite. It is recommended that while mastering this skill, the surgeon slow the motions down to the point of control and think about each step while maintaining alignment of needle, driver, countertraction, and tissues (Fig. 7-7). At the exit bite, the assistant instrument provides countertraction and the needle is released by the driver and regrasped further back toward the swage and pushed through the tissues. At this point it can be regrasped by the driver.

Suturing

Suture length should be kept to the absolute minimum required for the intended purpose. During laparoscopic suturing 8 cm is adequate for simple stitches. This allows ample room for the loops necessary for knotting, even in thick tissues. Urologic reconstruction can require the utilization of simple running or running locking sutures. These stitches require more length of intracorporeal suture material and careful attention to tension along the repair. A good rule of thumb is that twice the length of a linear incision in suture material is required. Here, as the needle is driven through the tissues, at each exit bite the assistant grasper is utilized to aid in pulling the running stitch through for the given length and the desired tension while the needle driver with the reloaded needle is utilized to provide counter pressure. The running suture should start 2 to 3 mm proximal to the incision and run to 2 or 3 mm beyond prior to tying each end. Locking is not particularly difficult but should also be carefully orchestrated and not started until the suture line's tension has been rechecked. It is far easier to tighten a running line of suture before it has been locked intracorporeally rather than after.

Knotting

The intracorporeal knot of most utility is the simple square knot. A square knot is two apposed half hitches, one atop the other. To synchronize the movements necessary to tie such a knot and eliminate wasted motions, each key movement must be identified and the entire sequence practiced. We have previously reported[22] the 12 steps in tying an intracorporeal square knot (Fig. 7-8). *Step one* is the starting position. A C shape is made in the suture with the right hand grasping the swaged end of the

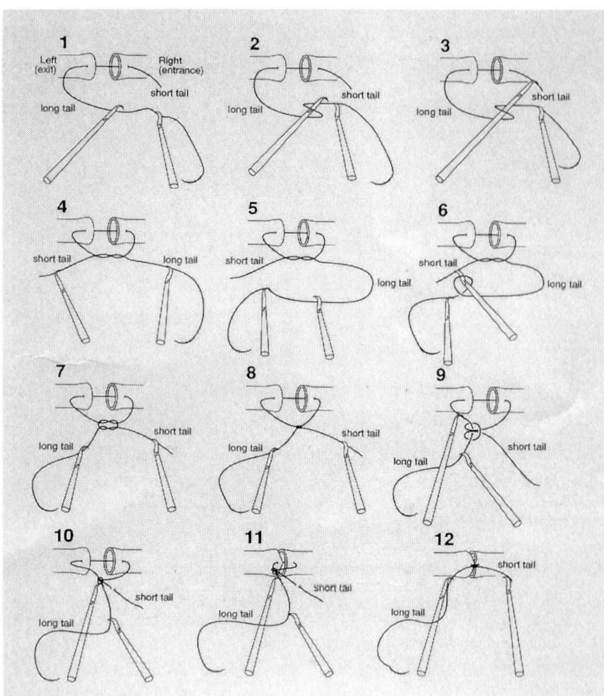

Figure 7-8 The 12 steps in choreographing the right and left hands for accomplishing fluid intracorporeal suturing and knotting (Courtesy of Dr. Z. Szabo).

suture and the left stabilizing the tail. *Step two*, the right hand only moves to create a loop around the tip of the left instrument. *Step three*, the right and left hands move together as the left instrument grasps the tail of the suture. *Step four*, the instruments are pulled in opposite directions paralleling the pull with the suture. *Step five*, the knot is adjusted to center the first half hitch directly above the laceration by placing more tension on the right- or left-hand grasp of suture. *Step six*, sets up throwing the second half hitch. The right grasps the swaged end and is rotated 180 degrees clockwise. *Step seven*, the left instrument releases the short tail and grasps the swaged end near the right grasper. *Step eight*, the right instrument releases the suture and is placed on top, directly in front of the left grasper *Step nine*, the left hand moves to create a loop around the right, which remains stationary. *Step ten*, the right and left instruments move together toward the short tail, which the right then grasps. *Step eleven*, both instruments are pulled in opposite directions parallel to the stitch. *Step twelve*, the two opposing half hitches are tightened against each other. A surgeon's knot can be incorporated by placing two loops around the left grasper during step two prior to tightening the first half hitch.

Intracorporeal Needles

The needle profile of choice for intracorporeal suturing has yet to be determined. In our study of intracorporeal bladder neck reconstructions we identified three configurations that facilitated intracorporeal suturing, a curved ⅜ needle, a "ski" configuration and an S shaped profile.[22] The anatomic limits of the retropubic space permit only a small ½ or ⅜ (RB-1 or TF) taperpoint-configured needle to allow eversion of knots when reconstruction is performed. Some investigators have advocated straight needles (SC-1, Ethicon; TS-20, Davis & Geck; Endosuture, WISAP; or ELW, U.S. Surgical). These have primary advantage on surface structures or when suturing with straight needle graspers.

Intracorporeal Sutures

Suturing under laparoscopic conditions creates unique influences on the choice of suture materials involving color and length. Surgical knots must hold, and the choice between a woven vs. monofilament or absorbable vs. nonabsorbable suture must be made with this in mind. For urologic applications, intracorporeal suturing with plain or chromic gut and polydioxanone have advantages with regard to the security of the half-hitch throws. Unfortunately the coloring of these suture materials is such that blood can obscure the specified ends crucial for the orchestrated movements required for knot-tying. Blood has a tendency to adhere to these suture materials, and strict attention to hemostasis is warranted. In addition, the coloration absorbs the light in all these materials except for the blue PDS. As multiple untied sutures are placed but not tied, as is required for complex end-to-end anastomoses, swage and tail ends become indistinct. Brightly colored, optically fluorescent colors are required to overcome this problem. Currently, dye materials that have been investigated to enhance visibility when exposed to xenon light have also demonstrated carcinogenic properties. Despite this, colors most efficacious for laparoscopic suturing include pink, yellow, green, and purple.[22]

Intracorporeal Suturing Techniques

Much effort has been expended developing innovative methods to circumvent the difficulties of intra-

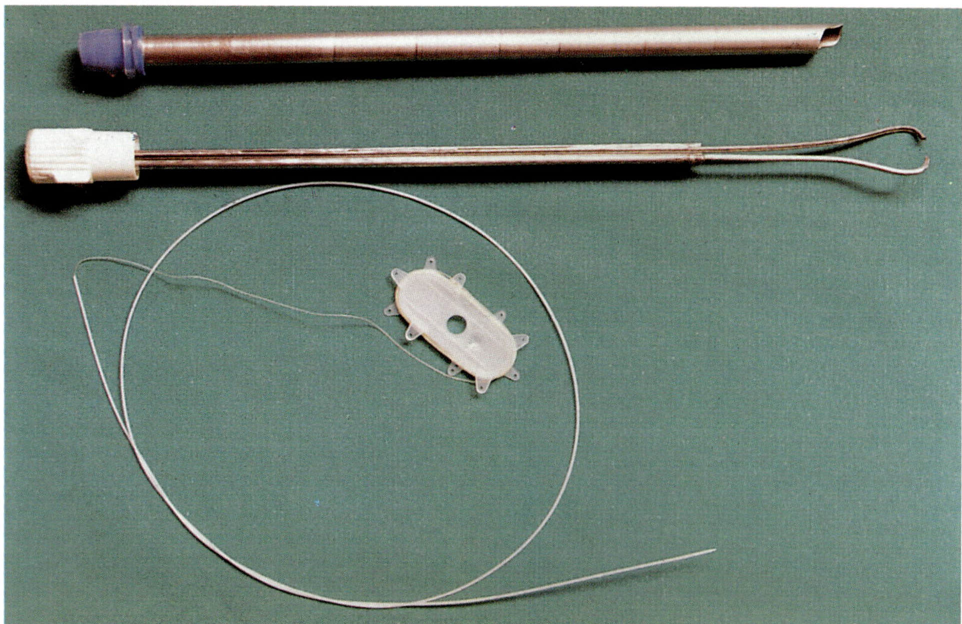

Figure 7-9 Suturescope from Gomes da Silva.

corporeal suturing and knotting.[23] Sheath systems that allow the needles and graspers to be positioned simultaneously have been described (Laparomed Suture Applier, Irvine, CA). Metal as well as absorbable clips for replacing intracorporeal knots are available. A suture scope has also been invented with a mechanism for aligning tissues and driving a long needle through two opposing tubular structures (Fig. 7-9).[24] Utilizing this device, an endoscopic ureteroneocystostomy has already been performed. The ultimate mechanical suturing device would be an automatic endoscopic sewing machine. Such a device has been developed and utilized clinically via a large colonoscope by Buess et al.[25]

Another approach to intracorporeal suturing is to take advantage of the magnified image and apply the techniques of microsurgery.[21,25,26] This of course requires bringing the laparoscope in close proximity to the area of interest. All of the intracorporeal skills discussed earlier must be precisely applied. Hemostasis is even more crucial during laparoscopic microsurgical suturing. Complex urologic anastomoses have been accomplished utilizing microsurgical techniques including urethravesical re-anastomosis, augmentation cystoplasties, and others.[26] The potential advantages of microsurgical reconstruction in urology include less need for long-term urinary diversion or drainage, less infiltration with scar tissue, and visually secure suture placement. With these techniques, spatial constraints and limited visual fields do not prevent the surgeon from even small anastomoses.

Laparoscopic Intracorporeal Stapling and Clipping

The primary applications of intracorporeal stapling and clipping have been discussed earlier. As with almost every laparoscopic instrument there are the considerations of reusable vs. disposable devices. Clip appliers come in both forms, but as of this writing the automatic staplers are single-patient-use items.

Clip Appliers

Clip appliers are primarily available from two manufacturers, Ethicon (Cincinnati, OH) and U.S. Surgical (Norwalk, CT), (Fig. 7-10). Clip appliers have several crucial features warranting careful scrutiny by the surgical consumer (Table 7-2). Titanium clip sizes range from 6.0 to 11.0 mm. Nondisposable clip appliers require multiple passages through the entrance trocar for multifiring, but have the advantage of a single initial purchase price versus the single-use disposable instruments. Nevertheless, the disposable clip appliers have features that are currently not available on the reusable devices (Fig. 7-

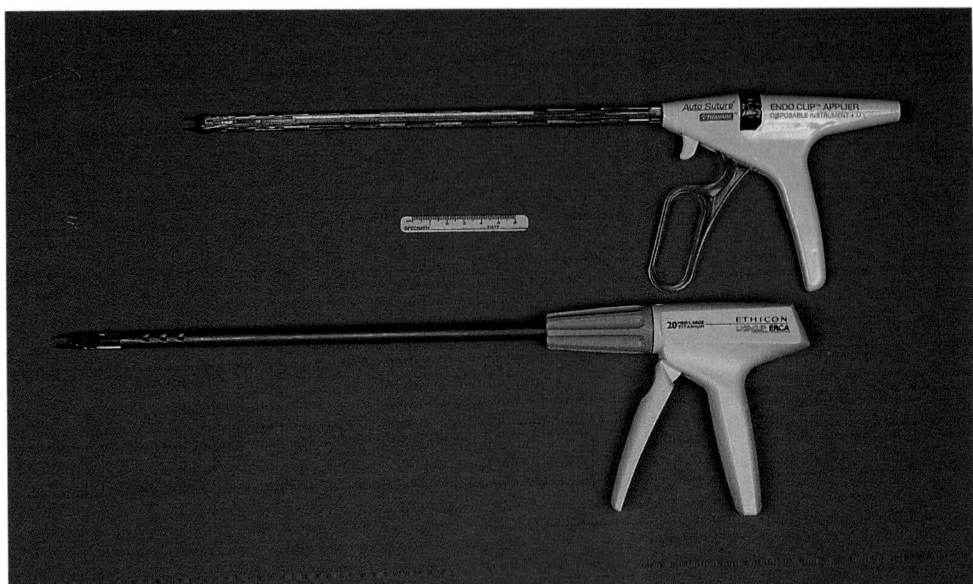

Figure 7-10 Two manufacturers' disposable clip appliers. U.S. Surgical (above) and Ethicon (below).

11). Disposable devices are multifire capable (20 clips) with rotatable shafts. The pistol grip can comfortably rest in the surgeon's palm, and the angle of application can be adjusted through 360 degrees. At present, all clip appliers are designed for placement through 10-mm portals. When a clip is deployed, the vessels should be carefully positioned by assisting graspers for alignment perpendicular to the jaws. Using multifire, disposable instruments, the clip should be loaded intracorporeally to avoid inadvertent dislodgement during passage through the flapper valves of the trocar. When the trigger is gently squeezed, the clip applier more firmly grasps the clip so that the exact deployment site can be selected. The trigger is then firmly squeezed. If too much force is used or too much tissue is taken, the delicate autoloading mechanisms can malfunction, precluding their further use.

Research work has also been performed upon the tissue reactivity of various types of clips.[13] All clips can potentially cause adhesion formation. In studies of metallic versus absorbable types of clips, no significant difference between the two was discerned. However, concerns about their reliability in maintaining hemostasis have been raised.[9] As such, the technique of vascular pedicle application deserves further discussion. Most investigators mention that more than one clip is necessary on major vascular structures. In addition, the clips are probably most secure if placed in an opposed fashion such that the

TABLE 7- 2 Endoscopic Clip Appliers

	Disposable Types	
	Endoclip	**Endopath**
MANUFACTURER	U.S. Surgical	Ethicon
NO. OF CLIPS	20	20
PORT SIZE	10 mm	10/11mm
CLIP SIZE	Medium, 6.0 mm Medium large, 8.9 mm Large, 11.0 mm	Medium large, 8.8 mm
SHAFT	360°	360°

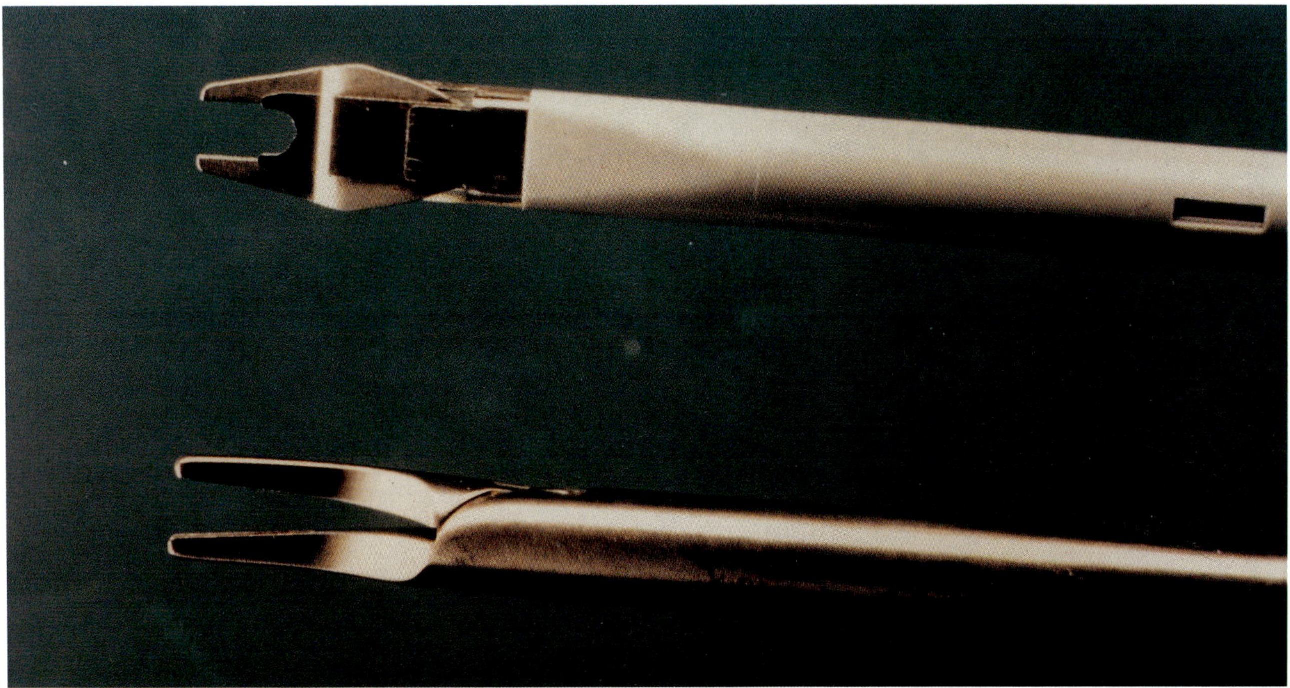

Figure 7-11 Disposable (above) and reusable (below) laparoscopic clip appliers (Ethicon, Cincinnati, OH).

open jaws are not facing the same direction. Electrocautery should not be used when dividing clipped vessels because conductance to the metallic structures could occur, resulting in possible necrosis that could result in sloughing of the vessels within the occluding clips. Finally, studies have been performed on the ability to perform CT and MR imaging following titanium clip application. Although they produce artifacts, they do so less than steel clips, yet more than absorbable ones.

Biting Clip Appliers

Clip appliers were initially designed to occlude and control vascular structures. The surgeon's interest in laparoscopic herniorrhaphy was the primary driving force for the availability of both reusable and disposable biting clip instruments. These must be applied carefully to take full advantage of the biting ends. Initially, the surgeon should have the two opposing tissue edges approximated with graspers. Next, the clip applier's trigger is pulled so as to just expose the biting ends. Each tip is carefully positioned to centrally locate the clip across the tissue edges. Finally, further tension upon the trigger produces the B configuration in an ideal location of the tissues to be approximated. These devices have been utilized for reperitonealization following transabdominal bilateral pelvic lymphadenectomy, fixation of mesh for hernia repairs, retracting viscera from the pelvis for high-dose radiation therapy, fixation of vesicourethral slings, and closure of mesenteric defects after bowel resection.[7,27–30] Another refinement of the biting clip applicator is the addition of a distal articulating segment. This additional degree of motion allows angulation upward to 40 degrees (Fig. 7-12). The surgeon can thus fixate materials such as mesh to the anterior abdominal wall or deep pelvic recess (i.e. Cooper's ligament) from a fixed access trocar.

Automatic Staplers

Automated stapling devices allow the rapid deployment of multiple, metallic staples to facilitate division and reapproximation of visceral structures (Fig. 7-13). These devices are available for laparoscopic, intracorporeal utilization with a variety of features (Table 7-3).

The Endo GIA 30 and Endopath 30 each deploy two triple rows of staples from the 30-mm blades. The staples are available in reloadable, color-coded cartridges: white, 2.5 mm: blue, 3.8 mm: and green, 4.8 mm. Staple size depends upon the thickness of

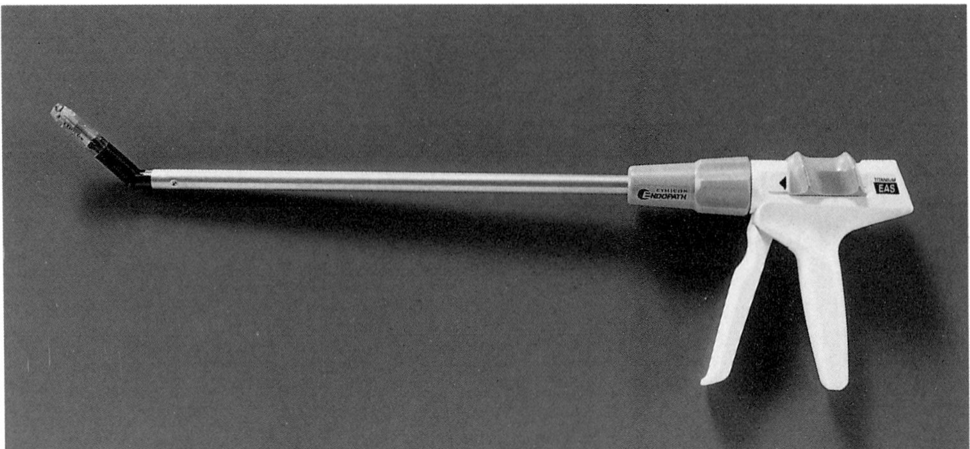

Figure 7-12 Biting, reticulated clip applier (Endopath, Ethicon, Cincinnati, OH).

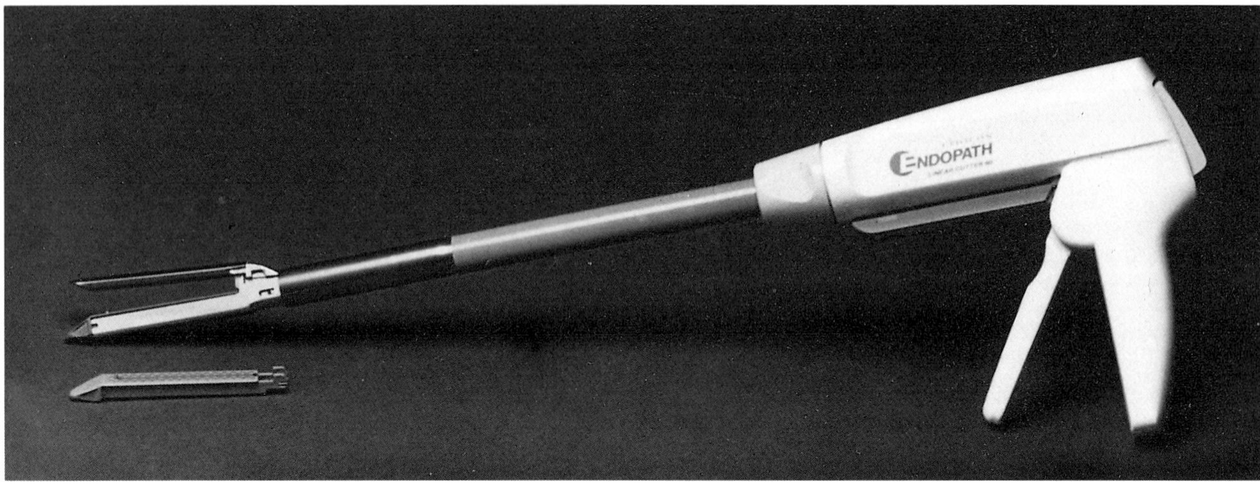

(a)

(b)

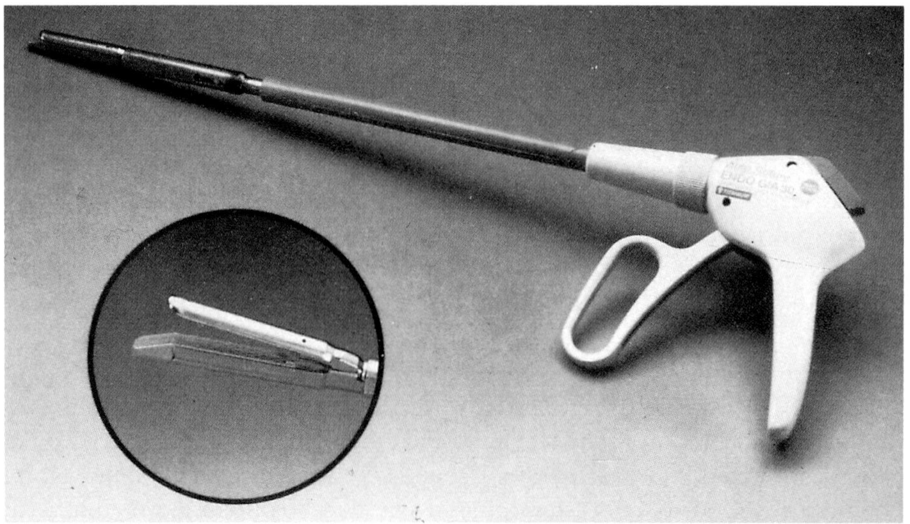

Figure 7-13 Intracorporeal automatic staplers: (a) Endopath, Ethicon, and (b) Endo GIA and Endo TA, U.S. Surgical.

TABLE 7-3 Endoscopic Linear Cutting Staplers

	Endo GIA 30	Endo GIA 60	Endopath 30	Endopath 60
Manufacturer	U.S. Surgical	U.S. Surgical	Ethicon	Ethicon
Port size	12 mm	15 mm	12 mm	12 mm
Length of staple line	30 mm	60 mm	30 mm	60 mm
Staple pattern	2 triple rows	2 triple rows	2 triple rows	2 double rows
Staple size (cartridge color)	2.5 mm (white) 3.8 mm (blue) 4.8 mm (green)		3.85 mm (blue) 4.85 mm (green)	
Reloads per instrument	3	3	3	3
Shaft	360°	360°	360°	360°
Special features	None	Pneumatic	Without cutting knife (4 rows)	Without cutting knife (4 rows)

tissues being reapproximated or divided. The white 2.5-mm staples are usually used on vascular structures because of their compressibility. The larger blue 3.8-mm and green 4.8-mm staples are more ideal for thicker visceral structures such as thickened ureter, small bowel, large bowel, or the bladder. An endoscopic sizer is available for tissue compression that will indicate which size staples will produce the best anastomosis or occlusion (Endogauge, U.S. Surgical).

Linear cutting staplers usually deploy three rows of staples on either side of the cutting blade. The one exception is the Endopath 60, which fires double rows. An important consideration in utilizing automated staplers is that the knife cuts short of the end of the staple line. Also, the staples are not loaded to the ends of the cartridges, making deployment length shorter than the 30 or 60 mm of the instrument. For this reason, when applying a linear cutting stapler, the ends should be seen protruding beyond the distal side of tissue prior to engaging the firing mechanisms. The actual placement and firing of an endoscopic stapler is similar to their open cousins.

Linear noncutting staplers are available in both 30- and 60-mm lengths. Theoretically, these staplers reapproximate tissues with less incorporation of tissue mass. The Ethicon Endopath 30 and Endopath 60 deploy four staple rows. The U.S. Surgical Endo TA is a pneumatically powered noncutting linear stapler that deploys three rows. The staples on all of the noncutting instruments are identical to their cutting relatives.

Conclusions

As operative laparoscopy continues to expand beyond its present limitations, suturing and stapling techniques will be mandatory skills in the armamentarium of the reconstructive laparoscopic surgeon.

References

1. Clarke HC: Laparoscopy: New instruments for suturing and ligation. *Fertil Steril* 23:274, 1972.
2. Ko S-T, Airan MC: Therapeutic laparoscopic suturing techniques. *Surg Endosc* 6:41, 1992.
3. Semm K: Operative Pelviscopy: Endoscopical Ligatures. WISAP manual.
4. Petrovsky B, Perelman M, Kuznichev A: Resection and plastic surgery of bronchi [transl]. Mir Publishing, p 202, 1968.
5. Steichen FM, Ravitch MM: Contemporary stapling instruments and basic mechanical suturing techniques. *Surg Clin North Am* 64(3):425, 1984.
6. Fowler DL, White RA: Laparoscopic-assisted sigmoid resection. *Surg Laparosc Endosc* 1:183, 1991.

7. Jacobs M, Verdeja JC, Goldstein HS: Minimally invasive colon resection (laparoscopic colectomy). *Surg Laparosc Endosc* 1:144, 1991.
8. Chiu AW, Chen MT, Huang WJS, Juang GD, Lu SH, Chang LS: Case report: Laparoscopic nephroureterectomy and endoscopic excision of bladder cuff. *Min Invas Therap* 1:299, 1992.
9. Kerbl K, Chandhoke PS, McDougall E, et al: Laparoscopic clips and staples: Vascular application. *J Endourol* 6:S142, 1992.
10. Kerbl K, Chandhoke PS, McDougall E, et al: Laparoscopic staples in the urinary tract: Bladder application. *J Endourol* 6:S144, 1992.
11. Kirker-Head CA, Steckel RR, Schwartz A, Williams R: Evaluation of surgical staples for ligation of the renal pedicle during nephrectomy. *Urol Res* 16:63, 1988.
12. Kozminski M, Partamian K, Moeller R, Remis R: Laparoscopic formation of an ileal loop conduit. *J Urol* 147:A780, 1992.
13. Grainger DA, Meyer WR, DeCherney AH, Diamond MP: Laparoscopic clips: evaluation of absorbable and titanium with regard to hemostasis and tissue reactivity. *J Reprod Med* 36:493, 1991.
14. Andrews S, Lewis JL: Minimal access suturing: An assessment of knot substitutes. *Min Invas Therap* 1:309, 1992.
15. Sugarbaker DJ, Mentzer SJ: Improved technique for hilar vascular stapling. *Ann Thorac Surg* 53:165, 1992.
16. Nelson MT, Nakashima M, Mulvihill SJ: How safe are laparoscopically placed clips? An in vitro and in vivo study. *Arch Surg* 127:718, 1992.
17. Mettler L, Semm K: Pelviscopic uterine surgery. *Surg Endosc* 6:23, 1992.
18. Reich H. Clarke C, Sekel L: A simple method for ligating with straight and curved needles in operative laparoscopy. *Obstet Gynecol* 79:143, 1992.
19. Cuschieri A, Shimi S, Nathanson LK: Laparoscopic reduction, crural repair, and fundoplication of large hiatal hernia. *Am J Surg* 163:425, 1992.
20. Marrero MA, Corfman RS: Laparoscopic use of sutures. *Clin Obstet Gynecol* 34(2):387, 1991.
21. McComb PF: A new suturing instrument that allows the use of microsuture at laparoscopy. *Fertil Steril* 57:936, 1992.
22. Bowyer DW, Moran ME, Szabo Z: Laparoscopic suturing in urology: a model for the lower urinary tract. *J Endourol* 6:S142, 1992.
23. Jansson OK, Zilling TL, Walther BS: Healing of colonic anastomoses: Comparative experimental study of glued, manually sutured, and stapled anastomoses. *Dis Colon Rectum* 34:557, 1991.
24. Gomes da Silva E: Suturoscope: A new device that allows endoscopic sutures to be performed with traditional threads. *Surg Endosc* 4:220, 1990.
25. Buess G, et al: Technique of transanal endoscopic microsurgery. *Surg Endosc* 2:71, 1988.
26. Moran ME, Bowyer DW, Szabo Z: Laparoscopic intracorporeal suturing: Microsurgical approach. *Min Invas Therap* 1:A71, 1992.
27. Boullier JA, Hagood PG, Parra RO: Endocavitary (Laparoscopic) pelvic lymphadenectomy with specific indications in urologic surgery. *Urology* 41(1):19, 1993.
28. Ger R. Monroe K, Duvivier R, Mishrick A: Management of indirect inguinal hernias by laparoscopic closure of the neck of the sac. *Am J Surg* 159:370, 1990.
29. Azziz R, Murphy AA, Rosenberg SM, Patton GW: Use of an oxidized, regenerated cellulose absorbable adhesion barrier at laparoscopy. *J Reprod Med* 36:479, 1991.
30. Dickson C, Boone T, Preminger GM: Laparoscopic urethral sling. *Min Invas Therap* 1:A105, 1992.

8

Complications of Laparoscopy

R. Ernest Sosa
Steve J. Shichman
John A. Boullier
Raul O. Parra

Introduction

Laparoscopic intervention is fraught with potential hazards and pitfalls.[1–6] Problems may arise from the time a patient is placed on the operating table until the late postoperative period. Invariably, some complications will occur. Prompt recognition of a problem and immediate application of corrective measures can minimize the associated morbidity.

Laparoscopic surgery poses challenges to the surgeon that are not encountered in open surgical techniques. First, for the surgeon, the operative site can only be viewed on the monitors. Despite the clarity and magnification of the image given by today's high resolution video equipment, only two dimensions can be appreciated, creating difficulty with depth perception during the performance of surgery on three-dimensional structures. Second, the organs of interest to the urologist are in the retroperitoneal space. Laparoscopic access to the extraperitoneal region commonly begins with entry into the abdominal cavity. The posterior peritoneum overlying the operative site must be identified and incised. This approach differs from the standard extraperitoneal pathway taken with open surgery and demands familiarization with different anatomic landmarks. Third, the hands cannot be introduced into the wound to serve as or in conjunction with retractors and other surgical instruments. Most important, the ability to palpate tissue for reconnaissance is lost. Fourth, laparoscopic instrumentation does not always resemble or have the capabilities of instruments we are accustomed to using in open surgery. For example, instruments for tissue retraction are, for the most part, prototypes. The surgeon must depend on gravity and decompression of the hollow viscera for adequate operative exposure. Taken together these factors represent a significant challenge for the surgeon in his or her transition from open to laparoscopic surgery. Careful patient selection and preparation will minimize complications.

Potential Problems of Access

During Insufflation

Introduction of the pneumoperitoneum needle is discussed in detail in Chap. 5. It is important to stress that the patient must be in the Trendelenburg position so as to move the bowels out of the lower abdomen for needle placement. A nasogastric tube and Foley catheter must decompress the stomach and bladder, respectively.[7–13] Correct needle placement should be confirmed before proceeding with insufflation. Improper placement of the needle into the subcutaneous tissues, properitoneal space, omentum, mesentery, bowel, stomach, bladder, or great vessels needs to be promptly identified and corrective measures instituted. If blood is aspirated through the pneumoperitoneum needle, serious consideration should be given to converting the procedure to a laparotomy. For this, the cannula should be left in place to tamponade the bleeding and to identify the site of injury during exploration.

If the patient has eructation or passes flatus during insufflation, evaluation for possible needle insertion into the stomach or bowel lumen should be undertaken. A syringe should be used to aspirate through the needle to reconfirm its placement. If correct needle position cannot be assured, then open trocar placement should be carried out and the needle entry path reviewed for evidence of injury to the stomach and bowel. Most visceral injuries due to small-caliber cannulas can be managed conservatively with a clear liquid diet, intravenous antibiotics, and close observation. Postoperative signs or symptoms or peritoneal inflammation or sepsis are indications for immediate surgical exploration.[7–9,14,15]

During Trocar Insertion

The first trocar is placed blindly, and as such the potential for complications is the greatest. To minimize the risk of injury to underlying structures, an adequate pneumoperitoneum must already have been established. After the initial trocar is inserted, the abdominal and pelvic organs should be examined. Immediate attention should be placed on the underlying viscera and retroperitoneum to rule out any obvious injury or evidence of an expanding mesenteric or retroperitoneal hematoma. Great vessel injury may not be visually dramatic as bleeding first occurs into the retroperitoneum, where it is incipiently concealed. Hemodynamic instability may be the first and only sign of a vascular injury. Trocar-induced injury requires a laparotomy for full evaluation and repair.[8,9,16–21] In patients with a prior history of abdominal surgery or in whom adequate pneumoperitoneum needle placement cannot be assured, it is prudent to perform a mini-laparotomy and Hasson trocar insertion.

All secondary trocars must be introduced under the visual guidance of the laparoscope-video unit. The abdominal wall is transilluminated at the planned trocar insertion site to assure that a vessel is not crossing at that location.[6] The skin incision must be ample enough to permit easy trocar introduction. It is our custom to spread the subcutaneous tissue with a curved clamp until the insinuation of the clamp tips on the parietal peritoneum is visually appreciated. We find that prior blunt dissection of the subcutaneous tissue and muscle tends to move vessels and muscle fibers out of the way of the penetrating trocar, reducing the risk for injury.

Once the secondary trocars are in place, the laparoscope-video unit is moved to a secondary port so that the umbilical trocar entry site may be evaluated for bleeding or injury to underlying viscera. All trocars are fixed to prevent uncontrolled excursions and unintended removal during the procedure. In and out trocar movements can dilate the tract, ruining the seal around the trocar. Carbon dioxide gas then escapes throughout the procedure, and the pneumoperitoneum may become inadequate to work safely. There are several commercially available trocar fixation devices. Alternatively, suture fixation of the trocar to the skin may be utilized.

Potential Problems during Surgery

Poor knowledge of the laparoscopic anatomy can result in an inefficient and dangerous dissection. It is important to identify the pertinent landmarks of each procedure. For example, in a laparoscopic pelvic lymph node dissection the obliterated umbilical artery, the crossing vas deferens, and the ureter can often be identified on the right side. The peritoneal incision is made lateral to the obliterated umbilical artery, avoiding the ureter. If the peritoneum is opened medial to the obliterated umbilical artery, errant dissection into the bladder is almost certain (Fig. 8-1). Careful blunt dissection lateral to the obliterated umbilical artery will permit prompt identification of the external iliac vessels and the obturator nerve.

Unattended instruments are a potential source of serious injury. Any time the surgeon's attention is diverted away from the monitor, all instruments should be removed. The insertion of all instruments into the abdominal cavity must be visually monitored to locate and safely guide them to the operative site. Retracting instruments are fixed into place and need only be visualized to readjust them. The surgical dissection, however, must be maintained at the center of the visual field.

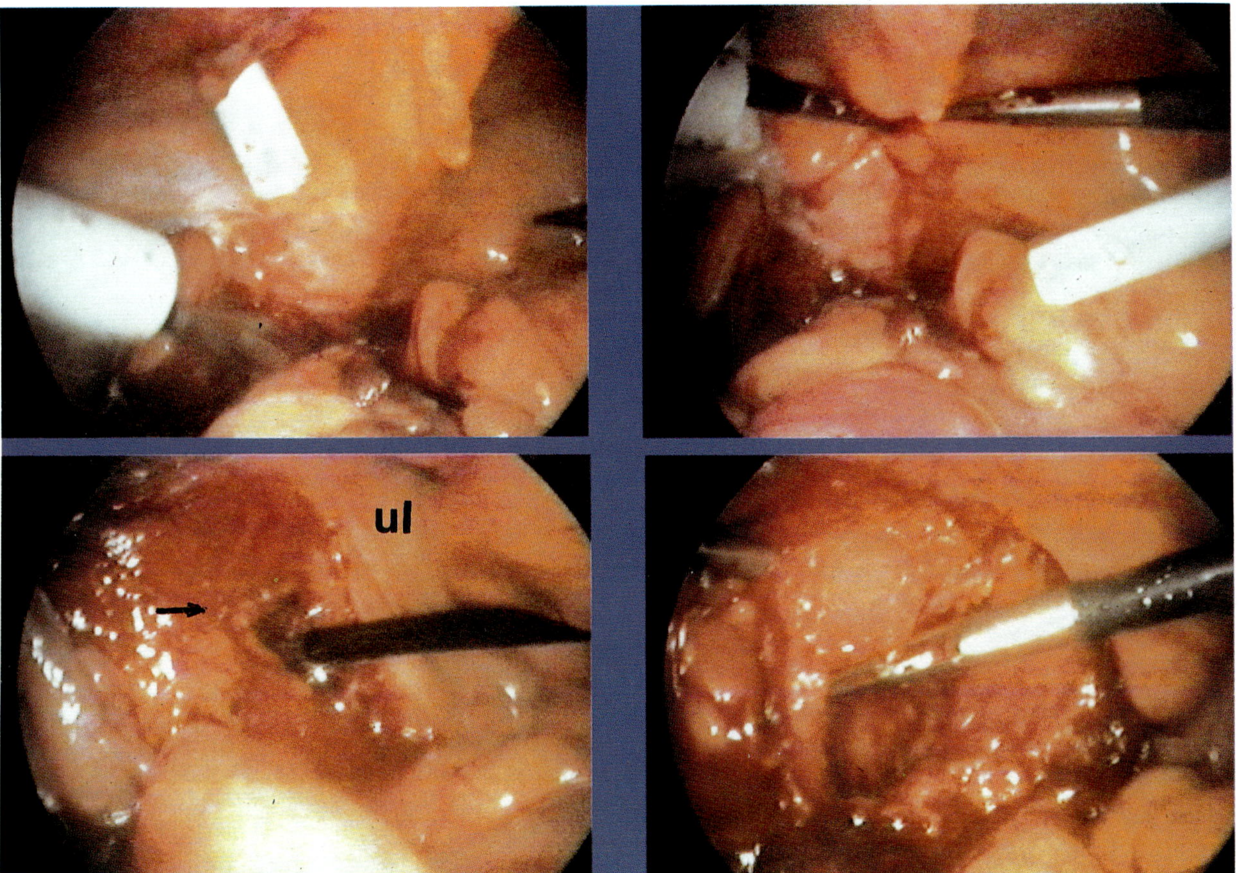

Figure 8-1 Sequence demonstrates right-sided pelvic node dissection (pictures captured retrospectively) of a bladder injury (arrow) created by inadvertently dissecting medial to the umbilical ligament (ul).

A major limitation of laparoscopic dissection is the inability to discern three dimensions on the video monitor. There is a loss of depth perception. This handicap can be minimized by advancing the camera close to the operating instruments. Movement of the instruments within the plane of the two dimensional field perceived on the video monitor affords an excellent appreciation of the full extent of the motion. Movements in the direction of the vector parallel to the camera are not appreciated well. Tactile sensation is minimal, further contributing to the difficulty the novice surgeon experiences during laparoscopic dissection.

Most hand instruments are equipped with monopolar electrosurgical capability. Prior to the start of surgery the patient should be properly grounded and the insulation in all the electrosurgical instruments should be intact. During electrocoagulation or cutting, the uninsulated portion of an instrument should be kept away from other conducting surfaces. The instrument should be placed precisely on the tissue being coagulated or cut, avoiding contact with neighboring tissues to prevent injury by unintended dissipation of electrical current. The voltage settings should follow the manufacturer's recommendation. Too high a voltage will cause immediate desiccation of tissue. Further application of electrical current will damage adjacent structures, as the current will seek the path of least resistance toward the grounding pad. This phenomenon can produce thermal injuries that are unnoticed during surgery (Fig. 8-2a). Thermal injuries may manifest in the postoperative period as sepsis (late perforation of a viscus), a urinoma (late perforation of the bladder or ureter), or a neuropathy (injury to a nerve)[10] (Fig. 8-2b). If the electrosurgical unit does not produce the desired effect on activation, its use should be immediately discontinued

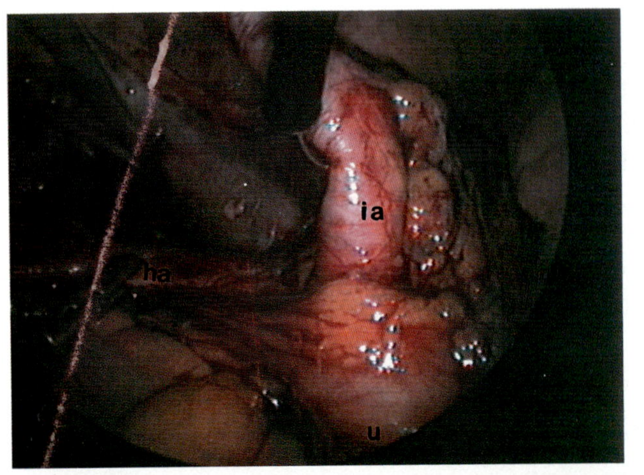

(a)

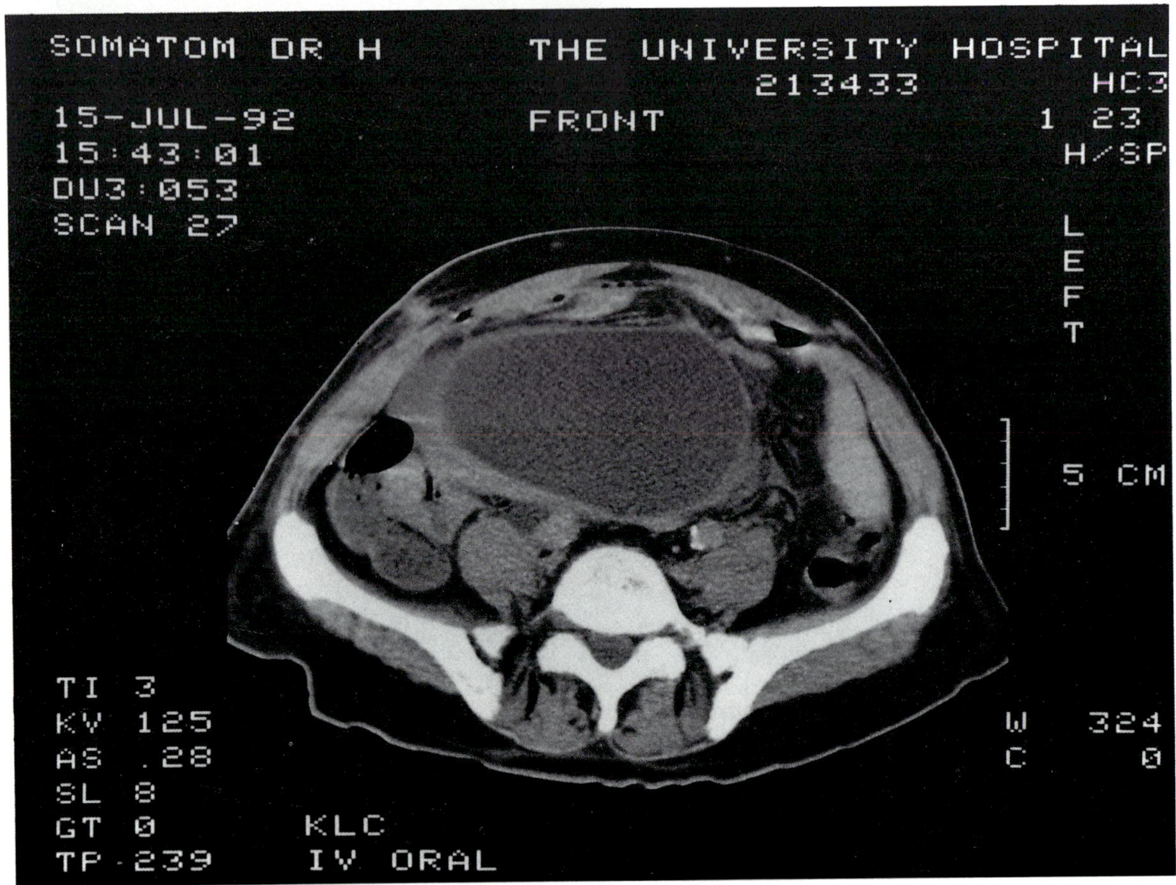

(b)

Figure 8-2 (a) The proximity of the ureter (u) crossing the iliac bifurcation (ia = iliac artery, ha = hypogastric artery) is demonstrated in this rightsided pelvic node dissection. Extreme care in the use of monopolar electrocautery is imperative in this vicinity to avoid a thermal injury to the crossing ureter. (b) Urinoma secondary to a delayed ureteral thermal injury incurred during a laparoscopic lymphadenectomy.

pending evaluation for loose connections, faulty insulation, or unrecognized contact with another metal instrument. The first reaction should not be to raise the voltage settings. The use of clips to secure vessels and lymphatics may decrease the need to resort to electrocautery for hemostasis.[6]

Hemorrhage from a large vessel, such as the iliac vein, encountered during dissection usually dictates immediate laparotomy.[18–21] Before opening the abdomen, an attempt should be made to secure the defect in the vessel using atraumatic graspers or clips. An open vessel will bleed dramatically once the pneumoperitoneum is released. The surgeon can elect to approach the injured vessel via an extraperitoneal or intraperitoneal approach, depending upon the anatomic location of the injury. If an extraperitoneal approach is used, such as an extended Gibson incision, the pneumoperitoneum is maintained to help minimize blood loss. If a transperitoneal route is selected, the insufflation should be discontinued. The laparoscope is then placed against the anterior abdominal wall at the midline to serve as a guide for the incision and protect the abdominal viscera from injury. The surgeon's aim is to get to the bleeding site as quickly as possible, surrendering the least amount of blood. Hemostasis should be established promptly, permitting time to start resuscitation and to secure appropriate instruments and help for the repair.

The pressure of the pneumoperitoneum can keep many small vessels collapsed, concealing evidence of injury. When the pneumoperitoneum is released, bleeding will commence. Prior to exiting the abdomen the intraperitoneal pressure should be reduced to < 8 mmHg. The operative site(s) should be irrigated and suctioned to inspect for bleeding. Any small vessels that are found bleeding should be controlled by electrocoagulation or by application of a clip. Failure to observe this simple precaution can result in serious blood loss.

Problems Related to the Pneumoperitoneum

Subcutaneous emphysema is frequently encountered during laparoscopy. The magnitude of this problem can range from a benign palpable crepitus in the tissues surrounding a trocar to dissection of the entire abdominal wall and upper body with large amounts of CO_2. The latter can lead to soft tissue distortion and hypercarbia.[22–32]

Immediate detection of subcutaneous emphysema during insufflation of the abdominal cavity indicates improper placement of the pneumoperitoneum needle. The needle should be removed immediately. Continued insufflation when the correct position of the needle tip has not been confirmed is a serious violation of proper laparoscopic technique and is potentially dangerous. Insufflation of the properitoneal space, for example, will push the anterior parietal peritoneum to the posterior wall, making subsequent access into the peritoneal cavity extremely difficult. Confirmation of the correct placement of the pneumoperitoneum needle in the abdominal cavity is a sine qua non before proceeding with the insufflation. Close monitoring of the insufflation pressures and percussion to confirm the presence of a four-quadrant pneumoperitoneum will help to verify correct needle placement.

Penoscrotal emphysema is frequently found in men at the conclusion of a laparoscopic pelvic lymph node dissection or varicocelectomy. Carbon dioxide dissects through the inguinal canal into the genital area. Treatment of this problem is simple. Prior to closure of the abdominal incisions, the scrotum and penis are gently squeezed to move the CO_2 back into the peritoneal cavity. Prophylactic wrapping of the scrotum and penis with stretch gauze (turban dressing) at the beginning of a case will prevent scrotal emphysema. However, some patients have postoperative discomfort and scrotal ecchymosis when the turban dressing is used.

Repeated side to side excursions of a trocar can loosen the peritoneal seal around the sheath, resulting in CO_2 dissection along the abdominal wall. Clinically, crepitus may be palpable from the trocar site to the patient's neck and face. Subcutaneous emphysema can be associated with hypercarbia and respiratory acidosis.[23] An increase in the tidal volume and in the respiratory rate can frequently eliminate the excess carbon dioxide, lessening the hypercarbia. No other intervention is usually necessary, as the crepitus and hypercarbia rapidly resolve following discontinuation of insufflation.[23,24,33,34]

Crepitus localized to the face, neck, and chest wall is likely to result from diffusion of CO_2 through the diaphragm or retroperitoneum. These findings may be an early sign of a pneumothorax, pneumomediastinum, or pneumopericardium. If these diagnoses are suspected, the pneumoperitoneum should be released immediately and evaluation should include assessment of vital signs, auscultation of heart and lungs, and a chest X-ray. Treatment generally consists of providing supportive measures to allow the CO_2 time to reabsorb. High insufflation pressures have been implicated as a risk factor for developing these potentially life-threatening problems. It is prudent to perform laparoscopic surgery at pressures ≤ 15 mmHg.[35–39]

An unexpected cause of hypotension may be overinsufflation of the abdomen. Excessive intraabdominal pressures may induce a vaso-vagal reflex, causing hypotension and bradycardia. Most case reports of vagal stimulation involve young women with firm abdominal musculature and less abdominal compliance. In the older patient, a more lax abdominal wall may render a protective effect. Nevertheless, the older urology patient is still at risk for vaso-vagal effect. Lowering the intraabdominal pressure eliminates the source of the problem, but supportive care and close monitoring are necessary. Atropine may be required to treat the bradycardia.[40–44]

Abdominal insufflation has been reported to have a cooling effect on the patient undergoing a lengthy procedure.[45] The CO_2 insufflated into the patient is below normal body temperature. Expansion of the compressed gas causes a significant absorption of heat. The patient's core temperature has been reported to drop at a rate of 0.3° C for each 50 L of CO_2 used. Alternatively, CO_2 induces peripheral vasoconstriction, which tends to reduce heat loss and increase the core body temperature. It is unclear which mechanism prevails. Careful monitoring of the patient's body temperature is important.

Carbon dioxide embolism is a rare but grave complication. Cardiovascular collapse results when a pocket of CO_2 gas obstructs right ventricular outflow. Early diagnosis and immediate initiation of therapeutic measures is essential for a successful outcome. The most sensitive method to detect CO_2 gas embolism is precordial Doppler ultrasonography. Unfortunately, this technology is not readily available in most operating rooms. Capnography is the next most sensitive method of detection. A rapid fall in end-tidal CO_2 occurs as the flow of CO_2-rich blood from the right side of the heart is prevented from entering the pulmonary circulation by the CO_2 "air lock." Trend recordings will reveal a drop in the height of the CO_2 peaks. Other signs that should heighten suspicion for CO_2 emboli include (1) a precipitous fall in blood pressure, (2) cardiac arrhythmias, (3) bilateral pulmonary rales, (4) an increase in pulmonary artery pressures, and (5) a mill-wheel murmur heard with an esophageal stethoscope. Treatment consists of immediate release of the pneumoperitoneum and placement of the patient in a steep Trendelenburg and left lateral decubitus position (Durant's maneuver) to raise the CO_2 bubble out of the pulmonary artery into the right ventricle. Attempts to aspirate the CO_2 bubble from the right side of the heart are made through a catheter passed into the right atrium. Once the patient is stabilized, hyperbaric oxygen treatment could be initiated to facilitate the resorption of the CO_2. Potential neurologic damage caused by obstruction of the cerebral blood flow requires initiation of additional measures such as steroid administration, diuresis, and hyperventilation to minimize the cerebral edema.[46–51]

Potential Problems with Trocar Removal

Although measures are taken to avoid injury to the abdominal wall vessels during trocar insertion, branches of the inferior epigastric artery and vein may be difficult to identify at the border of the rectus muscles or in obese patients. Inadvertent laceration of a vessel may be concealed by the tamponading effect of the trocar. At the end of a case, removal of all trocars must be performed under vision to look for and repair injured vessels.[16–21] A 5-mm laparoscope may be used through a small trocar to inspect the larger cannula insertion sites. Trocar sites ≥ 10 mm should be closed under visual surveillance to assure that the underlying bowel and omentum are not involved by the suture. The last trocar is removed over the 5-mm laparoscope. The laparoscope is slowly withdrawn while the puncture site is assessed for bleeding.

Injured vessels at trocar sites must be controlled as soon as they are identified. During surgery blood can drip down the laparoscope, obscuring visibility. In the postoperative period, injured abdominal wall vessels are a relatively frequent source of significant morbidity. Hemorrhages can be of sufficient severity to require transfusions and/or re-exploration. If the bleeding vessel is visible on the inside of the abdominal wall, laparoscopic directed sutures may be placed intracorporeally. In thin patients, percutaneous sutures may suffice to establish hemostasis. One technique calls for the introduction of a long, straight needle into the abdominal cavity alongside the injured vessel. The suture is grabbed internally by the needle, brought out of the trocar site, and tied, compressing the bleeding vessel. Another technique that may be helpful to tamponade a large bleeding abdominal wall vessel calls for the insertion of a Foley catheter through the trocar site. The balloon is inflated and traction is applied.

Postoperative Problems

Pain

Patients experience minimal pain following laparoscopic surgery. In most instances oral narcotics, such as acetaminophen with codeine preparations, are adequate to relieve their discomfort. Rarely, one or two doses of a parenteral narcotic may be necessary in the immediate postoperative period. If the patient complains of severe abdominal pain or requires narcotics for more than 48 hours, the surgeon should be suspicious of an undiagnosed complication. A thorough history and physical examination should be performed looking for signs or symptoms of an ileus, bowel obstruction, visceral perforation, or wound infection.

Minor abdominal discomfort may be due to peritoneal irritation from trapped CO_2 and its by-product, carbonic acid. This potential cause of postoperative discomfort can be minimized by expressing as much CO_2 as possible from the abdominal cavity at the conclusion of the procedure.

Shoulder pain can usually be attributed to referred diaphragmatic irritation caused by carbon dioxide trapped in the subdiaphragmatic space. This can usually be relieved by having the patient lie either in the prone position with his or her buttocks raised or in the lateral decubitus position with the painful side down. These maneuvers place the subdiaphragmatic space in a dependent position, allowing the trapped gas to rise off the diaphragm. Various studies evaluating the role of local anesthetics in the abdominal cavity to prevent CO_2-induced pain are currently underway.[52]

Complications Associated with Initial Experience

A recent report reviewed 372 laparoscopic pelvic lymph node dissections comprising the laparoscopic experience at 8 institutions.[2] Fifteen percent of the patients experienced a complication. Seven required immediate exploration to repair a complication. Delayed laparotomy was necessary in an additional 6 patients. Twenty-five percent of the complications were recognized intraoperatively (14/55), with the remainder diagnosed postoperatively. In addition, in 16 patients the lymph node dissection could not be completed by laparoscopy.

The complications reported by this group included vascular injury in 11 patients. The inferior epigastric vessels and branches were the most frequently injured. Visceral organ injury occurred in 8 patients. Injury to the bowel, bladder, and ureter was recognized intraoperatively in 4 patients. In the remaining 4 the diagnosis was made postoperatively. Five patients experienced deep vein thrombosis. There were wound infections in 4 patients. Seven patients had problems related to the gastrointestinal tract. A temporary ileus afflicted 5 patients, while 2 patients required exploration for small bowel obstruction. Hypercarbia was observed in 2 patients. Finally, 7 men went into urinary retention postoperatively.

In the overall initial laparoscopic experience with 221 patients at St. Louis University, including procedures ranging from laparoscopic varicocelectomy to cystoprostatectomy, a total of 33 complications (15.8%) were encountered (Table 8-1).[53]

The adverse effects seen with each type of operation are listed in Table 8-2. Discounting the procedures performed less than ten times, pelvic lymphadenectomies were associated with the highest rate of significant complications (9.3%). Varicocelectomies were linked with few major complications but a 14.3% rate of minor problems.

In 13 patients adjuvant surgical intervention was required (Table 8-3). Five patients required celiotomy. In 1 patient, what appeared to be a large artery was transected during a difficult dissection of a nonfunctional kidney that had been previously explored. Pressure was promptly applied with laparoscopic forceps and an immediate laparotomy performed (Fig 8-3). An intraperitoneal bladder perforation occurred early in our experience as a result of dissection medial to the obliterated umbilical artery during a pelvic lymphadenectomy. This was immediately diagnosed and was repaired openly. Three other patients required delayed celiotomy for a cecal perforation, a bowel obstruction secondary

TABLE 8-1 Early Laparoscopic Surgical Experience at St. Louis University

Procedure	Success	
Varicocelectomy	90/91	(98.9%)
Lymphadenectomy	96/98	(97.9%)
Diverticulectomy	3/3	(100%)
Cystectomy	3/4	(75%)
Repair bladder rupture	1/1	(100%)
Nephrectomy	8/9	(88%)
Lymphocelectomy	4/4	(100%)
Renal cyst unroofing	2/2	(100%)
Orchiectomy	2/2	(100%)
Bladder neck suspension	3/3	(100%)
CAPD catheter revision	4/4	(100%)
Total	216/221	(97.7%)

The age ranged from 12 to 81 (mean 42.5).

TABLE 8-2 Complication by Procedure

	Major	Minor
Varicocelectomy	Anesthetic (1)	Shoulder pain (7) Hydrocele (2) Scrotal emphysema (1) Wound ecchymosis (1) Wound infection (1) Genitofemoral nerve (1)
Total	1/91 (1.1%)	13/91 (14.3%)
Lymphadenectomy	Lymphocele* (4) Bladder perforation (1) Ureteral transection* (1) Cerebrovascular accident (1) Bowel obstruction* (1) Cecal perforation* (1)	Lymphocele, incidental (5) Shoulder pain (2) Ecchymosis (2) Epigastric artery (1) Prolonged ileus (2)
Total	9/96 (9.3%)	7/96 (7.3%)†
Diverticulectomy	0	Urine extravasation (1)
Total		1/3 (33%)
Cystectomy		Medial umbilical ligament (1)
Total		1/3 (33%)
Nephrectomy	Vascular injury (1)	
Total	1/9 (11%)	
Total	11/217 (5.0%)	22/217 (10.1%)†
Total (Major and Minor)	33/217 (15.2%)†	

† excluding incidentally found lymphoceles
* Extended node dissection

TABLE 8-3 Summary of Surgical Interventions

Adjuvant Surgical Intervention	13/217 (5.9%)
Celiotomy	5 (2.3%)
Immediate	2
Delayed	3
Laparoscopy	4 (1.8%)
Immediate	1
Delayed	3
Other surgery	4 (1.8%)
Percutaneous drainage	1
Hydrocelectomy	1
Incision/Drainage wound	2

to herniation through a trocar site, and a urinoma resulting from an unsuspected ureteral injury.

Four complications were treated by laparoscopic intervention. A medial umbilical ligament was transected proximally without ligation. It was immediately clipped without significant blood loss. Four symptomatic lymphoceles developed in men who had extended node dissections with partial retroperitonealization. Three of these lymphoceles were marsupialized laparoscopically.

Four complications required some other type of surgical intervention: percutaneous drainage of a lymphocele (1), hydrocelectomy in a patient following a varicocelectomy (1), and incision and drainage of superficial wound infections at trocar sites (2). Five cases were not completed as planned. Finally, the data was examined by category or type of complication (Table 8-4).

Complications of Laparoscopic Surgery Decrease with Experience

The experience at the 9 different centers just described attest to the difficulties encountered in ini-

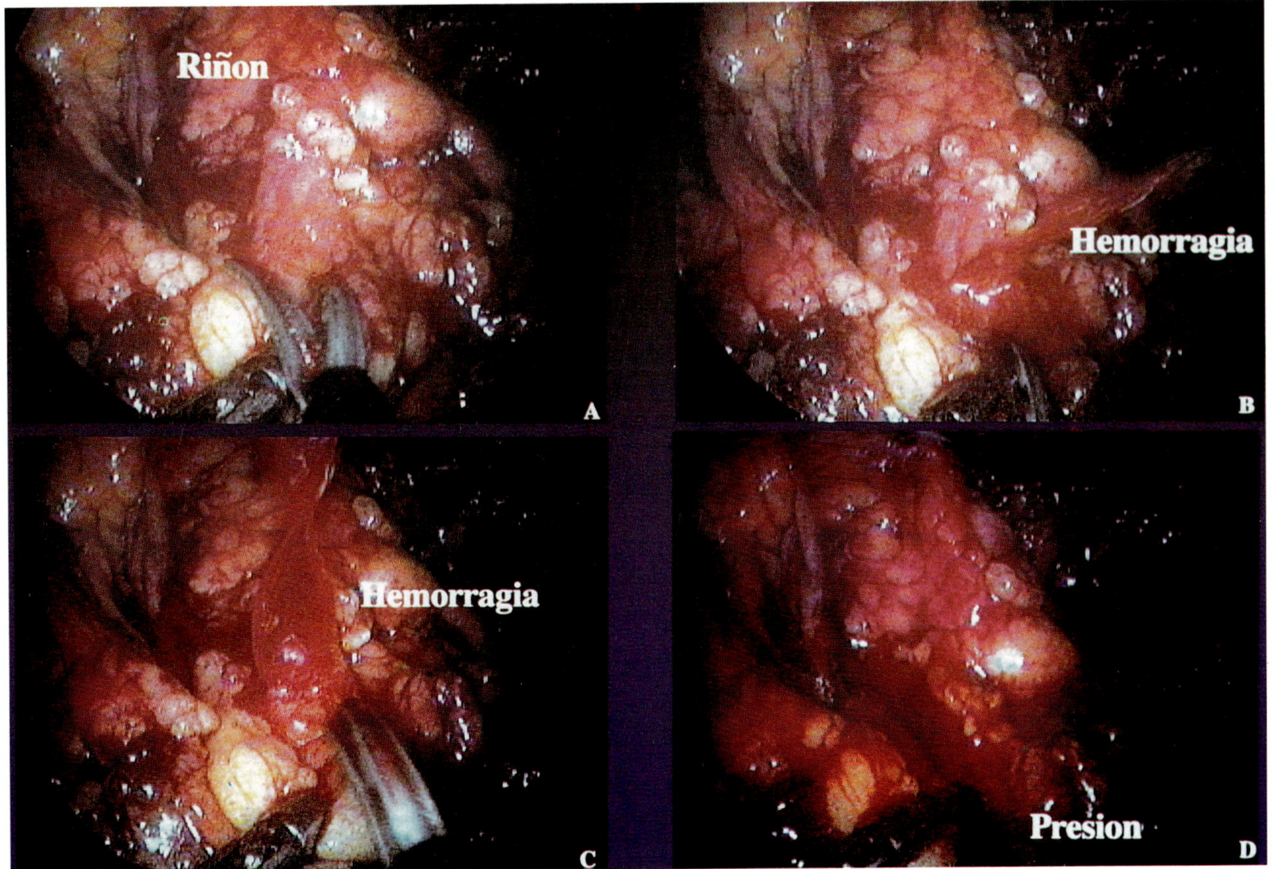

Figure 8-3 (a) Laparoscopic left nephrectomy in a case with severe perirenal fibrosis. (b, c) A polar renal artery has been inadvertently transected. (d) Pressure applied, allowing control of the bleeding vessel.

TABLE 8-4 Complications by Category

Complication (No.)	Intervention
Vascular	
Epigastric artery (1)	Fulguration
Medial umbilical ligament (1)	Laparoscopic clip ligation
Renal vessel (1)	Celiotomy/spontaneous occlusion
Superficial ecchymosis (4)	Observation
Viscus	
Bowel injury (1)	Celiotomy/cecostomy
Bladder perforation (1)	Celiotomy/closure
Ureter transection (1)	Celiotomy/psoas hitch
Bowel obstruction (1)	Celiotomy/ileal resection
Urine extravasation (1)	Foley drainage
Prolonged ileus (2)	NPO
Lymphatic	
Lymphocele (symptomatic) (4)	Laparoscopic marsupialization (3) Percutaneous drainage (1)
Lymphocele (asymptomatic) (5)	Observation
Infection	
Wound infection (2)	Local treatment
Anesthetic	
Pulmonary edema (1)	Mechanical ventilation
Pneumoperitoneum	
Cerebrovascular accident (1)	Supportive
Shoulder pain (9)	Analgesia
Scrotal/Miscellaneous	
Hydrocele (2)	Hydrocelectomy (1) Observation (1)
Subcutaneous emphysema (1)	Observation
Nerve	
Genitofemoral (1)	Observation

tiating laparoscopic surgery. Gomella et al.[54] contrasted the outcome of laparoscopic urologic surgery (for the most part pelvic lymph node dissections and varicocele ligations) performed during two different periods of time at 6 medical centers. There were 114 patients in Group I (GP I), all undergoing laparoscopic intervention before October 1991. Group II (GP II) was composed of 148, all undergoing surgery between October 1991 and September 1992. Major complication rates decreased from 10.5% (GP I) to 6% (GP II); minor complications remained unchanged at 10%. Transfusion rates decreased from 5.2% to 2%, and laparotomy rates decreased from 2.6% to 2%. There were no deaths in either group.

Operating time for pelvic lymph node dissections decreased from a mean of 162 minutes to 125 minutes, and hospital stay declined from 45.6 hours to 39.3 hours. The transfusion rate for this procedure dropped from 5.2% to 1.5% and the laparotomy rate from 2.9% to 1.5%.

Proper patient selection and preparation is imperative to minimize the risk of complications. Improved instrumentation and the continued experience of a laparoscopy team will contribute to better patient outcomes and lessen complication rates.

References

1. Kavoussi LR, Sosa RE, Capelouto C: Complications of laparoscopic surgery. *J Endourol* 6(1):95–98, 1992.
2. Kavoussi LR, Sosa E, Chandhoke PJ, et al: Complications of laparoscopic pelvic lymph node dissection. *J Urol* 149:322–325, 1993.
3. Semm K: *Operative Manual for Endoscopic Abdominal Surgery*. Chicago, Year Book Medical Publishers, 1987.
4. Sosa RE, Weingram J, Poppas D, Lyons J: Physiologic considerations in laparoscopic surgery in urology. *J Endourol* 6:85–87, 1992.
5. Monk TG, Weldon BC: Anesthetic considerations for laparoscopic surgery. *J Endourol* 6:89–93, 1992.
6. Sosa RE, Poppas DP, Schlegel PN, Lyons JM: Laparoscopic surgery in urology. In: *Campbell's Urology* 6th ed. Edited by Walsh PC, Retik AB, Stamey TA, Vaughn ED. Philadelphia, WB Saunders, Update 2, 1992.
7. Reynolds RC, Pauca AL: Gastric perforation, an anesthesia-induced hazard in laparoscopy. *Anesthesiology* 38:84–85, 1973.
8. Yuzpe AA: Pneumoperitoneum needle and trocar injuries in laparoscopy. *J Reprod Med* 35:485–490, 1990.
9. Penfield AJ: Trocar and needle injuries. In: *Laparoscopy*. Baltimore, Williams & Wilkins, pp 236–241, 1977.
10. Hershlag A, Loy RA, Lavy G, DeCherney AH: Femoral neuropathy after laparoscopy. *J Reprod Med* 35:575–576, 1990.
11. Prentice JA, Martin JT: The Trendelenberg position: Anesthesiologic considerations, in *Positioning in Anesthesia and Surgery*, Philadelphia, WB Saunders, pp 127–145, 1987.
12. Jones MJ, Mitchell RW, Hindocha N: Effect of increased intra-abdominal pressure during laparoscopy on the lower esophageal sphincter. *Anesth Analg* 68:63–65, 1989.
13. Roberts CJ, Goodman NW: Gastro-esophageal reflux during elective laparoscopy. *Anaesthesia* 45:1009–1011, 1990.
14. Thompson AG, Wheeless CR: Gastrointestinal complications of laparoscopy sterilization. *Obstet Gynecol* 41:669–676, 1973.
15. Milliken RA, Milliken GM: Gastric perforation during laparoscopic examination: Report of a case. *Anesth Analg* 53:239–240, 1974.
16. Pring DW: Inferior epigastric hemorrhage: An avoidable complication of laparoscopic clip sterilization. *Br J Obstet Gynecol* 90:480–482, 1983.
17. Green LS, Loughlin KR, Kavoussi LR: Management of epigastric vessel injury during laparoscopy. *J Endourol* 6(2):99–101, 1992.
18. Baadsgaard SE, Bille S, Egeblad K: Major vascular injury during gynecologic laparoscopy: Report of a case and review of published cases. *Acta Obstet Gynecol Scand* 68:283–285, 1989.
19. Lynn SC, Katz AR, Ross PJ: Aortic perforation sustained at laparoscopy. *J Reprod Med* 27:217–219, 1982.
20. Peterson HB, Geenspan JR, and Ory HW: Death following puncture of the aorta during laparoscopic sterilization. *Obstet Gynecol* 59:133–134, 1982.
21. Borten, M: Vascular complications in laparoscopic complications: Prevention and management: Philadelphia, BC Decker, pp 298–326, 1986.
22. Kent RB: Subcutaneous emphysema and hypercarbia following laparoscopic cholecystectomy. *Arch Surg* 126:1154–1156, 1991.
23. Sosa RE, Weingram J, Stein B, et al: Hypercarbia in laparoscopic pelvic lymph node dissection. *J Urol* 147:246A, 1992.
24. Seed RF, Shakespeare TF, Muldood MJ: Carbon dioxide homeostasis anesthesia for laparoscopy. *Anaesthesia* 25:223–230, 1970.
25. Wilcox S, Vandon D: Alas, poor Trendelenberg and his position! *Anesth Analg* 67:574–578, 1988.
26. Rasmussenk JP, Dauchot PJ, Depalma RG, et al: Cardiac function and hypercarbia. *Arch Surg* 113:1196–1200, 1978.
27. Kubal K, Komatsu T, Sanchala V, et al: Trendelenberg position used during venous cannulation increases myocardial oxygen demand. *Anesth Analg* 63:239, 1984.
28. Schiller WR: The Trendelenberg position. In: *Positioning in Anesthesia and Surgical Requirements*. Edited by Martin, JT. Philadephia: WB Saunders, pp 87–89, 1978.
29. Heinonen J, Takki S, Tammisto T: Effect of the Trendelenberg tilt and other procedures on the position of endotracheal tubes. *Lancet* 1:850–853, 1969.
30. Kavoussi LR, Clayman RV: Urologist at work: Trocar fixation during laparoscopy. *J Endourol* 6:71–72, 1992.
31. Schwimmer WB: Electrosurgical burn injuries during laparoscopy sterilization. Treatment and prevention. *Obstet Gynecol* 44:526–530, 1974.

32. Bard PA, Chen L: Subcutaneous emphysema associated with laparoscopy. Letter to the Editor. *Anesth Analg* 71:100–106, 1990.
33. Wittgen CM, Andrus CH, Fitzgerald SD, et al: Analysis of the Hemodynamic and Ventilatory Effects of Laparoscopic Cholecystectomy. *Arch Surg* 126:997–1000, 1991.
34. Johannsen G, Andersen M, Juhl B: The effect of general anesthesia on the hemodynamic events during laparoscopy with CO_2 insufflation. *Acta Anaesthesiol Scand* 33:132–136, 1989.
35. Hussain NH: Bilateral pneumothorax associated with laparoscopy: A case report of a rare hazard and a review of the literature. *Anaesthesia* 28:75–81, 1973.
36. Batra MS, Driscoll JJ, Coburn WA, et al: Evanescent nitrous oxide pneumothorax after laparoscopy. *Anesth Analg* 62:1121–1123, 1983.
37. Nicholson RD, Berman ND: Pneumopericardium following laparoscopy. *Chest* 76:605–607, 1979.
38. Herrerias JM, Ariza A, Garrido M: An unusual complication of laparoscopy: Pneumopericardium. *Endoscopy* 12:254, 1980.
39. Knos GB, Sung YF: A pneumopericardium associated with laparoscopy. *J Clin Anesth* 3:56–59, 1991.
40. Ostman PL, Pantie-Fisher FH, Faure EA, et al: Circulatory collapse during laparoscopy. *J Clin Anesth* 2:129–132, 1990.
41. Carmichael DE: Laparoscopy-cardiac considerations. *Fertil Steril* 22:69–70, 1971.
42. Lee CM: Acute hypotension during laparoscopy: A case report. *Anesth Analg* 54:142–143, 1975.
43. Shifren JL, Adelstein L, Finker JN: Asystolic cardiac arrest: A rare complication of laparoscopy. *Obstet Gynecol* 79:840–841, 1992.
44. Brantley JC, Riley PM: Cardiovascular collapse during laparoscopy: A report of two cases. *Am J Obstet Gynecol* 159:735–737, 1988.
45. Ott DE: Laparoscopic hypothermia. *J Laparosc Surg* 1:127–131, 1991.
46. Deplater RMH, Jones IMC: Non-fatal carbon dioxide embolism during laparoscopy. *Anaesth Intensive Care* 17:359–360, 1989.
47. Diakun TA: Carbon dioxide embolism: Successful resuscitation with cardiopulmonary bypass. *Anesthesiology* 74:1151–1153, 1991.
48. Greville, AC, Clements EA, Erwin DC, et al: Pulmonary air embolism during laparoscopic laser cholecystectomy. *Anaesthesia* 46:113–114, 1991.
49. Root B, Levy MN, Pollack S, et al: Gas embolism after laparoscopy delayed by "trapping" in portal circulation *Anesth Analg* 57:232–237, 1978.
50. Yacoub OF, Cardona I, Coverler LA, et al: Carbon dioxide embolism during laparoscopy. *Anesthesiology* 57:533–535, 1982.
51. Clark C, Weeks DB, Gudson JP: Venous carbon dioxide embolism during laparoscopy. *Anesth Analg* 56:650–652, 1977.
52. Helvacioglu A, Weis R: Operative laparoscopy and postoperative pain relief. *Fertil Steril* 57:548–552, 1992.
53. Parra RO, Hagood PG, Boullier JA, Cummings JM, Mehan DJ: Complications of laparoscopic urologic surgery: Experience at St. Louis University. *J Urol* 151:681–684, 1994.
54. Gomella L, Lotfi MA, Stone NN, Sosa RE, Shichman S, Albala D, Manyak M, Kozminski M: Laparoscopic urologic surgery: Improvement in outcome. *J Urol* 149:418A, 1993.

SECTION TWO

Operative Laparoscopy

9

Laparoscopic Varicocelectomy

Donald J. Mehan

Introduction

Ligation of the internal spermatic veins to correct hypofertility in the male has become a well-established and accepted means of treating male factor infertility. Since Tulloch's initial report in 1952, numerous studies have pointed to the efficacy of internal spermatic vein ligation in the treatment of the infertile male.

Various surgical and nonsurgical approaches have been advocated to interrupt the dilated pampiniform venous plexus, including the classic inguinal (Ivanissevich), the retroperitoneal (Palomo), inguinal and subinguinal mini-incisions using magnification, and percutaneous embolization.[1] All of these measures have their adherents, advantages, and disadvantages.

The ready accessibility of the internal spermatic veins cephalad to their exit from the retroperitoneal space via the internal inguinal ring makes their obliteration via the laparoscope quite simple. The anatomy is clear, and if a few simple rules are followed, laparoscopic clipping is not only safe, but quick and readily mastered.

Surgical Indications and Evaluation

Criteria for laparoscopic varicocelectomy are the same as those for any other varicocele procedure.[2,3] We require an established barren state of at least 6 but preferably 12 months. There should be no overwhelming female factor that would mitigate the result of any successful varicocele procedure. Other male factors should be eliminated by history and physical examination and appropriate laboratory studies.

Varicoceles are demonstrable on physical examination with the patient undressed, standing in a comfortably heated room performing the Valsalva maneuver. The incidence of bilateral occurrence has been variably reported.[4,5] We see varicoceles as a bilateral feature in slightly over 80 percent of our cases. Some authors use Doppler or ultrasound studies to aid in the diagnosis, but we have not found this to be necessary.[6,7]

At least two semenograms are obtained that are within laboratory variation. In our clinic, we seldom recommend surgery if the sperm density is greater than 40 million sperm per mL unless there is a marked asthenospermia with significant dead and immobile forms. Azoospermia in patients is not an absolute contraindication of surgery unless the serum follicle stimulating hormone (FSH) is significantly elevated (twice normal) or the azoospermia is believed due to obstructive factors. All patients with oligospermia (sperm densities less than ten million sperm per mL) have serum gonadotropins and testosterone determinations to eliminate cases of intrinsic gonadal failure.

The standard contraindications for all laparoscopic procedures also hold for spermatic vein ligations. There has been no problem in doing laparoscopic varicocelectomies in patients who have had prior appendectomies (two cases), herniorrhaphies (three cases), and orchidopexies (one case).

Surgical Technique

The technique is simple.[8–10] Once induction of general anesthesia is obtained and the bladder catheterized, a minilap incision is made immediately inferior to the umbilicus as described in Chap. 5. Doing this adds to the safety of the operation eliminating the concerns of a "blind stick," and in our experience adds nothing to the time of surgery. Once open, an 11-mm Hasson-type trocar is passed safely into the peritoneal cavity, its position assured, and inflation with CO_2 begun. After reaching 15 mm Hg pressure, careful inspection is made of the peritoneal contents to be certain there is no trauma or other significant lesion. Placement of the two lateral trocars in each anterior axillary line is done visually to assure a safe trocar passage. A 10-mm trocar is placed on the left and a 5-mm trocar on the right (Fig. 9-1). Although these can be reversed to suit the needs of the surgeon, I prefer to operate on the patient's left. These three trocar sites offer excellent operative visibility and maneuverability and allow for easy performance of bilateral procedures. We have found it beneficial to have the patient's arms at his side and to have at least 20 to 30 degrees of Trendelenburg.

Often, particularly on the left, adhesions from the bowel to the peritoneal wall are present, obscuring vision (Fig. 9-2). These can be taken down quite readily with the endoshears and have not constituted a problem. The anatomy can then be reviewed. The

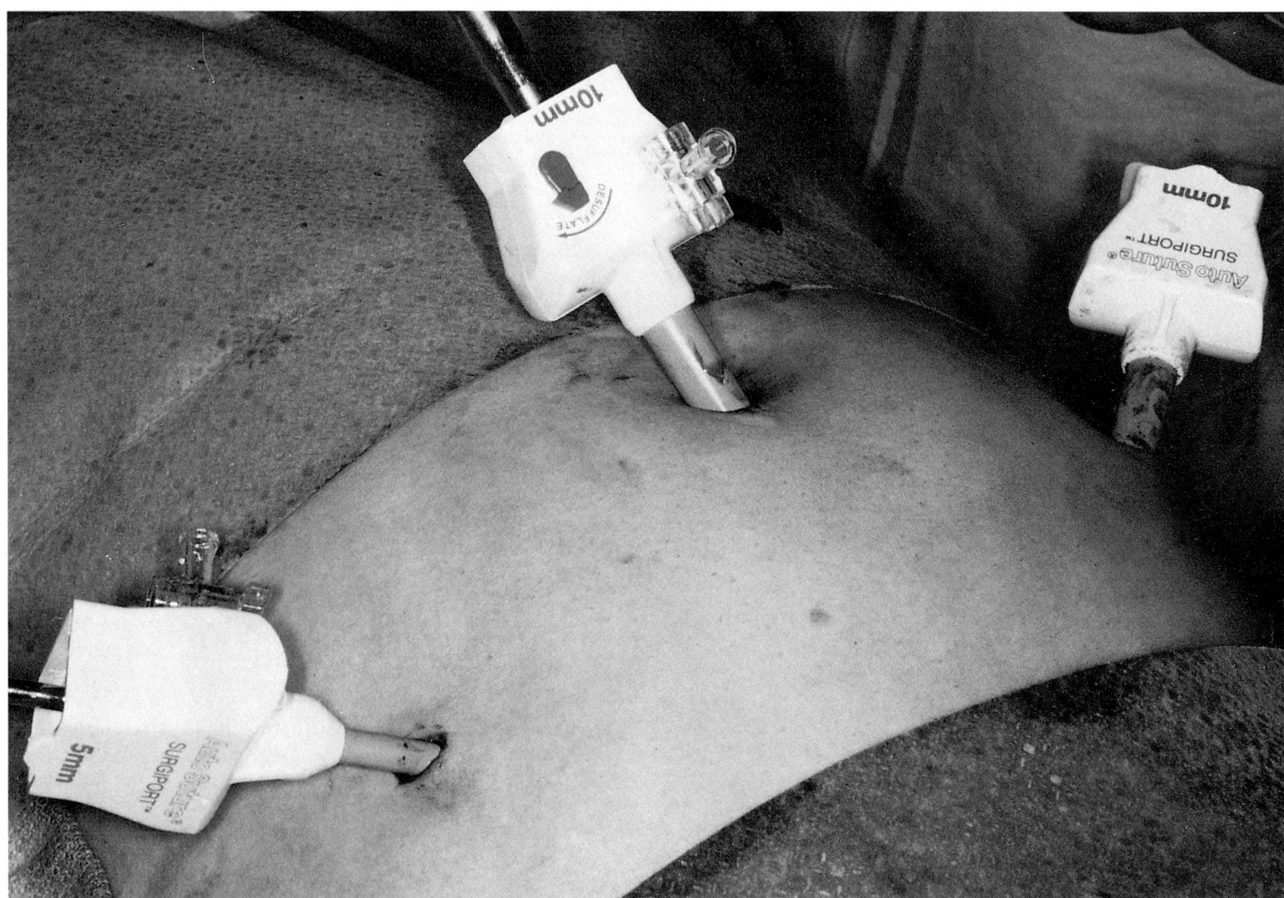

Figure 9-1 Position of the three ports. Two 10-mm and one 5-mm cannulas.

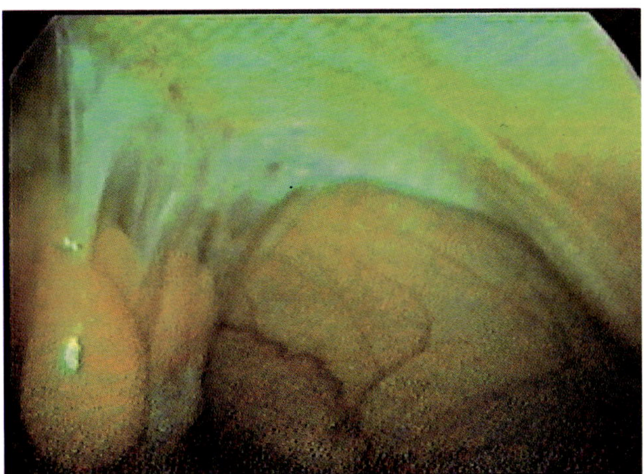

Figure 9-2 Adhesions of sigmoid to anterior abdominal wall.

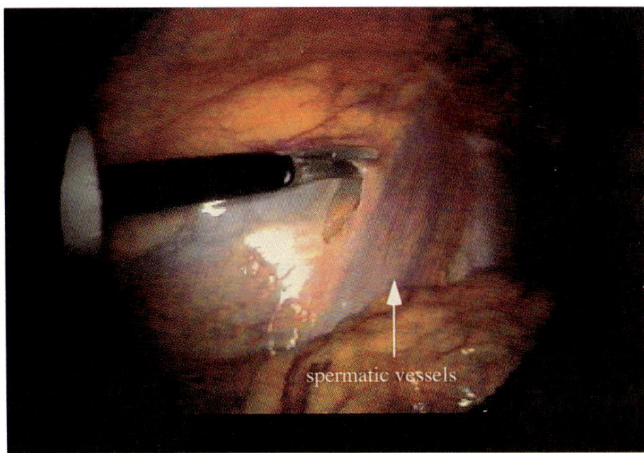

Figure 9-4 Incision in parietal peritoneum lateral to the left spermatic vessels.

internal ring is identified with the vas exiting and coursing medially. The spermatic vascular bundle can be seen below and cephalad to the ring. The median umbilical ligament and the bladder with the catheter balloon in place is medial to the vascular bundle (Fig. 9-3). Sometimes pulsations from the iliac vessels medial to and below the spermatic bundle are seen.

(a)

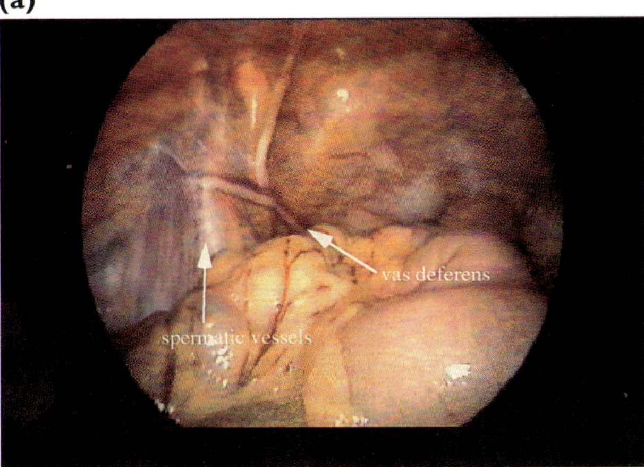

(b)

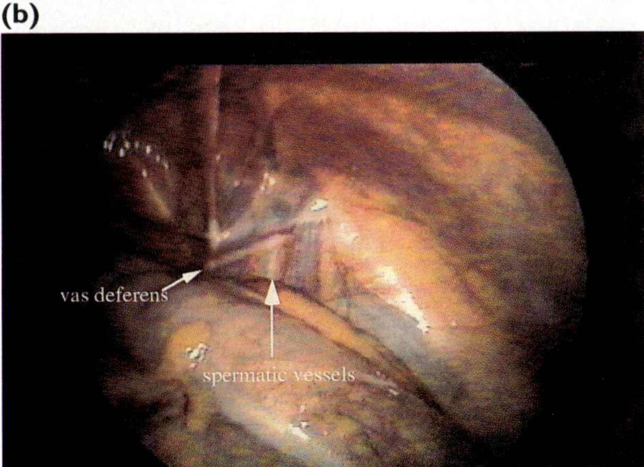

Figure 9-3 (a) Left-sided anatomy. (b) Right-sided anatomy. Prominent vas exiting from internal ring.

After identification of the internal ring, the vas, and the spermatic vascular bundle, a parallel incision is made in the parietal peritoneum, cephalad to the internal ring and vas and lateral to the vascular bundle. If these landmarks are adhered to, the dissection is in a perfectly safe area and adequate exposure is obtained to perform the spermatic vein ligation. A 1-in. incision is made in the parietal peritoneum. We have not found it helpful to open the peritoneum medially or to "T" the incisions (Fig. 9-4). Using a Petelin right angle dissector, the spermatic vascular bundle can be freed from beneath the peritoneum. To facilitate this, the assistant grasps the medial edge of the peritoneum and holds it up while the operator then sweeps the vascular bundle up into the wound space (Fig. 9-5). Once the bundle

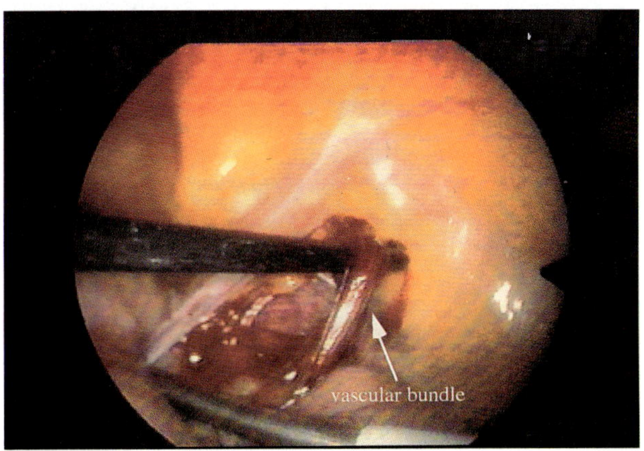

Figure 9-5 Vascular bundle is identified and isolated.

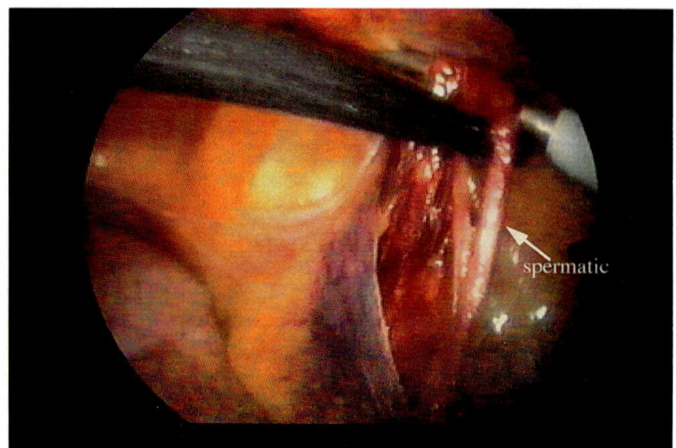

Figure 9-6 Assistant holding vascular bundle with straight probe. Separation of artery from vein can be seen.

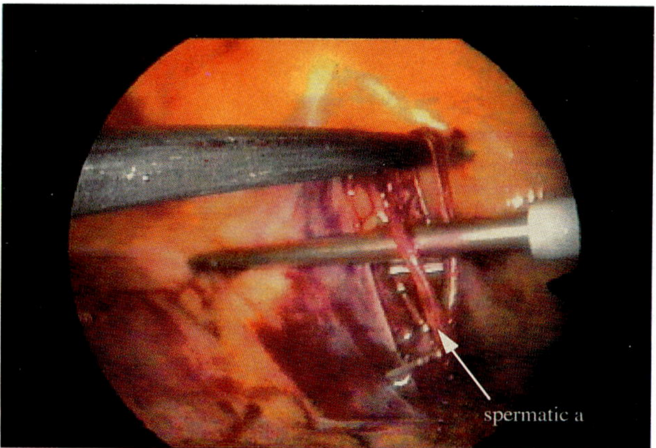

Figure 9-8 Complete separation of major vein—clipping in progress.

is freed, the assistant then places a straight probe under the bundle. At that time the pulsating spermatic artery can usually be seen. Again, with the Petelin dissector, the artery is separated from the major venous bundle. When this is accomplished, the assistant repositions the probe under the venous bundle, holding it free from the artery (Fig. 9-6), allowing the surgeon to place four clips, two distal and two proximal, on the spermatic vein. Once this has been done, the spermatic vein is transected, avoiding any injury to the artery (Fig. 9-7). We believe the artery should be spared in all cases, although some authors have questioned whether this is absolutely necessary (Fig. 9-8).

(a)

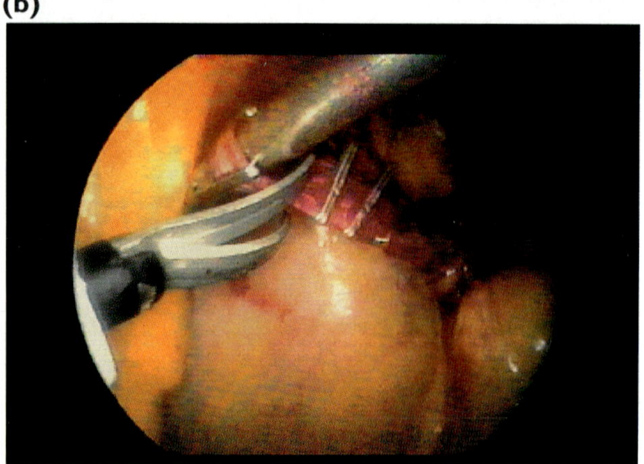

(b)

Figure 9-7 (a) Vein separated clearly from artery with proximal clips in place. (b) Division of veins with endoshears.

Multiple spermatic arteries are not common but must be looked for, as we have seen them in 2 percent of our patients. As a general rule, if the dissection is precise, careful, and meticulous, the artery will not become spastic and can be identified. The use of a Papaverine drip may help should identification of the artery become difficult due to spasm. We used this technique early in the course of the series, but once operative technique had been mastered this maneuver was rarely required. An operative Doppler is available should one wish to use it.[6] With experience and care, however, visualization of the artery should pose no problem, and we have not found it necessary to use an operative Doppler.

After incising the major venous bundle, attention is directed to the possibility of additional veins or, more precisely, a vein intimately associated with the artery. The assistant can place his probe under the artery, and the operator can safely dissect any associated vein from the artery (Fig. 9-9). In almost all cases, we have found a vein immediately adjacent to the artery and feel its transsection is mandatory for an adequate operation. Once dissected from the artery, the vein may be clipped and transected. In most cases three veins are seen, although as many as five have been identified and transected.

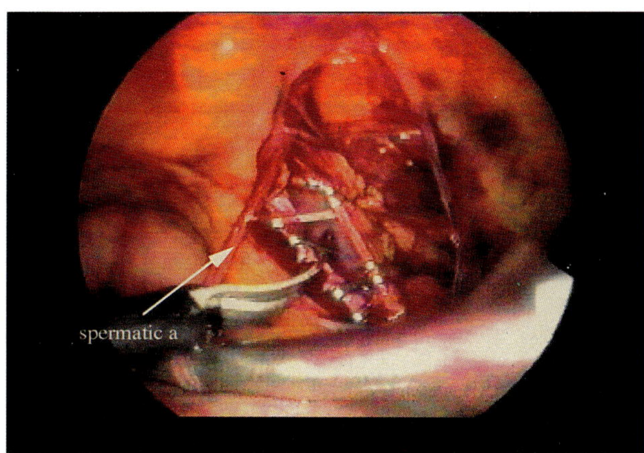

Figure 9-9 Vein transected. Note additional spermatic vein adjacent to artery.

Some authors describe using a Yag laser to control minor venous bleeding. We have found a combination of cautery and clipping to be quite adequate.

If indicated, the contralateral side can be handled in a similar fashion without the placement of additional ports. The surgeon can operate on a rightsided varicocele with equal ease standing on the left side using a 10-mm trocar. Once satisfied that all veins have been transected, a careful inspection is made of the operative sites, to confirm that there is no bleeding and the artery is pulsating (Fig. 9-10).

The peritoneal contents are again examined. The lateral trocars are removed under direct vision to be certain there is no bleeding at the trocar site. In two instances, when bleeding has occurred, this was handled either by direct cautery or the placement of a suture through the skin. Desufflation is accomplished through the midline trocar and then it, too, is removed. Vicryl sutures of 2-0 are placed in the fascia in the midline, and a subcuticular stitch closes the skin and subcutaneous tissue. No fascial sutures are placed in the lateral incisions, which are closed only with a subcutaneous stitch.

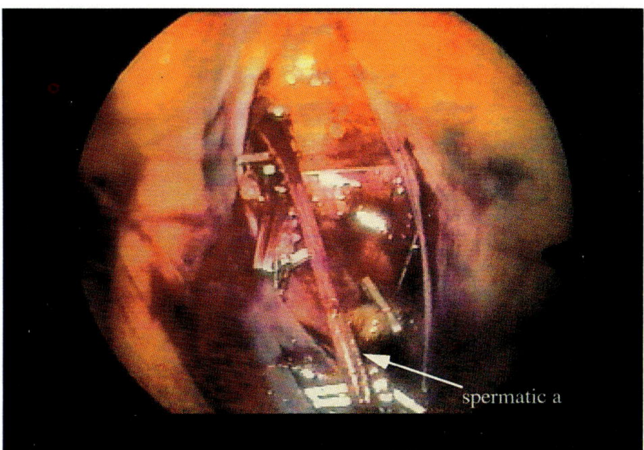

Figure 9-10 Dissection and transection completed. Note multiple cut veins and the preservation of the artery.

Infiltration with a local anesthetic agent such as Marcaine can be performed. In addition, upon completion of anesthesia, 60 mg of Toradol may be given intramuscularly. We have found this combination to significantly reduce the postoperative pain associated with laparoscopic procedures.

Once the patient is awake from anesthesia, the Foley is removed and he is discharged within 2 to 3 h. He is given a prescription for ten 10-mg Toradol tablets, although five to seven of them will usually suffice. Patients are discharged the day of surgery and are told to rest. Following that they may resume whatever activity they wish. Some patients have played golf or bowled the first or second day post-op, and all patients have either returned to work or could have returned to work within 72 h of surgery. There have been no major complications, and morbidity has been minimal. One hydrocele developed, an incidence of less than 2 percent. Some patients have complained of mild transient testicular swelling and soreness, but this has been of a minimal nature and has not posed any problems.

In our personal series of over 100 patients operated on for infertility, 72 have complete follow-up and 30 pregnancies have occurred, an incidence of 41.6 percent. Sixty-four percent of patients in the entire series experienced a significant improvement in the semenogram. Of those patients achieving a pregnancy, 76 percent showed a significant improvement in the semenogram. No recurrences have been seen to date.[11] These results are comparable to or better than those reported in most series.

Conclusion

We feel the laparoscopic varicocelectomy is a suitable alternative to open varicocele surgery. A large number of urologists perform varicocele ligations through the classic inguinal or Ivanissevich approach. If these surgeons have a facility with the laparoscope, it is possible to master this technique rapidly, saving their patients significant postoperative distress and allowing them to return to work in less than 72 hours.

References

1. Palomo A: Radical cure of varicocele by a new technique: Preliminary report. *J Urol* 61:604, 1949.
2. Howards SS: Varicocele. *Fertil Steril* 41:356, 1984.
3. Amelar RD, Dubin L: Infertility in the male. In: *Practice of Surgery (Urology).* Edited by Kendall R, Karafin L. Philadelphia: Harper & Row, vol 2, chap 21, p 43, 1984.
4. World Health Organization. The influence of varicocele in parameters of fertility in a large group of men presenting to infertility clinics. *Fertil Steril,* 57:1289, 1992.
5. Cockett ATK, Takihara H, Consentino MJ: The varicocele. *Fertil Steril,* 41:5, 1984.
6. Laughlin KR, Brooks DC: The use of a Doppler probe in laparoscopic surgery. *J Laparoendosc Surg* 2(3):191, 1992.
7. McClure RD, Hricak H: Scrotal ultrasound in the infertile man: Detection of subclinical unilateral and bilateral varicoceles. *J Urol* 135:711, 1986.
8. Hagood P, Mehan D, Worischeck J, Andrus C, Parra R: Laparoscopic varicocelectomy: Preliminary report of a new technique. *J Urol* 147:73, 1992.
9. Donavon J, Winfield H: Laparoscopic varix ligation. *J Urol* 147:77, 1992.
10. Mehan D, Andrus C, Parra R: Simultaneous laparoscopic varicocelectomy and removal of an intra scrotal atrophic testicle. *Surg Laparosc Endosc* 2(4):327, 1992.
11. Mehan DJ, Andrus CH, Parra RO: Laparoscopic internal spermatic vein ligation: Report of a new technique. *Fertil Steril* 58:1263, 1992.

10

Laparoscopic Pelvic Lymphadenectomy

John A. Boullier
Raul O. Parra

Introduction

The use of laparoscopic approach for the dissection of the pelvic lymph nodes was first reported as a staging procedure for cervical cancer.[1] Shortly after this Schuessler and colleagues reported on their experience with transperitoneal laparoscopic pelvic lymphadenectomy in the staging of prostate cancer.[2] Since these initial reports, numerous papers have been published reporting experience with the technique;[3–8] others have addressed the relative efficacy,[3,9,10] morbidity,[11] and cost of the procedure.[12] In this chapter we will discuss the indications for this procedure; the various recommended approaches, with emphasis on our current technique; intraoperative and postoperative complications; and possible future applications with regard to new treatment modalities for pelvic malignancies.

Indications

The value of a laparoscopic pelvic lymph node dissection (LPLND) prior to definitive radiation therapy for prostate or bladder cancer is unequivocal. Likewise, the staging of prostate cancer via this approach prior to a radical perineal prostatectomy has inherent appeal. The relative morbidity of this combination alone and with respect to the current most commonly employed combination of open dissection followed by radical retropubic prostatectomy has been the subject of several recent studies.[13–16]

Indications for the laparoscopic approach prior to a radical retropubic prostatectomy are not well defined. Its advantage in patients with positive lymph node metastasis, the elimination of a more extensive and potentially morbid incision, is clear. How to select such patients preoperatively is decidedly less obvious.[17] The use of clinical or biochemical parameters as well as imaging modalities to determine nodal involvement has proven less than reliable.[18–23] Advanced clinical stage and/or pathological grade appear more predictive of lymphatic involvement. Donahue and associates[24] in their review of 4,492 patients found that clinical stages B-2 and C were associated with a 43 percent incidence of positive pelvic nodes. The histopathologic grading of prostatic adenocarcinoma using the Gleason system[25] has been shown in separate reports by Kramer and associates,[26] the uro-oncology research group,[27] and Osterling and colleagues[28] to correlate with pelvic node involvement in 28 percent to 93 percent of patients with poorly differentiated cancers. Nevertheless, utilizing staging and histological grade for selecting patients for LPLND would result in a significant number of individuals with negative nodes.

Incorporating the predictive value of preoperative prostate specific antigen (PSA) with these two parameters has proven a useful refinement. Most patients with carcinoma of the prostate are found to have levels of serum PSA over 4 ng/dL.[29] In studies correlating preoperative PSA values with final pathological stage, increasing serum levels of PSA have been demonstrated to closely parallel progressive pathological stages.[30,31] Unfortunately, appreciable overlap exists between each stage and no specific PSA level is able to dependably discriminate confined disease from more advanced prostatic cancer. Nevertheless, we believe certain levels of preoperative PSA can be used as a warning of the possibility of lymph node involvement. In Lange's series,[32] 59 percent of the men in whom the serum PSA level was over 10 ng/dL were found to have positive seminal vesicles or lymph nodes. These findings increased to 66 percent and 65 percent when levels were between 10 and 20 or over 20 ng/dL, respectively. Such data suggested that LPLND prior to retropubic prostatectomy in patients with advanced clinical stage, poorly differentiated tumors, elevated serum PSA, or elevated serum prostate acid phosphatase (PAP) and a negative bone scan, (stage D-0) might prove efficacious.

Two studies have addressed this issue.[33,34] While the design of the two studies differed, both identified a preoperative PSA of 20 or more as a significant predictor of nodal metastasis. Parra and colleagues[33] data suggested PSA to be the single best predictor of nodal involvement, but Wolf and coworkers found a parameter of clinical stage, a digital rectal examination suggesting uncontained tumor, as the single most valuable indicator of metastasis. Both papers found a combination of preoperative parameters to be most consistently predictive: PSA and clinical stage,[33] and PSA and Gleason score.[34] Such data has limited the use of LPLND prior to radical retropubic prostatectomies. While we continue to recommend an LPLND prior to a retropubic prostatectomy in patients with a PSA > 20 ng/mL, a Gleason score ≥ 8, or clinical stages B2 or C, we would more frequently recommend a LPLND followed by a radical perineal prostatectomy. Conversely, we no longer perform pelvic lymph node dissections in patients with clinical stage A1 or B1 and a PSA < 10 ng/mL with Gleason score < 7.

Although few LPLNDs for the staging of bladder cancer have been formally reported, its utility prior to definitive treatments other than cystectomy seems obvious. The technique may also prove useful in the staging of penile carcinoma. The confirmation of pelvic metastasis by a LPLND in patients with palpable inguinal lymphadenopathy could eliminate the significant morbidity of an unindicated bilateral inguinal lymphadenectomy. Finally, although rare, the staging of urethral carcinoma by this technique could potentially spare patients with nodal metastasis the morbidity of a probable unsuccessful exenteration procedure.

Preoperative Studies

As stated earlier, we believe patients who are candidates for a laparoscopic pelvic lymphadenectomy should be those at the greatest risk of having metastatic disease. As such, they are the patients most likely to benefit from the full metastatic workup characteristic of their particular malignancy. In the case of prostate cancer, those patients who fulfill our criteria for LPLND are evaluated preoperatively with a bone scan, chest x-ray with tomograms, and a liver panel. We do not perform a pelvic computerized tomography study. We no longer evaluate patients who are clinical stage A1 or B1 with well or moderately differentiated cancers (Gleason score less than 7) and PSAs less than 10. It is currently our policy to proceed directly to definitive treatment in these patients without a formal examination of the pelvic lymph nodes.

Preoperative Preparation

Studies and treatments specific to the performance of a laparoscopic procedure are as outlined in Chap. 2.

Patient Positioning

The patient is positioned in a modified lithotomy position with the buttocks elevated. The arms are positioned at the patient's side to allow maximum movement by the operating team. The table is placed in approximately 45 degrees of Trendelenburg.

Pneumoperitoneum and Trocar Placement

The technique for a LPLND involves the induction of a pneumoperitoneum of 12 to 15 mm Hg with carbon dioxide via a Veress needle or Hasson cannula inserted through a minilaparotomy incision. We have found the technique described by Mitchell and colleagues to be simple and yet efficacious for this purpose.[35] The initial trocar is then introduced transumbilically and consists of a 10- or 11-mm port through which the camera lens is passed. After a thorough inspection of the peritoneal cavity for the presence of adhesions or any other underlying pathology, two to four additional trocars are then placed under direct visual control. Numerous trocar arrangements have been advocated, the four-point "diamond" placement and the fan configuration (five trocars) being the most frequently cited.[36] We feel that the fewer the trocars, the better. We utilize two 11-mm trocars positioned one third of the distance from the umbilicus to the iliac crest bilaterally (Fig. 10-1). We prefer the use of bilateral 11-mm ports because it allows untroubled introduction of the endoclip applier and ready removal of lymphatic tissue once the dissection is completed. Also, alterations in the site of the camera may be made without changing to a smaller lens. An additional 5-mm trocar may be positioned in the midline 2 to 3 cm above the pubis if extra retraction becomes necessary.

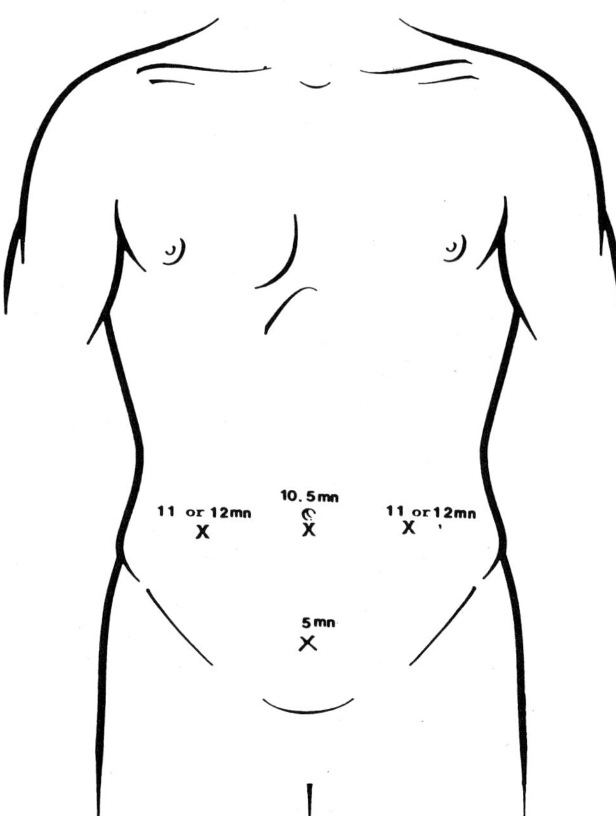

Figure 10-1 Trocar positions for laparoscopic pelvic lymph node dissection (LPLND).

Procedure

Pertinent Anatomic Landmarks

Once access has been obtained, the pertinent pelvic landmarks are readily visualized. Central to the procedure is the identification of the umbilical ligaments or obliterated umbilical arteries on either side of the bladder (Fig. 10-2). In obese patients the external iliac vessels are often obscured by the overlying peritoneum, but they may often be recognized by their pulsations. In thin individuals they are sometimes readily visible through the peritoneal layer (Fig. 10-3). The internal ring is identified with the spermatic vessels and vas deferens coursing through its opening as a constant landmark. Placing the patient in the Trendelenburg position aids in the cephalad displacement of loops of bowel, tilting the table to the contralateral side may further displace the visceral contents. It is often necessary to perform adhesiolysis—particularly on the left side, where it is not uncommon to find adhesions between the sigmoid colon and the peritoneum, most often thought to be secondary to diverticular disease.

Initial Dissection

Access to the pelvis is obtained via a peritoneotomy medial and cephalad to the internal ring and lateral to the umbilical ligament. Although others have utilized the KTP laser[2] to incise the peritoneum, we prefer the use of electrocautery scissors. In either instance the incision is extended proximally for several centimeters (Fig. 10-4). The vas deferens is encountered during the extension of the incision and divided (Fig. 10-5). An inverted V peritoneotomy, which is proported to result in an increase in nodal yield, has been recommended.[37]

Limited Dissection

Our limits of dissection consist of the area delineated by the pubic rami distally, the bifurcation of the common iliac artery proximally, the external iliac

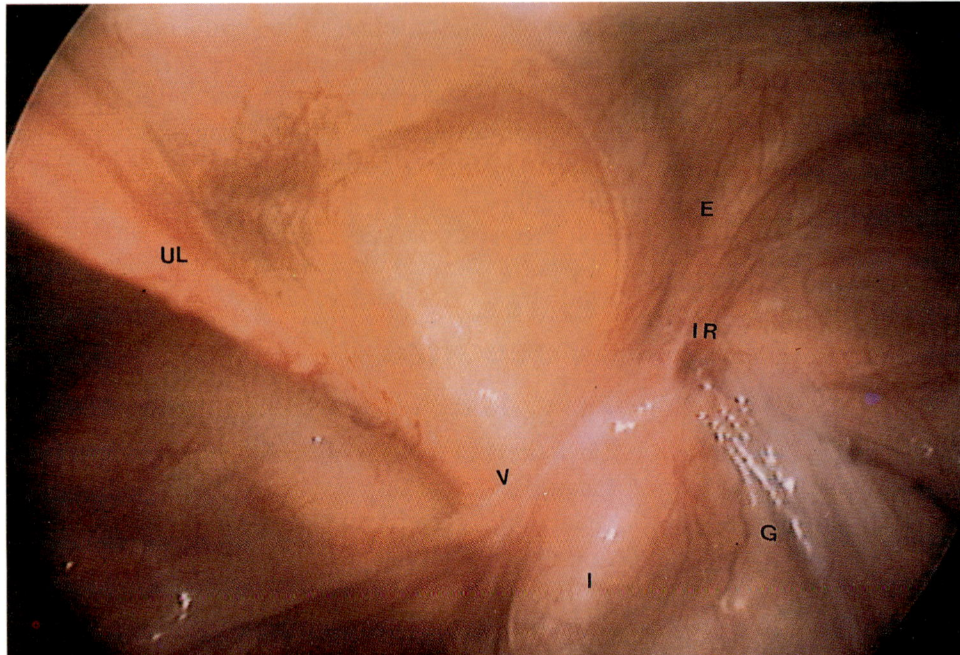

Figure 10-2 Pertinent pelvic landmarks of LPLND: IR, internal ring; UL, umbilical ligament; V, vas deferens; E, epigastric vessels; G, gonadal vessel; I, iliac artery.

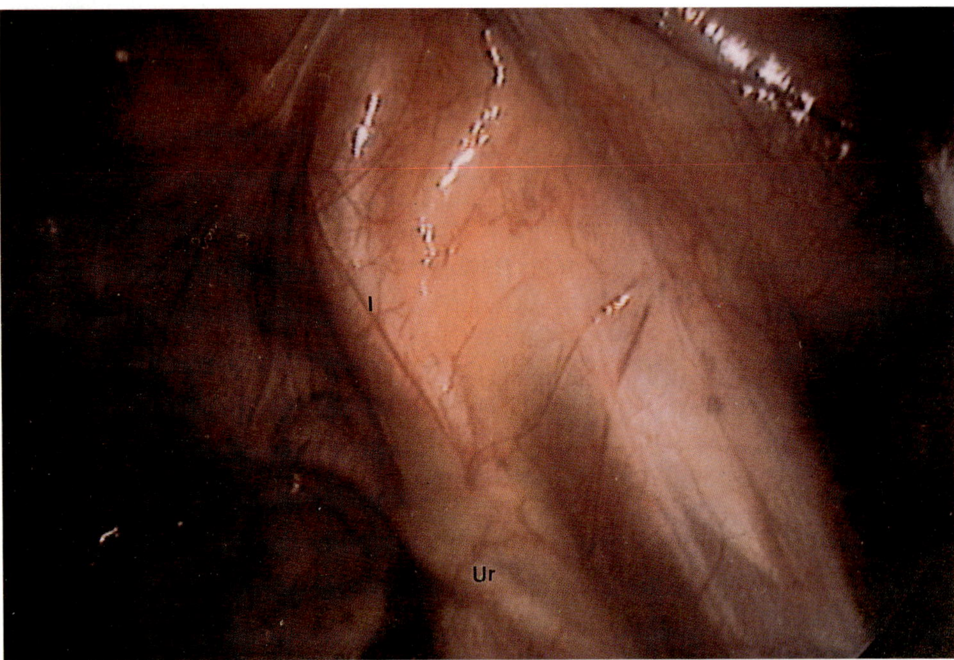

Figure 10-3 Pertinent proximal anatomical landmarks: UR, ureter; I, iliac artery.

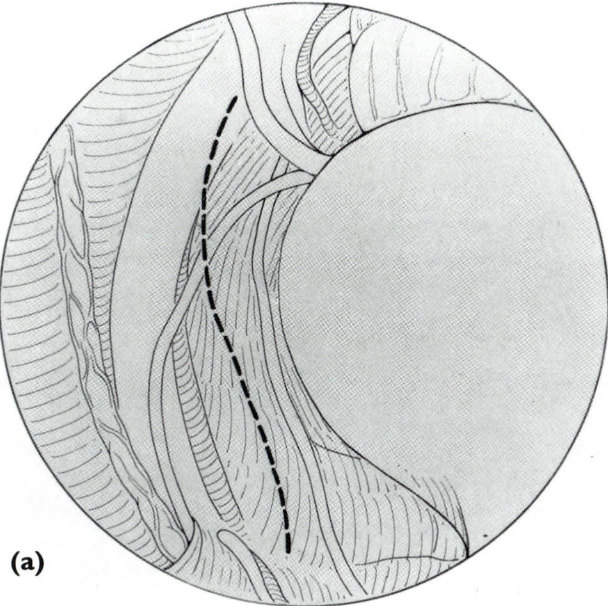

(a)

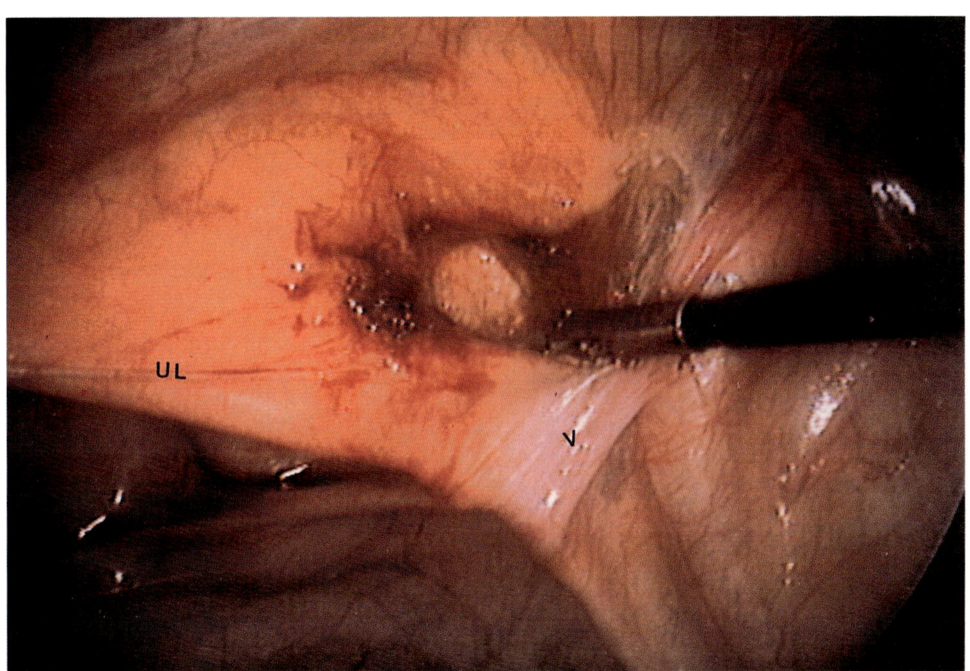

(b)

Figure 10-4 (a) Line drawing of peritoneal incision lateral to umbilical ligament. (b) Initiation of peritoneotomy: UL, umbilical ligament; V, vas deferens.

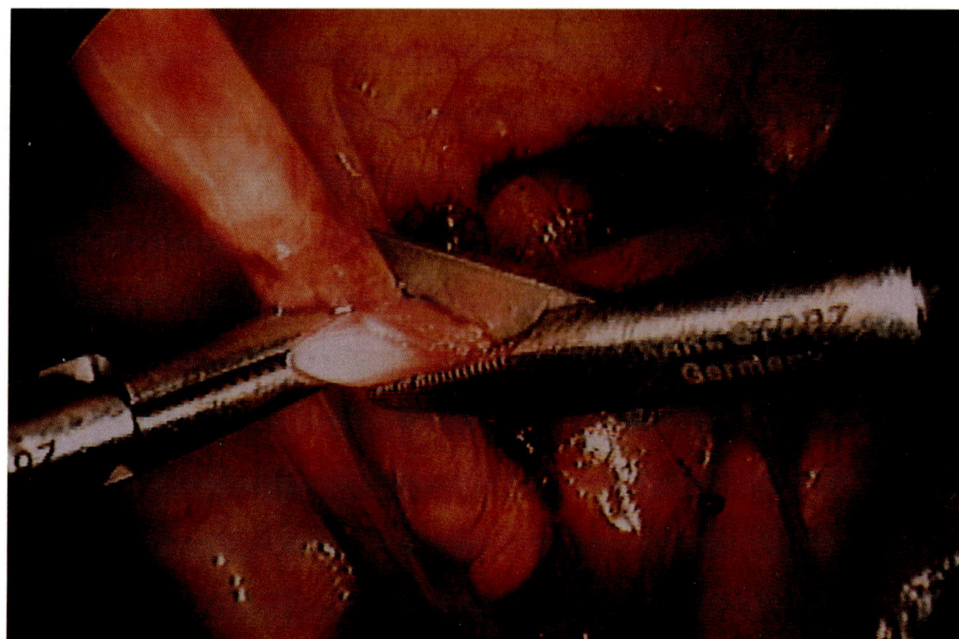

(a)

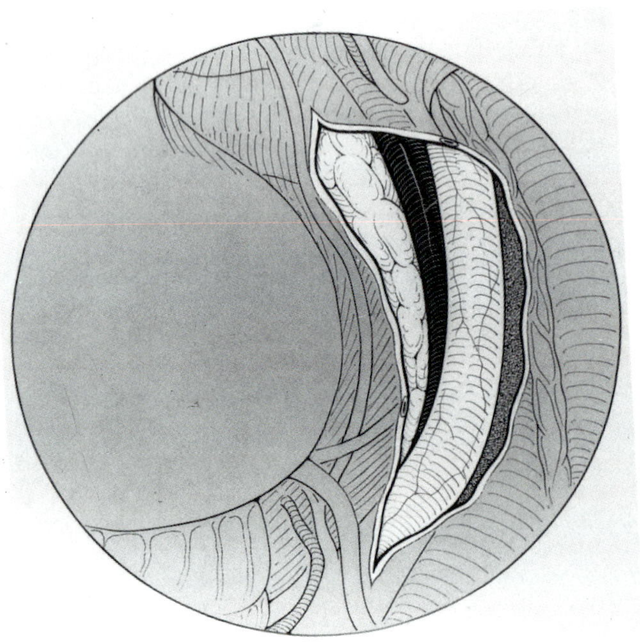

(b)

Figure 10-5 (a) Performance of vasectomy aids in visualization of the nodal packet. (b) Line drawing of exposure of obdurator nodal packet following vasectomy.

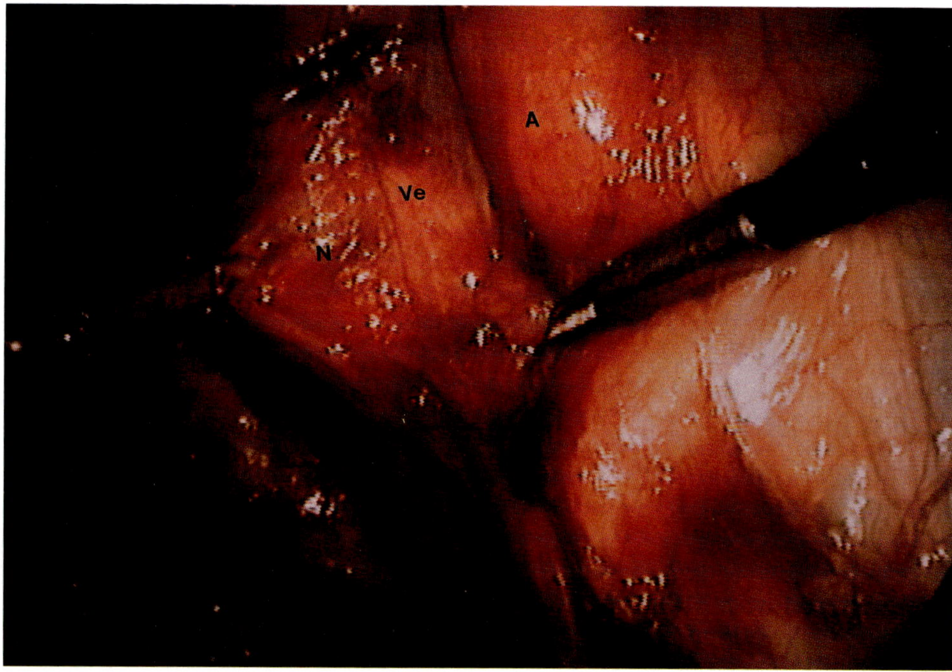

Figure 10-6 The obdurator nodal packet is grasped at the level of the pubic rami and placed under tension: N, nodal packet; Ve, external iliac vein; A, external iliac artery.

artery laterally, and the umbilical ligament medially. The dissection commences distally at the pubic rami and proceeds proximally toward the juncture of the hypogastric and external iliac arteries (Fig. 10-6). Care is taken to remain lateral to the umbilical ligament in order to avoid a potential bladder injury. All the areolar node-bearing tissue within this zone is carefully dissected with a combination of blunt and sharp maneuvers (Fig. 10-7). The obturator fossa is skeletonized of all lymphatic tissue, allowing clear visualization of the obturator nerve and vessels following excision of the nodal packet (Fig. 10-8). A similar dissection is carried out on the contralateral side, followed by removal of the specimens via the corresponding 11-mm trocar. The use of a lap sack to facilitate removal of the dissected tissue has been reported,[38] but we have not found this time-consuming added step necessary. Once the dissections are completed the areas are irrigated and examined for hemostasis.

Extended Dissection

Some surgeons advocate a more extensive dissection including the external as well as the common iliac arteries, particularly on the right.[39,40] The necessity and rationale for such a dissection awaits the results of further studies. We are partisans of a bilateral extended dissection when a patient is thought to be at high risk for nodal metastasis and the obturator and hypogastric frozen sections are reported negative. Nonetheless, preliminary evidence suggests that morbidity is significantly increased by extended dissections, particularly when performed in conjunction with a radical retropubic prostatectomy.

Complications

Reports of the morbidity of large series of LPLNDs have appeared. Lang and colleagues assessed the intraoperative and early postoperative complications in their first 50 patients and found a 14 percent occurrence, significantly different from the 4 percent occurence in their second 50 patients.[41] In a multicenter study Kavoussi and colleagues reported a 15 percent complication rate in 372 patients.[42] In another multicenter experience Kozminski and colleagues had a 21 percent rate of major (10.5%) and minor (10.5%) complications in 105 cases with a 2.6 percent laparotomy rate.[43] In our initial series of 96 patients we experienced a major and minor complication rate of 9.3 percent and 7.3 percent respectively, for a total complication rate of 16.6 percent.[44] Intraoperative morbidity encountered has ranged from bladder perforation requiring prolonged catheter drainage to ureteral and vascular injuries prompting immediate celioto

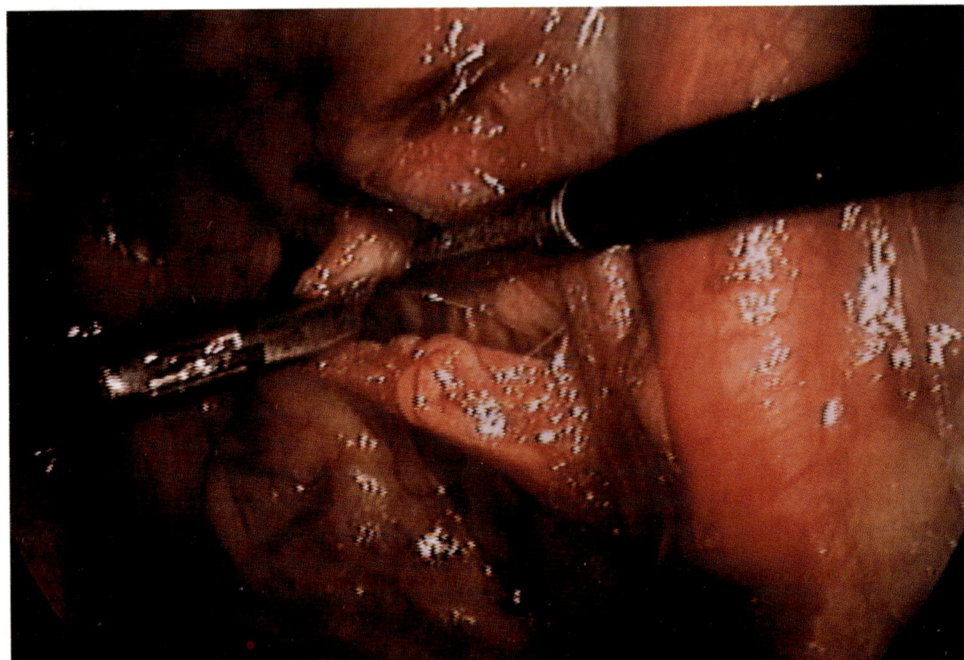

(a)

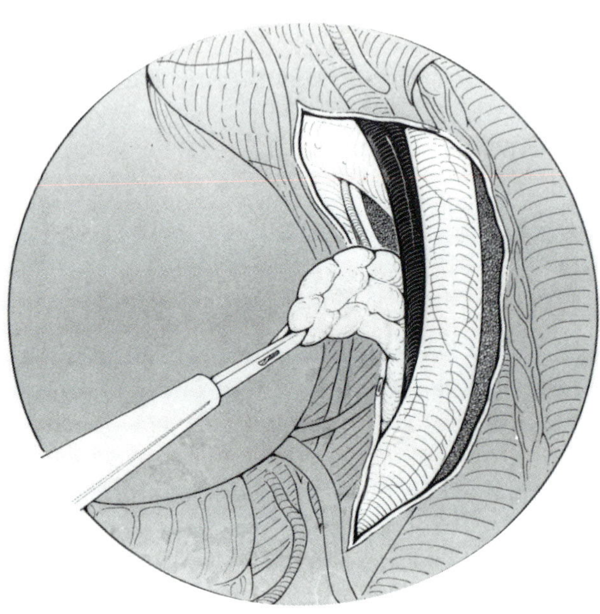

(b)

Figure 10-7 (a & b) Demonstration of distal to proximal dissection of obdurator lymph nodes.

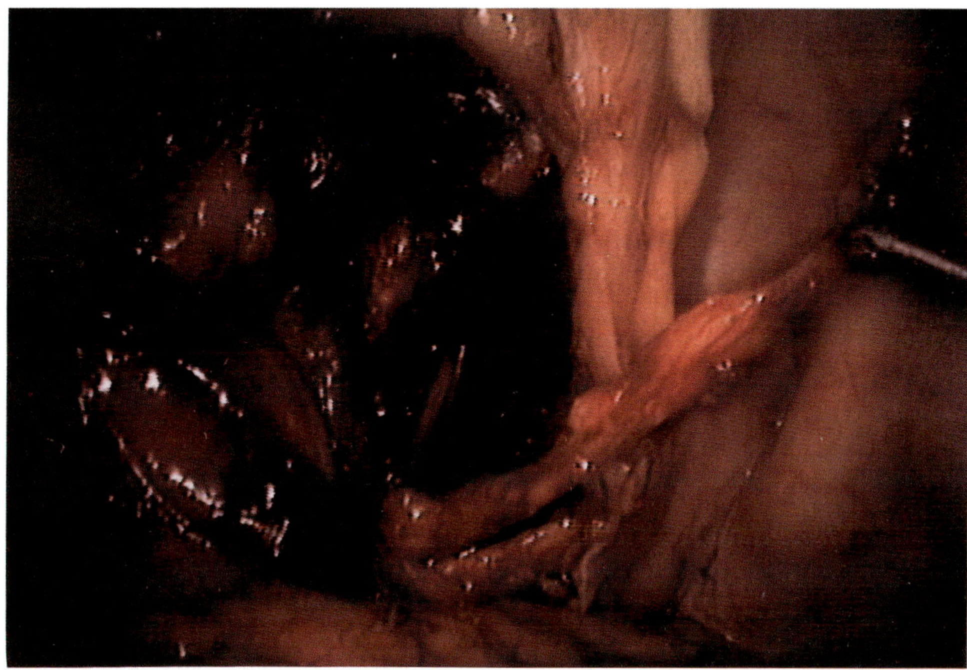
(c)

Figure 10-7 (c) Removal of the nodal packet.

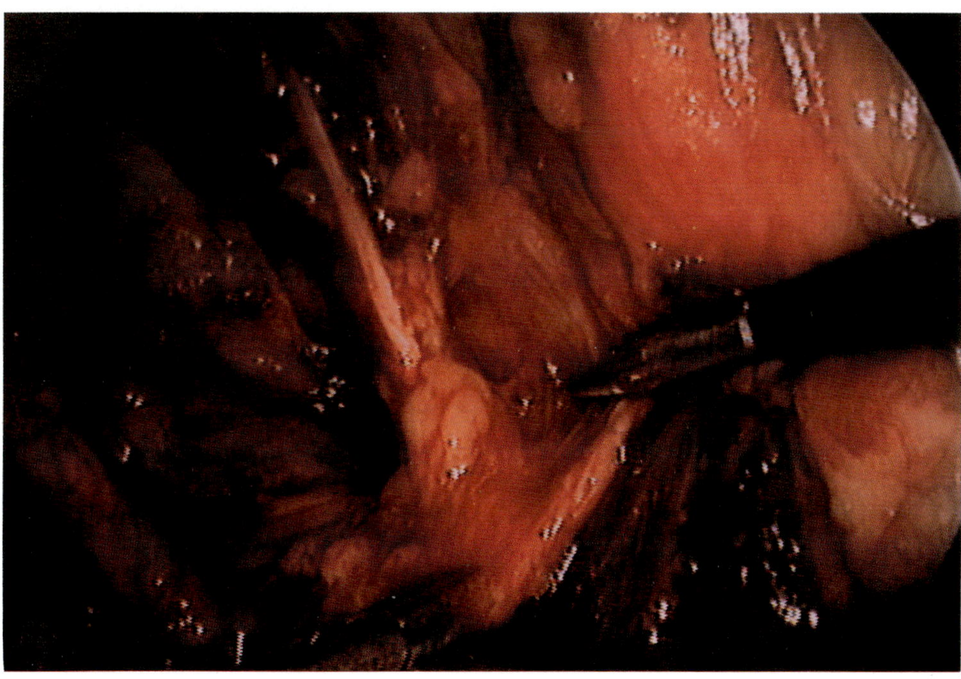
(d)

Figure 10-7 (d) Lymph tissue at the level of the iliac bifurcation.

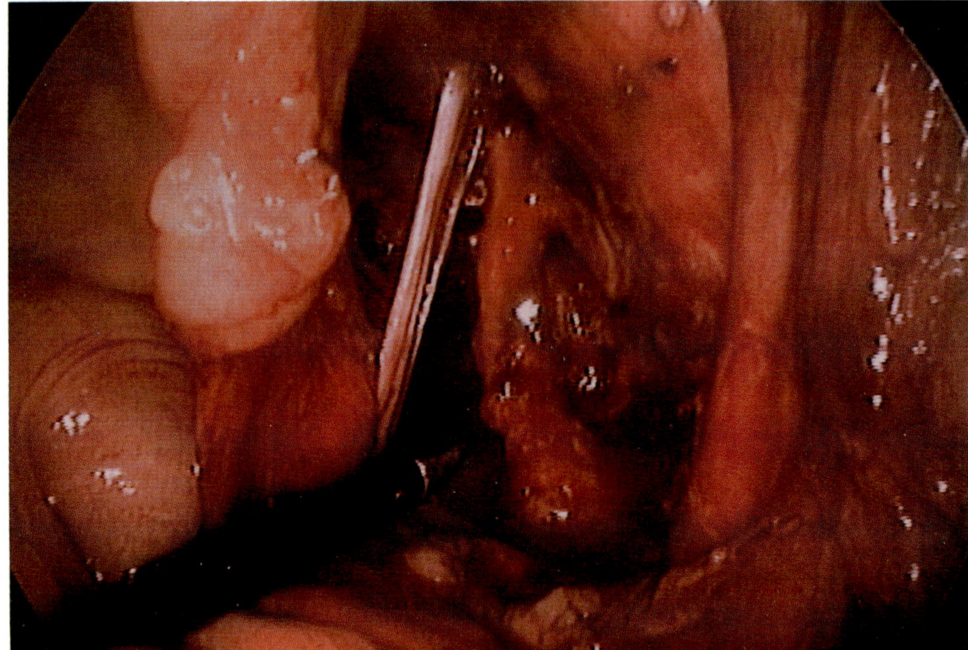

(e)

Figure 10-7 (e) Removal of remaining lymph tissue at the iliac bifurcation is facilitated by medial retraction of the obdurator nerve.

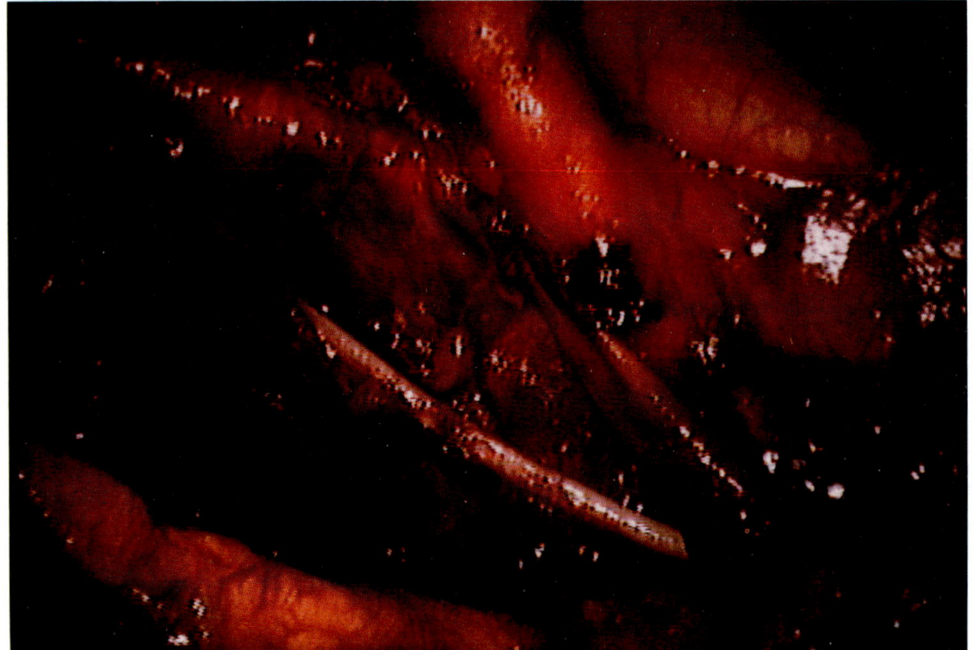

(a)

Figure 10-8 (a) Completed obdurator lymph node dissection.

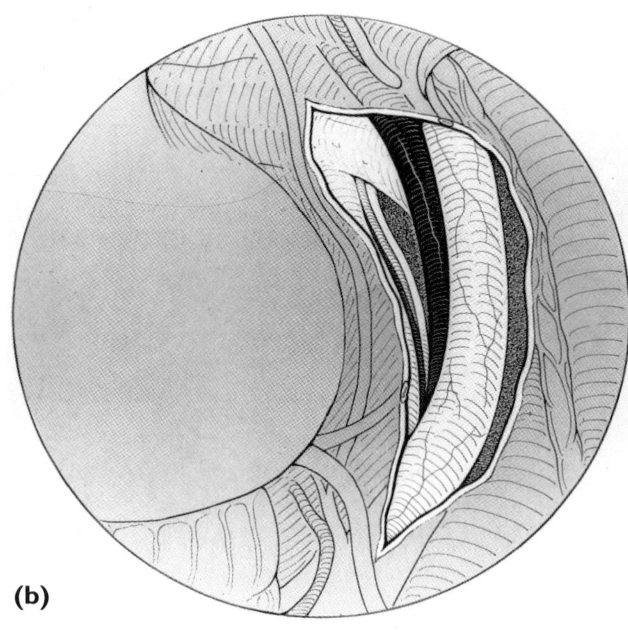

(b)

Figure 10-8 (b) Completed obdurator lymph node dissection.

my. Reported postoperative morbidity has included urinary retention, deep vein thrombosis, pelvic lymphoceles, and abscess formation. The combined complication rate of the above studies is approximately 16 percent which compares favorably with the rate reported by McDowell and colleagues for open dissection.[39]

It is universally accepted that this technique has a steep learning curve. It is generally agreed, however, that operative time and complications decrease with experience.

References

1. Querleu D, LeBlanc E, Castelain B: Laparoscopic pelvic lymphadenectomy in the staging of early carcinoma of the cervix. *Am J Obstet Gynecol* 164:579, 1991.
2. Schuessler WW, Vancaillie TG, Reich H. Griffith DP: Transperitoneal endosurgical lymphadenectomy in patients with localized prostate cancer. *J Urol* 145:988, 1991.
3. Parra RO, Andrus CH, Boullier JA: Staging laparoscopic pelvic lymph node dissection: Comparison of results with open pelvic lymphadenectomy. *J Urol* 147:875, 1992.
4. Rioja Sanz C, Blas-Marin M, Rioda Sanz L: Laparoscopic pelvic lymphadenectomy in the staging of prostate cancer. *Eur Urol* 24 S2:19, 1993.
5. Madsen MR, Holm-Nielsen A: Laparoscopic lymphadenectomy. Preliminary experience. *Scand J Urol Nephrol* 27:215, 1993.
6. Lang GS, Ruckle HC, Hadley HR, Lui PD, Stewart SC: One hundred consecutive laparoscopic pelvic lymph node dissections: Comparing complications of the first 50 cases to the second 50 cases. *Urology* 44:221,1994.
7. Prasad DR, Parr NJ, Fowler JW: Laparoscopic pelvic lymphadenectomy—Early results. *Br J Urol* 73:271, 1994.
8. Doublet JD, Gattegno B, Thibault P: Laparoscopic pelvic lymph node dissection for staging of prostatic cancer. *Eur Urol* 25:194, 1994.
9. Rukstalis DB, Gerber GS, Vogeizang NJ, Haraf DJ, Straus FH, Chodak GW: Laparoscopic pelvic lymph node dissection: A review of 103 consecutive cases. *J Urol* 151:670, 1994.
10. Guazzoni G. Montorsi F. Bergamaschi F. et al: Open surgical revision of laparoscopic pelvic lymphadenectomy. *J Urol* 151:930, 1994.
11. Kerbl K, Clayman RV, Petros JA, Chandhoke PS, Gill IS: Staging pelvic lymphadenectomy for prostate cancer: A comparison of laparoscopic and open techniques. *J Urol* 150:396, 1993.
12. Toxel S. Winfield HN: Comparative financial analysis of laparoscopic versus open pelvic lymph node dissection for men with cancer of the prostate. *J Urol* 151:675, 1994.

13. Melman A, Gladshteyn M, Stifelman M: Celioscopic lymphatic excision and radical perineal prostatectomy: A strategy for the treatment of prostatic cancer. *Prog Urol* 3:197, 1993.

14. Levy DA, Resnick Ml: Laparoscopic pelvic lymphadenectomy and radical perineal prostatectomy: A viable alternative to radical retropubic prostatectomy. *J Urol* 151:905, 1994.

15. Lerner SE, Fleischmann J. Taub HC, Chamberlin JW, Kahan NZ, Melman A: Combined laparoscopic pelvic lymph node dissection and modified belt radical perineal prostatectomy for localized prostatic adenocarcinoma. *Urology* 43:493, 1994.

16. Parra R0, Boullier JA, Rauscher JA, Cummings JM: The value of laparoscopic lymphadenectomy in conjunction with radical perineal or retropubic prostatectomy. *J Urol* 151:1599, 1994.

17. Danella JF, DeKernion JB, Smith RB, Steckel J: The contemporary incidence of lymph node metastasis in prostate cancer: Implication for laparoscopic lymph node dissection. *J Urol* 149:1488, 1993.

18. Morgan CL, Calkins RF, Cayalcanti EJ: Computed tomography in the evaluation, staging and therapy of carcinoma of the bladder and prostate. *Radiology* 140:751, 1981.

19. Biondetti PR, Lee JK, Ling D, et al: Clinical stage B prostatic carcinoma: Staging with MR imaging. *Radiology* 162:325, 1987.

20. Hricak H. Dooms GC, Jeffrey RB, et al: Prostatic carcinoma: Staging by clinical assessment, CT, and MR imaging. *Radiology* 162:331, 1987.

21. Partin AW, Carter HB, Chand DW, et al: Prostate specific antigen in the staging of localized prostate cancer: Influence of tumor differentiation, tumor volume and benign hyperplasia. *J Urol* 143:747, 1990.

22. Osterling JE: Prostate specific antigen: A critical assessment of the most useful tumor marker for adenocarcinoma of the prostate. *J Urol* 145:9007, 1991.

23. Flanigan RC, Mohler JL, King CT, et al: Preoperative lymph node evaluation in prostatic cancer patients who are surgical candidates: The role of lymphangiography and computerized tomography scanning with directed fine needle aspiration. *J Urol* 134:84, 1985.

24. Donohue RE, Mani JH, Whitesel JA, et al: Intraoperative and early complications of staging pelvic lymph node dissection in prostatic adenocarcinoma. *Urology* 35:223, 1990.

25. Gleason DF, Mellinger GT, The Veterans Administration Cooperative Urological Research Group: Prediction of prognosis for prostatic adenocarcinoma by combined histological grading and clinical staging. *J Urol* 111:58, 1974.

26. Kramer SA, Spahr J. Brendler CB, et al: Experience with Gleason histopathologic grading in prostatic cancer. *J Urol* 124:223, 1980.

27. Paulson DF, Uro-Oncology Research Group: Predictors of lymphatic spread in prostatic adenocarcinoma. *J Urol* 123:697, 1980.

28. Osterling JE, Brendler CB, Epstein Jl, et al: Correlation of clinical stage, serum prostatic acid phosphatase and preoperative Gleason grade with final pathological stage in 275 patients with clinically localized adenocarcinoma of the prostate. *J Urol* 138:92, 1987.

29. Catalona WJ, Smith DS, Ratliff TL, et al: Measurement of prostate-specific antigen in serum as a screening test for prostate cancer. *N Engl J Med* 324:1156, 1991.

30. Hudson MA, Bahnson RR, Catalona WJ: Clinical use of prostate-specific antigen in patients with prostate cancer. *J Urol* 142:1011,1989

31. Lange PH, Ercole CJ, Lightner S, et al: The value of serum prostate specific antigen determination before and after radical prostatectomy. *J Urol* 141:873, 1989.

32. Lange PH: Prostate-specific antigen for staging prior to surgery and for early detection of recurrence after surgery. *Urol Clin North Am* 17:813, 1990.

33. Parra RO, Andrus CH, Boullier JA: Staging laparoscopic pelvic lymph node dissection. Experience and indications. *Arch Surg* 127:1294, 1992.

34. Wolf JS Jr, Shinohara K, Kerlikowske KM, Narayan P. Stoller ML, Carroll PR: Selection of patients for laparoscopic pelvic lymphadenectomy prior to radical prostatectomy: A decision analysis. *Urology* 42:680, 1993.

35. Mitchell MB, Stiegmann V, Mansour A: Improved technique for establishing pneumoperitoneum for laparoscopy. *Surg Laparosc Endosc* 1:198, 1991.

36. Tobin MS, Kavoussi LR: Current role of laparoscopy in the management of prostate cancer. *Advances in Urology* 7:33, 1994.

37. See WA, Cohen MB, Winfiel HN: Inverted V peritoneotomy significantly improves nodal yield in laparoscopic pelvic lymphadenectomy. *J Urol* 149:772, 1993.

38. Kavoussi LR, Clayman RV: Organ entrapment system for removing nodal tissue during laparoscopic pelvic lymphadenectomy. *J Urol* 147:879, 1992.

39. McDowell GC, Johnson JW, Tenney DM, Johnson DE: Pelvic Iymphadenectomy for staging clinically localized prostate cancer. *Urology* 25:476, 1990.

40. Schuessler WW, Pharand D, Vancaille TG: Laparoscopic standard pelvic node dissection for carcinoma of the prostate: Is it accurate? *J Urol* 150:898, 1993.

41. Lang LS, Ruckle HC, Hadley HR, Lui PD, Stewart SC: One hundred consecutive laparoscopic pelvic lymph node dissections: Comparing complications of the first 50 cases to the second 50 cases. *Urology* 44:221, 1994.

42. Kavoussi LR, Sosa E, Chandhoke PJ, et al: Complications of laparoscopic pelvic lymph node dissection. *J Urol* 149:322, 1993.

43. Kozminski M, Comella L, Stone NN, et al: Laparoscopoic urologic surgery, outcome assessment. *J Urol* 147:245A, 1992.

44. Parra RO, Hagood PG, Boullier JA, Cummings JM, and Mehan DJ: Complications of laparoscopic urologic surgery: Experience at St. Louis University. *J Urol* 151:681, 1994.

11

Laparoscopic Anti-Incontinence Surgery

Michael E. Moran
Sidney Radomski

Introduction

The correction of urinary incontinence is replete with a plethora of surgical approaches but no one operation has proven capable of successfully re-establishing continence in all patients.

Accepted procedures for stress incontinence due to hypermobility can be classified as transabdominal, transvaginal, or a combination of both. Although popular in the past, Kelly plication and anterior colporrhaphy have very poor long-term success rates and are not recommended as the sole procedure to treat stress incontinence.[1,2] In 1949, Marshall-Marchetti and Krantz reported on a transabdominal suspension approach in which sutures were placed through periurethral and vaginal wall tissues at the bladder neck and then through the periosteum of the symphysis pubis.[3] The sutures were then tied, and this resulted in elevation of the bladder neck. In 1961, Burch described a similar transabdominal procedure in which sutures were placed through the vaginal wall at the bladder neck and through Cooper's ligament along the pubic bone.[4] Several modifications have occurred since then.

Multiple needle suspension techniques via the transvaginal approach exist. The Stamey, Raz, Pereyra, and Gittes procedures are perhaps the best known.[5–7] All of these methods involve placing sutures into the "periurethral" tissues around the bladder neck through the vagina and then transferring the ends retropubically with a long needle and tying it over the rectus fascia to elevate the bladder neck and urethra.

Since long-term follow-up in the reported literature is sparse, concerns that the efficacy of these procedures diminishes with time have been raised.[8] Randomized studies comparing different types of surgery are few, and it remains unclear which technique produces the best lasting results. The Marshall-Marchetti-Krantz has a success rate between 57 percent and 98 percent,[9–15] and that quoted for the Burch procedure is between 63 percent and 100 percent.[12,16–25] The needle suspension procedures have a success rate between 65 percent and 94 percent.[5,7,14–20,24,26,27]

Stress incontinence due to a "drain pipe" urethra is best treated with either a sling procedure or an artificial sphincter and consequently will not be discussed further in this chapter.[28–30]

The question remains whether laparoscopic approaches to antiincontinence surgery offer any advantage to this current surgical list. The available series for review are small, and follow-up remains short. Practical comparison to the many open operative techniques is not yet possible. Inherently, any new operative approach should have potential advantages over the standard treatments. Therefore, laparoscopic anti-incontinence procedures must be scrutinized carefully prior to acceptance.

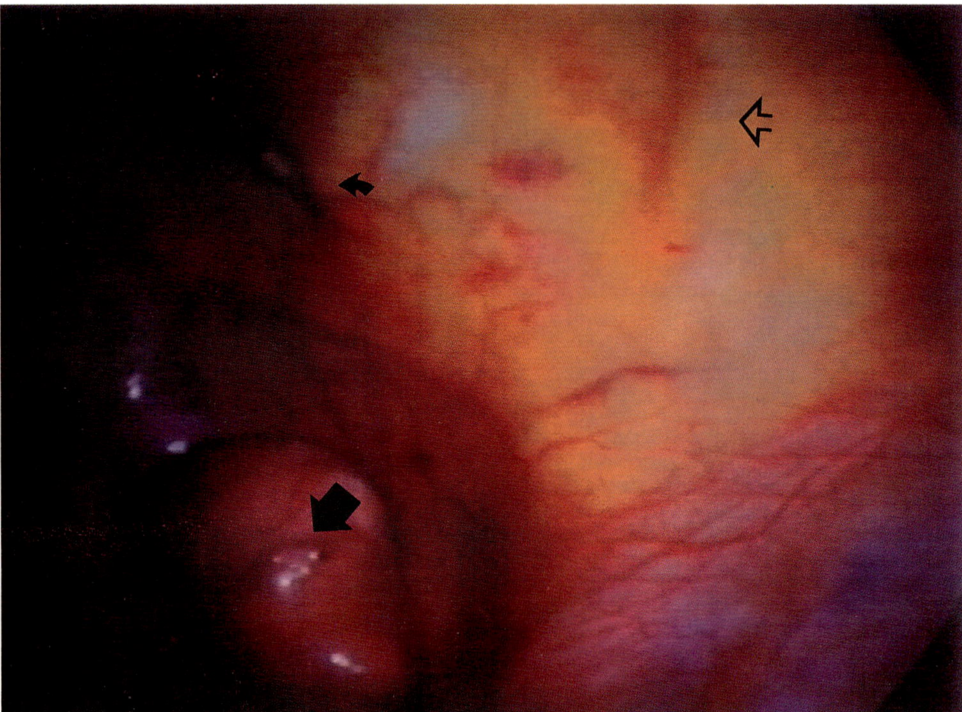

Figure 11-1 Anatomical landmarks in a human female. The view is from a 30 degree scope angled from the patient's right via the umbilical portal. A large uterine fibroid is apparent dorsally (*arrow*); the urachus (within the median umbilical fold, *open arrow*) and the left medial umbilical fold (obliterated umbilical artery, *curved arrow*) are readily identified.

Indications and Contraindications

Indications and contraindications are the same for laparoscopic anti-incontinence surgery as they are for their open counterparts. Coagulation disorders, recent myocardial infarctions, and active urinary tract infections must be recognized and treated appropriately prior to performing this type of surgery. Previous abdominal or pelvic surgery has been a relative contraindication for laparoscopic surgery. However, open techniques for access and retroperitoneal approaches can make these challenging cases possible.

Applied Anatomy

Transperitoneal Approach to the Space of Retzius

Once successful entry has been accomplished and the abdomen has been inspected systematically to exclude inadvertent access injury, landmarks are identified for the surgeon's orientation. Both males and females have readily discernable median umbilical folds with variable amounts of loose fatty areolar tissues. These folds contain the urachus and variable numbers and sizes of veins, especially close to the umbilicus. The medial umbilical folds are lateral and represent the peritoneum covering the medial umbilical ligaments (the obliterated fetal umbilical arteries) (Fig. 11-1). The vessels within these ligaments, though vestigial, can certainly bleed if not carefully addressed. Paired lateral umbilical folds covering the origin of the inferior epigastric arteries can also be appreciated in some individuals. Bladder and bladder neck surgery require access to the retropubic space of Retzius through this fold. Once into the retropubic space, the anatomy is similar to that described below.

Pre-peritoneal Approach to the Space of Retzius

There are no standardized methods of developing a dissection plane in the retropubic space. Several techniques have been described. A small suprapubic incision has allowed blunt finger dissection in this space prior to placement of a Hasson trocar and pneumoinsufflation. Another technique requires the placement of a Veress needle via a small infraumbilical incision directly into this space with insufflation, followed by placement of a large trocar and an operating laparoscope for visualized development of this potential space (Fig. 11-2). Others have described the placement of a low-pressure balloon system to less traumatically develop an insufflant cavity. The major advantages to this approach include elimination of the risk of injuring abdominal viscera other than the bladder and avoidance of transperitoneal dissection, thereby minimizing the potential for adhesion formation. Disadvantages

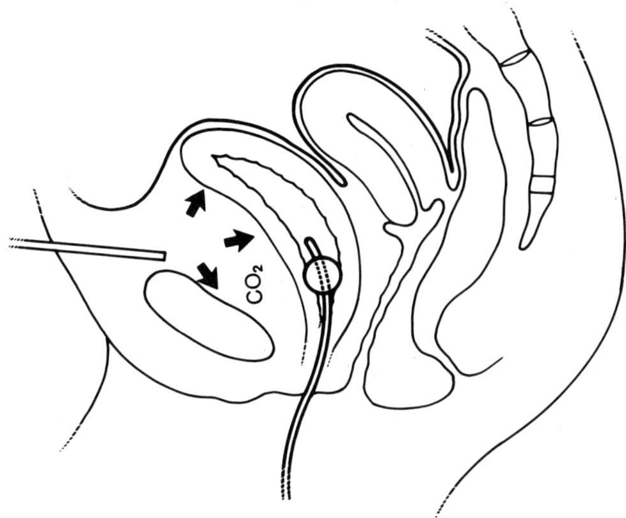

Figure 11-2 Preperitoneal insufflation technique of Chapple (Photo courtesy of Dr. Chapple).

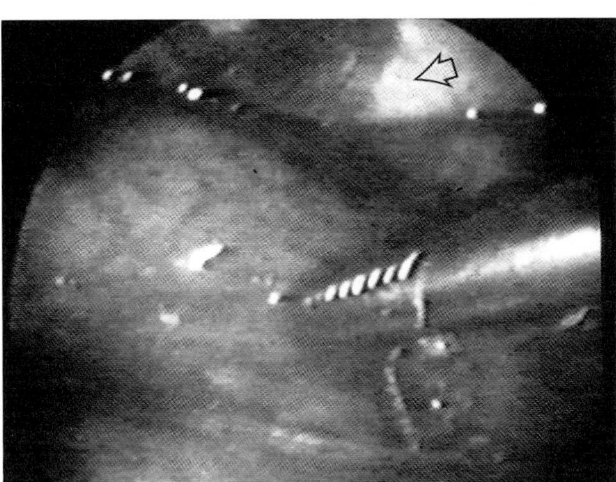

Figure 11-3 Preperitoneal laparoscopic view. Pubic symphysis is above (*arrow*) and the urethrovesical junction is being pointed to by the dissector.

include the possibility for increased hypercarbia (theoretical) and the risk of inadvertent injury to the inferior epigastric vessels or bladder during the development of the insufflant cavity. Anatomical landmarks are the pubic symphysis in the caudad midline and the inferior epigastric vessels laterally (Fig. 11-3).

Anatomic Approach to Laparoscopic Bladder Neck Surgery

To begin with, it is important to stress the laparoscopic impression of the depth of dissection required to reach the vesical neck and pelvic floor (Fig. 11-4). The magnified image creates the illusion of some distance when, in fact, it is mere centimeters from the start of the dissection (Fig. 11-4b). Bladder dissection should be avoided until the correct landmarks have been identified and the retropubic plane has been started. More than one series recommends inflating the bladder partially at this point to identify the anterior wall (Fig. 11-4c). A finger placed within the vagina also helps identify the pelvic floor (Fig. 11-4c and d). In some instances, pelvic floor musculature is thin but should be identified with motion of the assisting finger. Inferiorly, the urethra becomes adherent to the inferior ramus of the symphysis. In most instances the actual distance to the external meatus at this point is less than 1 cm. Lateral dissection from the bladder neck is necessary to identify Cooper's ligament. Cooper's ligament is the lateral deep pectineal portion of the inguinal ligament that curves around the pelvic tubercle. These ligamentous fibers originate from the lower margins of the external oblique, which rolls back onto itself. The internal oblique and the transversus derive some of their origin from the lateral portions of this ligament. Cooper's ligament medially may give rise to fibers reflected up to the linea alba, and the external oblique may insert here.

Although not essential for most bladder work, the lateral obturator fossa's anatomy has crucial elements of concern to the laparoscopic surgeon. The course of the obturator nerve and its trajectory through the obturator fossa prior to exiting the foramen may have consequences. Bilateral obturator injuries have been reported from dorsal lithotomy positioning by stretching this nerve across bone at the exit site of the obturator foramen. (Fig. 11-5).[31]

More important are the vessels accompanying the obturator nerve or lying within the obturator fossa. Major hemorrhage can result from the inadvertent division of these vessels during dissection or placement of ligatures. Specific risk areas have been described. There are occasional anastomotic branches between the epigastric and obturator arteries that run close to Cooper's ligament. Anomalous venous branching to the external iliac vein is likewise common. These branches tend to be located at the lateral portion of Cooper's ligament and can be encountered during the Burch procedure, especially if the needle traverses the ligament with an upward-outward trajectory. An accessory obturator vein can also wind its way from medial to lateral across the obturator nerve close to the endopelvic fascia, lateral to Cooper's ligament.

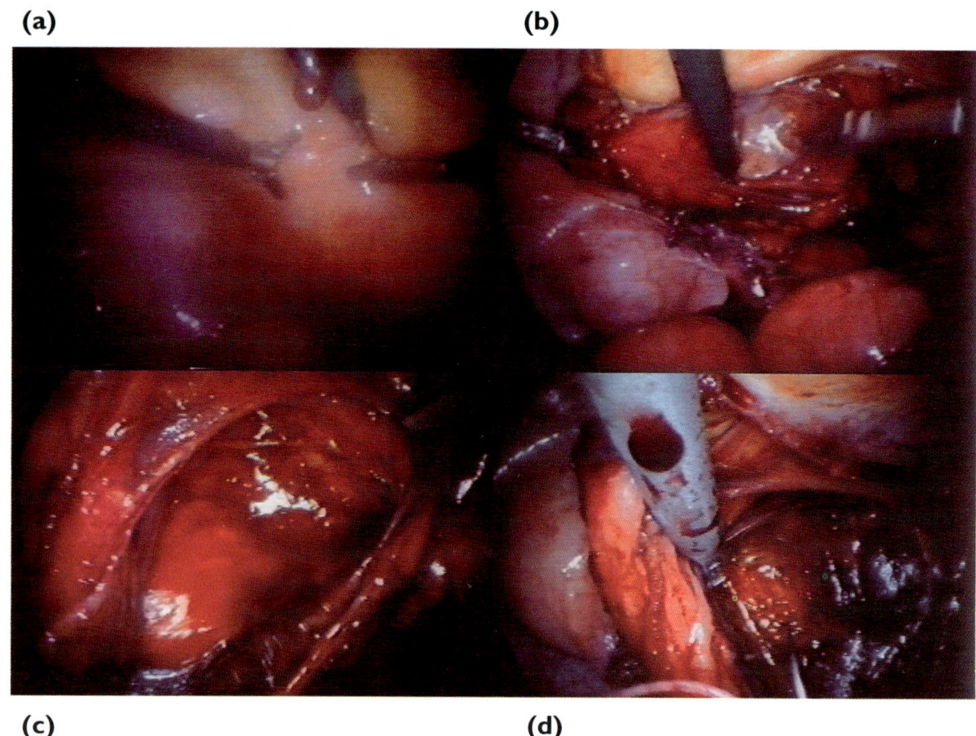

Figure 11-4 Transabdominal approach for retropubic bladder neck suspension. (a) Right sided approach shown, urachus to the left and medial umbilical fold in the right grasper. (b) Opening of the space of Retzius, dissection is deeper than expected. (c) Bladder slightly insufflated with 250 mL of sterile water and finger is pushing up on the vaginal wall. (d) Suture is passed intra-abdominally while finger distracts the vaginal wall ventrally.

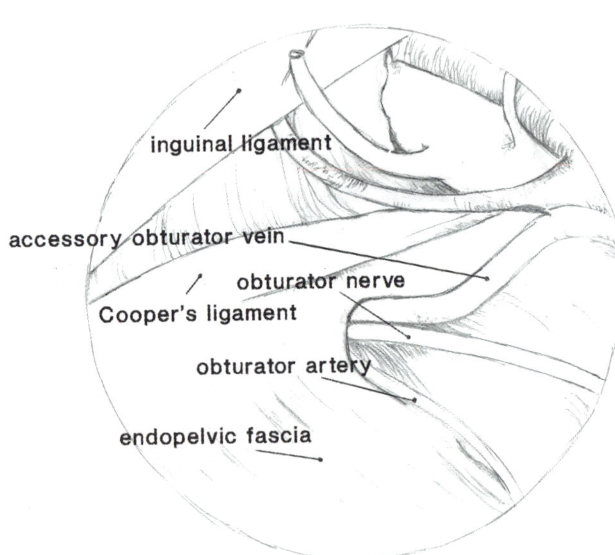

Figure 11-5 Cooper's ligament in laparoscopic perspective to the obturator fossa.

Transperitoneal Technique

Early clinical and laboratory work for laparoscopic anti-incontinence surgery utilized the transperitoneal approach. To date, laparoscopic Marshall-Marchetti-Krantz procedures,[32,33] Burch colposuspension,[34] needle colposuspensions,[35] and pubobladder neck slings[36,37] have all been described. In addition, laparoscopic electroneuromodulation devices have been successfully implanted.[38]

In all reported series, the patients are placed supine with partial or low lithotomy positioning. The arms are routinely tucked bilaterally to allow maximal lateral table mobility for the surgeon and the assistant (Fig. 11-6). The abdomen and the vagina are prepped because placement of a finger along the anterior vaginal surface is crucial during dissection and suspension techniques. The patient is placed in the Trendelenburg position. Access is accomplished by the creation of a pneumoperitoneum via the techniques described in Chap. 5. Insufflation is carried to 14 to 15 mm Hg routinely, although less pressure can be utilized. A 10-mm portal is then positioned via the access incision for the visual placement of the remaining working ports. Schuessler and co-workers employ three ancillary portals to perform the laparoscopic Marshall-Marchetti-Krantz (LMMK) procedure: a 10-mm trocar above the symphysis pubis, and two lateral 5-mm trocars halfway between the anterior superior iliac spines and rectus abdominus muscles. Another consideration should be the placement of 10-mm lateral ports if large curved needles are to be used or if larger instruments need to be introduced (Fig. 11-7a). Once the laparoscopic portal is positioned, a thor-

Figure 11-6 Patient positioning; key is dorsal lithotomy position with arms tucked to patient's side. Access and surgery is facilitated by slight Trendelenburg positioning.

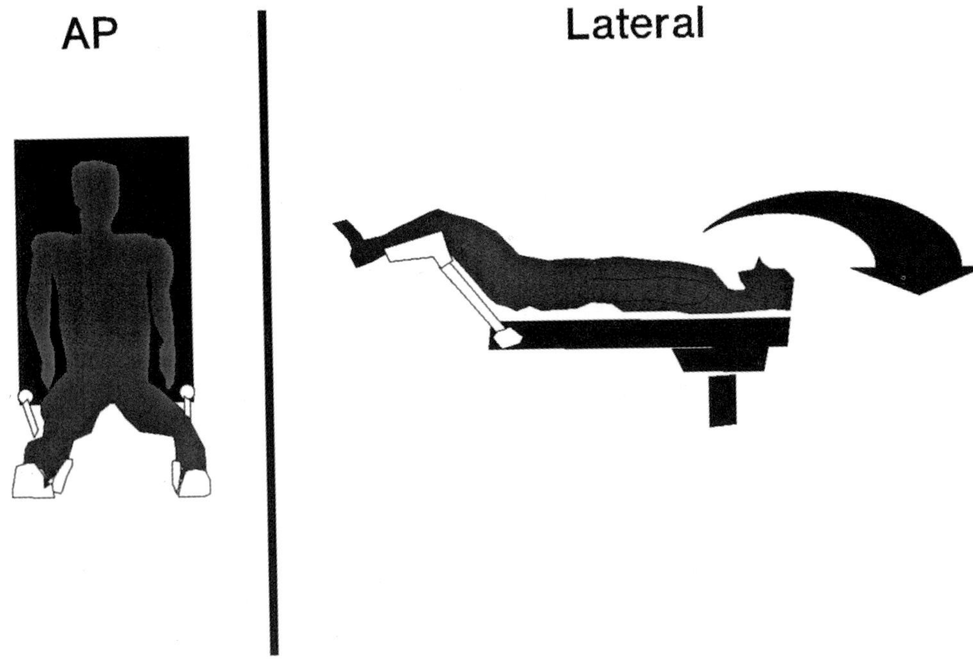

(a)

Laparoscopic Anti-incontinence Surgery
Trocar Placement
primary portal size 10-11 mm.
secondary ports size 5 mm.

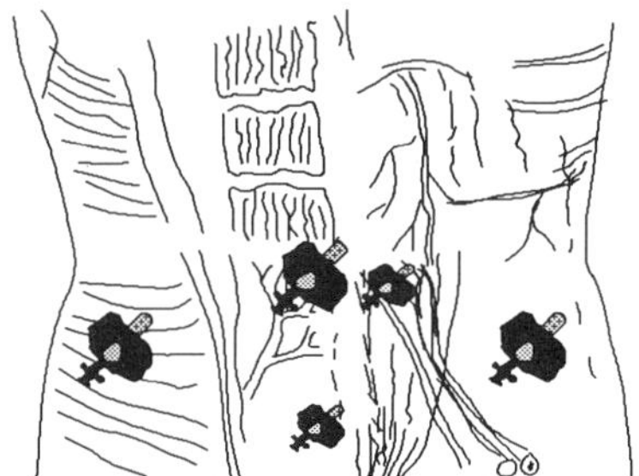

(b)

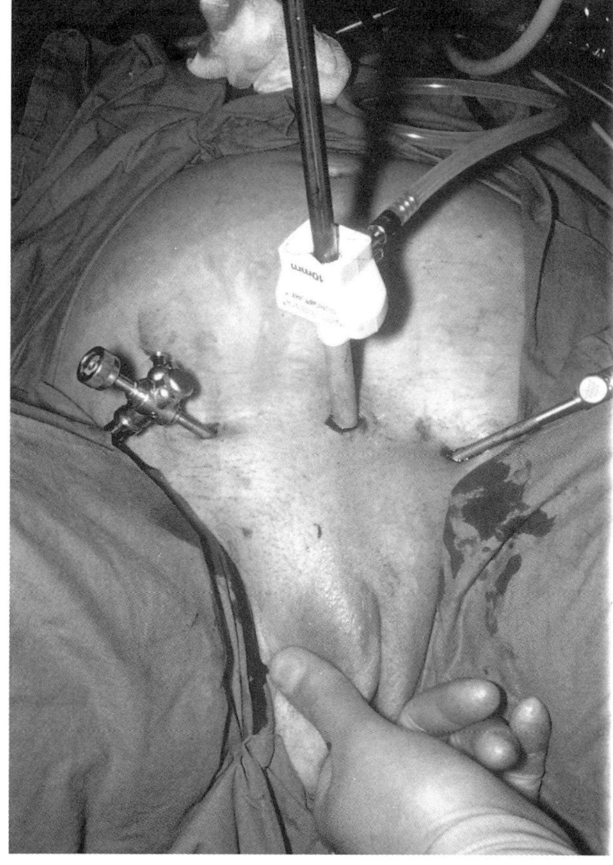

Figure 11-7 (a) Location and positioning of trocars for transperitoneal bladder neck suspensions. (b) Location of trocars for laparoscopic needle suspension technique of Chapple (Photo courtesy of Dr. Chapple).

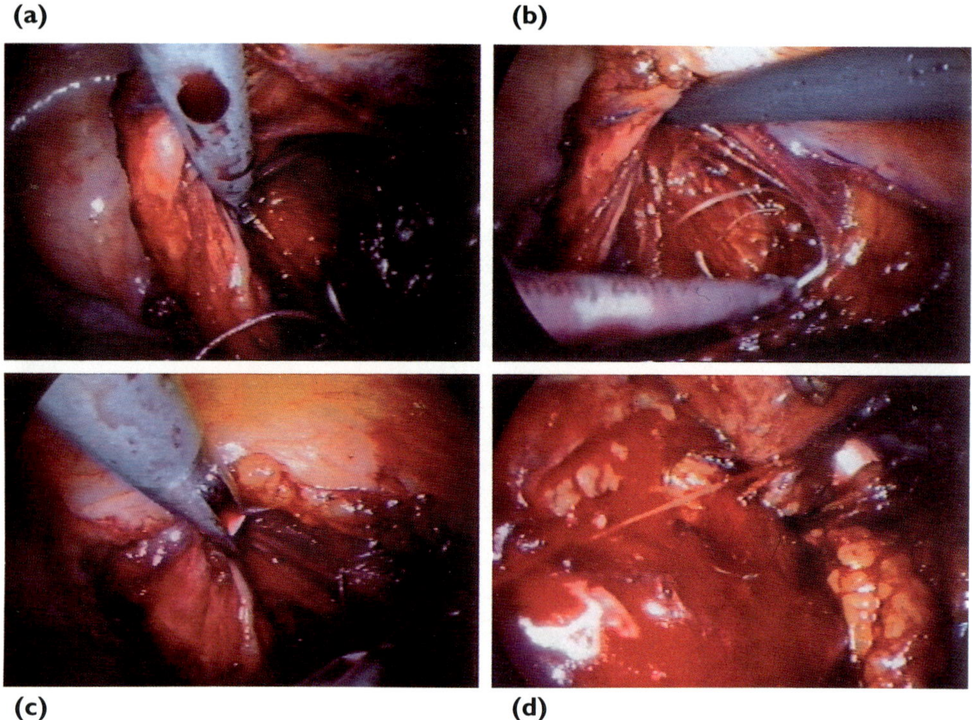

Figure 11-8 Intracorporeal sutured Burch bladder neck suspension. (a) Bladder neck identified by downward displacement of Foley catheter. (b) Whip-stitch placed through ventrally displaced vaginal tissues. (c) Cooper's ligament identified and needle shown prior to driving through the medial aspect of this ligament. (d) Completion of the bladder neck suspension by intracorporeal tying of the stitch.

ough inspection of the abdominal viscera is made and all trocars and underlying bowel are inspected for integrity. The prevesical space of Retzius is then opened with electrocautery scissors. At this point it is important to mention that the bladder can be inadvertently injured. Harewood points out that this is best avoided by insufflating the bladder with 250 mL of sterile water (or saline) prior to further dissection,[35] although this can be difficult in incontinent patients with the pneumoperitoneum above 10 mm Hg.

The San Antonio group begins the dissection in the midline with a blunt grasper holding the bladder down and away from the plane of dissection.[33] The pubic symphysis is identified, and the posterior arch is dissected. Meticulous hemostasis is necessary in order to identify the bladder and bladder neck for subsequent suspension. The Melbourne group places two 5-mm working trocars laterally after the laparoscopic portal is positioned for the needle colposuspension. Two incisions are made into the retropubic space, each at the medial umbilical folds extending toward the midline and the urachus. Dissection is then carried down to the symphysis. In either instance, dissection and identification can be facilitated by the placement of a finger into the vagina and lifting upward.

Radomski and his group begin the dissection just medial to the medial umbilical fold and just above the lateral aspect of the bladder neck. They then carry the dissection down to Cooper's ligament for a Burch colposuspension.[34] By approaching Cooper's ligaments laterally, the dissection may then proceed directly onto the bladder neck and vaginal wall below the symphysis pubis. Cooper's ligament is carefully dissected, and the same procedure is carried out on the contralateral side. The intracorporeal suspension utilizes the Szabo-Berci suturing set (Karl Storz, Culver City, CA) and a no. 1 Vicryl on a J-shaped curved needle (Fig. 11-8a). Suture length is kept to the minimum to facilitate throwing of the intracorporeal knots, 8 to 10 cm. The suture is placed through the elevated vaginal wall (Fig. 11-8a) and a second, whip-stitch suture is placed (Fig. 11-8b) prior to suturing to Cooper's ligament above the bladder neck (Fig. 11-8c and d). The knot is tied intracorporeally and cinched to approximate the vagina to Cooper's ligament (Fig. 11-8d).[39] Three or more simple throws are then completed. This technique is identical to that performed during open Burch colposuspension. Cystoscopy has been recommended at the conclusion of the suture placement to insure against inadvertent bladder injury.

Harewood, in addition to the three trocars makes a 5-cm transverse suprapubic incision for rectus needle suspension.[35] Laparoscopically, the urachus and periurethral tissues are left intact in order to prevent scarification. The Stamey needle is then passed

TABLE 11-1 Data from initial series on operative times, catheterization requirements, and complications

Series	Surgery Time	Catheterization Time	Hospital Stay	Complications
Schuessler 1992	65 min (35–175)	2.2 days (1–35)	1.3 days	Urinary retention = 9% 3 conversions to open (2 technical suturing, 1 bladder perforation)
Radomski 1993	120 min	2.2 days	1.6 days	Urinary retention = 0 1 conversion to open (bladder perforation)
Chapple 1992	120 min	NA	NA	Urinary retention = 0 conversion to open (not reported)
Harewood 1992	112.5 min (90–180)	1 day	4.6 days (2–12)	Urinary retention = 0 conversion to open = 0 bladder perforation = 1 prolonged ileus =1

in the manner described originally (two passes for each side), and the suture is tied through a silicon button on the anterior rectus fascia.[5] Tension on the suture is observed via the laparoscope so that during the knot tying the vaginal wall does not elevate or descend.

All methods of laparoscopic bladder neck suspensions have been associated with complications (Table 11-1), ranging from urinary retention to inadvertent bladder injuries. Open laparotomy was required in 4 of 44 patients in the initial series found in Table 11-1.

Laparoscopic Extraperitoneal Colposuspension

The extraperitoneal approach to the genitourinary organs offers distinct advantages. There is no potential risk of inadvertent visceral injury by access techniques and less need for retraction and dissection of the abdominal organs. Early experience with retroperitoneal dissection techniques were primarily limited to pelvioscopy for limited one-sided lymphatic sampling procedures.[40] More recently, full bilateral pelvic lymphadenectomies have been accomplished.[41,42] The major drawbacks of working in these potential spaces are the necessity to identify and avoid crossing vascular bundles (i.e., the inferior epigastrics) and establishing room enough to work on a given region. There have also been references to increased risks of hypercarbia from insufflating these potential spaces with carbon dioxide gas.[43]

Despite these drawbacks, laparoscopic colposuspension has been successfully performed clinically by the retroperitoneal approach.[44] A needle is positioned transcutaneously into the retropubic space and care taken not to penetrate through to the bladder. Once the potential space is accessed, insufflation with carbon dioxide proceeds and trocars are then placed. Three trocars aid the laparoscopically guided, vaginally placed, and tied sutures (Fig. 11-7b). Careful attention is paid to dissecting in the midline down to the pubic symphysis prior to any lateral dissection. Identification of the bladder neck is thus expeditiously accomplished even in patients who have had previous antiincontinence procedures.

Conclusions

Laparoscopy is a burgeoning area in the urologist's armamentarium that deserves further attention. As with all new surgical techniques, critical review is necessary before determining the exact role laparoscopy will have in our day-to-day management of urinary incontinence. The potential for minimal access performance of established open procedures cannot be questioned. Questions arise with regard to the risks inherent in the laparoscopic alternatives and whether the results are the same, better, or worse. Steep learning curves have been the rule for most operative laparoscopic procedures. For anti-incontinence surgery, few centers are beyond these initial experiences. As technology improves, it might well be expected that all types of anti-incontinence techniques could be accomplished.

References

1. Lose J, Jorgensen L, Mortenson SO, et al: Voiding difficulties after colposuspension. *Obstet Gynecol* 69:33–38, 1987.
2. Stanton SL, Cardoza LD: Results of the colposuspension operation for incontinence and prolapse. *Br J Obstet Gynecol* 86:693–697, 1979.
3. Marshall VF, Marchetti AA, Krantz KE: The correction of stress incontinence by single vesicourethral suspension. *Surg Gynecol Obstet* 88:509–512, 1949.
4. Burch JC: Cooper's ligament urethrovesical suspension for stress incontinence. *Am J Obstet Gynecol* 100:764–774, 1968.
5. Stamey TA: Endoscopic suspension of the vesical neck for urinary incontinence. *Surg Obstet Gynecol* 136:547–554, 1973.
6. Raz S: Modified bladder neck suspension for female stress incontinence. *Urology* 17:82–85, 1981.
7. Pereyra AJ, Lebherz TB: Combined urethrovesical suspension and vaginourethroplasty for correction of urinary stress incontinence. *Obstet Gynecol* 30:537–546, 1967.
8. Kelly MJ, Leach GE: Long term results of bladder neck suspension procedures. *Probl Urol* 5(1):94–105, 1991.
9. Goodno JA, Powers TW: Modified retropubic cystourethropexy. *Am J Obstet Gynecol* 154:1211–1216, 1986.
10. Mainprize TC, Drutz HP: The Marshall-Marchetti-Krantz procedure: A critical review. *Obstet Gynecol Surg* 43:724–729, 1988.
11. McDuffie RW, Listin RB, Blundon KE: Urethrovesical suspension (Marshall-Marchetti-Krantz): Experience with 204 cases. *Am J Surg* 141:297–298, 1981.
12. Milani R. Scalambrino S. Quadri G. et al: Marshall-Marchetti-Krantz procedure and Burch colposuspension in the surgical treatment of female urinary incontinence. *Br J Obstet Gynecol* 92:1050–1053, 1985.
13. Parnell JP, Marshall VF, Vaughan ED: Primary management of urinary stress incontinence by the Marshall-Marchetti-Krantz vesicourethropexy. *J Urol* 127:679–682, 1982.
14. Riggs JS: Retropubic cystourethropexy: A review of two operative procedures with long-term follow-up. *Obstet Gynecol* 68:98–105, 1986.
15. Spencer JR, O'Conor VJ, Schaeffer AJ: A comparison of endoscopic suspension of the vesical neck with suprapubic vesicourethropexy for treatment of stress urinary incontinence. *J Urol* 137:411–415, 1987.
16. Bergman A, Ballard CA, Koonings PP: Comparison of three different surgical procedures for genuine stress incontinence: Prospective randomized study. *Am J Obstet Gynecol* 160:1102–1106, 1989.
17. Bergman A, Koonings PP, Ballard CA: Primary stress urinary incontinence and pelvic relaxation: Prospective randomized comparison of three different operations. *Am J Obstet Gynecol* 161:97–101, 1989.
18. Bhatia NN, Bergman A: Modified Burch versus Pereyra retropubic urethropexy for stress urinary incontinence. *Obstet Gynecol* 66:255–261, 1985.
19. Fowler JE: Experience with suprapubic vesicourethral suspension and endoscopic suspension of the vesical neck for stress urinary incontinence in females. *Surg Gynecol Obstet* 162:437–441, 1986.
20. Green DF, McGuire EJ, Lytton B: A comparison of endoscopic suspension of the vesical neck versus anterior urethropexy for the treatment of stress urinary incontinence. *J Urol* 136:1205–1207, 1986.
21. Grant D, O'Conor VJ: Long-term results of suprapubic vesicourethropexy. *J Urol* 107:610–612, 1972.
22. Mundy AR: A trial comparing the Stamey bladder neck suspension procedure with colposuspension for the treatment of stress incontinence. *Br J Urol* 55:687–690, 1983.
23. Park S, Miller EJ: Surgical treatment of stress urinary incontinence: A comparison of the Kelly plication, Marshall-Marchetti-Krantz, and Pereyra procedures. *Obstet Gynecol* 71:575–579, 1988.
24. Pow-Sang JM, Lockhart JL, Suarez A, et al: Female urinary incontinence: Preoperative selection, surgical complications and results. *J Urol* 136:831–833, 1986.
25. Stanton SL, Cardozo LD: A comparison of vaginal and suprapubic surgery in the correction of incontinence due to urethral sphincter incompetence. *Br J Urol* 51:497–499, 1979.

26. Hilton P: A clinical and urodynamic study comparing the Stamey bladder neck suspension and suburethral sling procedures in the treatment of genuine stress incontinence. *Br J Obstet Gynecol* 96:213–220, 1989.
27. Leach GE, Raz S: Modified Pereyra bladder neck suspension after previously failed anti-incontinence surgery: Surgical technique and results with long-term follow-up. *Urology* 23:359–362, 1984.
28. Blaivas JG, Olson CA: Stress incontinence: Classification and surgical approach. *J Urol* 139:727–731, 1988.
29. McGuire EJ, Lytton B: The pubovaginal sling in stress urinary incontinence. *J Urol* 119:82–84, 1978.
30. Webster GD, Perez LM, Khoury JM, Timmons SL: Management of type III stress urinary incontinence using artificial urinary sphincter. *Urology* 39:499–503, 1992.
31. Pelligrino MJ, Johnson EW: Bilateral obturator nerve injuries during urologic surgery. *Arch Phys Med Rehabil* 69:46, 1988.
32. Vancaillie TG, Schuessler WW: Laparoscopic bladder-neck suspension. *J Laparoendosc Surg* 1:169–173, 1991.
33. Albala DM, Schuessler WW, Vancaillie TG: Laparoscopic bladder neck suspension. *J Endourol* 6:137–141, 1992.
34. Radomski SB, Herschorn S. Gleshner N. Stewart R, Adanja D: Laparoscopic Burch procedure: A porcine model. AUA Combined Northeastern and New England Section Meeting, Toronto, Canada, Abstract #34, 1992.
35. Harewood LM: Laparoscopic needle colposuspension for genuine stress incontinence. *J Endourol* 6(4):S145, 1992.
36. Moran ME, Radomski SB, Stone AR: Laparoscopic Pubo-bladder neck sling: An animal model. *Min Invas Ther* 1:46, 1991.
37. Dickson C, Boone T, Preminger GM: Laparoscopic urethral sling. *J Endourol* 6(4):S170, 1992.
38. Moran ME, Radomski SB, Roach M, Stone AR: Celioscopic neuromodulation: Porcine lumbar sympathetic model. *Min Invas Ther* 1:53, 1991.
39. Szabo Z, Bowyer DW, Moran ME: Operative laparoscopy in urology: Intracorporeal suturing of the lower urinary tract. *J Urol* 147:A782, 1992.
40. Hald T, Rasmussen F: Extraperitoneal pelvioscopy: a new aid in staging of lower urinary tract tumors. A preliminary report. *J Urol* 124:245–248, 1980.
41. Ferzli G, Trapasso J, Raboy A, Albert P: Extraperitoneal endoscopic pelvic lymph node dissection. *J Laparoendosc Surg* 2:39–44, 1992.
42. Shafik A: Extraperitoneal laparoscopic lymphadenectomy in prostatic cancer: Preliminary report of a new approach. *J Endourol* 6:113–116, 1992.
43. Sosa RE, Weingram J, Stein B, et al: Hypercarbia in laparoscopic pelvic lymph node dissection. *J Urol* 147(4):246A, 1992.
44. Chapple CR, Osborne JL: Laparoscopic colposuspension—a new procedure. *J Urol* 147(4):280A, 1992.

12

Laparoscopic Bladder Surgery

Raul O. Parra
Paul G. Hagood

Introduction

Numerous pathologies of the urinary bladder requiring surgical intervention are amenable to an endocavitary (laparoscopic) approach. Some feasible applications are listed in Table 12-1. Many of these procedures have already been described in case reports and reviews.[1–6] In general, the advances made in laparoscopic surgery have resulted in notable decreases in patient morbidity and hospital stay.[7–11]

Our experience with diverticulectomies[1] and simple cystectomies[2] has demonstrated not only the efficacy, but also the comparative advantage of the laparoscopic approach. Obviously the potential for decreased morbidity and convalescence that is attributed to these approaches is not to be underestimated. This chapter will examine the indications for and the techniques essential to performing a simple cystectomy, diverticulectomy or partial cystectomy and repair of traumatic bladder rupture. The potential for more complex extirpative bladder surgery will also be explored. Bladder neck suspension procedures are considered in Chap. 11.

TABLE 12-1 Laparoscopic Bladder Procedures

Extirpative
Laser palliation of bladder cancer
Excision of urachal cyst and fistula
Partial cystectomy
Diverticulectomy
Cystectomy (with and without urinary diversion)
Nephroureterectomy with a cuff of bladder
Laser ablation of endometriosis involving bladder or ureters
Reconstructive
Coloposuspension
Augmentation cystoplasty/autoaugmentation
Repair of intraperitoneal bladder rupture
Ureteroneocystotomy

Cystectomy

Indications

On occasion, supravesical urinary diversion with omission of a cystectomy is performed. Difficult problems such as neurogenic bladder, obstinate incontinence, surgically uncorrectable outlet obstruction, and intractable symptoms due to tuberculosis, interstitial cystitis, fistula, and radiation have all been treated by diversion without cystectomy.

The urine-deprived bladder that is left behind can be the source of malignant transformation[12–18] or other significant complications. Eigner and Freiha encountered complications directly related to the bladder in 24 of 30 patients previously diverted without bladder removal.[19] A review of our own experience and scrutiny of the literature[19–27] provided information on a total of 777 patients with cutaneous urinary diversions done for a variety of condi-

TABLE 12-2 Pyocystis in the Retained Bladder

	Pyocystis		Cystectomy	
Series	No./Total	(%)	No./Total	(%)
Retik[20]	10/86	(11)	10/86	(11)
Holland[21]	3/37	(8)	2/37	(5)
Engel[22]	22/102	(21)	22/102	(21)
Schmidt[23]	25/130	(19)	9/76	(6)
Guerrier[24]	24/128	(18)	24/128	(18)
Stewart[25]	23/76	(30)	9/76	(11)
Richie[26]	2/32	(6)	2/32	(6)
Stevens[27]	27/113	(24)	11/113	(9)
Eigner[19]	20/30	(67)	4/30	(13)
Parra[2]	9/44	(20)	7/44	(15)
TOTAL	**164/777**	**(21)**	**99/777**	**(12)**

tions. Pyocystis developed in 164 of the 777 patients (21.1 %). Ninety-nine (12.7%) required removal of the bladder (Table 12-2). However, cystectomy is a major operation associated with significant morbidity and prolonged convalescence. Giving consideration to decreasing the morbidity is a legitimate concern, especially in this group of patients already familiar with major surgery.

Possible contraindications to this procedure besides those for general laparoscopy[28] are previous pelvic radiation and the presence of an ongoing bladder or upper tract infection. Relative contraindications include a history of peritonitis, extensive adhesions, a history of bowel obstruction, dilated loops of bowel, and large vascular aneurysms.

Preoperative Evaluation

At a minimum, the patient should have a cystogram performed. Paraplegic patients should be questioned as to the possibility of autonomic dysreflexic events. Any infectious history should be examined in detail.

Patient Preparation

For some laparoscopic techniques, such as a varicocelectomy[7] or lymphadenectomy,[10] most patients can be admitted on the day of surgery. More complex endocavitary procedures must be viewed as major surgery, and proper patient preparation is essential. We prefer a mechanical bowel preparation with 2 to 4 L of Golitely the day prior to surgery. If possible, admission the day before surgery will assure compliance with the bowel prep and adequate hydration. This preparation reduces distension of the intestines, which aids in exposure of the pelvis and reduces the risk of visceral puncture during the procedure. Sterilization of the bladder and urine is imperative to limit the morbidity should urine or bladder contents be spilled intraperitoneally. In the female, a vaginal prep with a bactericidal agent is important to minimize the risk of infection should the vagina be violated while dissecting the posterior vesicovaginal plane. Furthermore, broad spectrum prophylactic parenteral antibiotics are routinely administered 2 h prior to laparoscopy.

Finally, a detailed informed consent is obtained. The discussion should include a review of all alternatives, both surgical and conservative. Obviously, the patient must be aware that the procedure is new, but based upon sound principles that can be readily applied to his or her own condition. Emphasis on the complications unique to laparoscopy should be made. The potential for conversion to an open procedure must be discussed.

Anesthesia

In all bladder surgery we feel general endotracheal anesthesia is necessary. The use of local anesthesia has been described for some short laparoscopic cases,[29] but in our opinion, this burdens the patient with unnecessary risk and discomfort. Surgery that involves the potential for extensive adhesiolysis and complex extirpation can extend to hours. Conversion to an open procedure is always a possibility, and an exploratory laparotomy cannot be delayed for the induction of general anesthesia. Positive pressure ventilation is essential to provide adequate

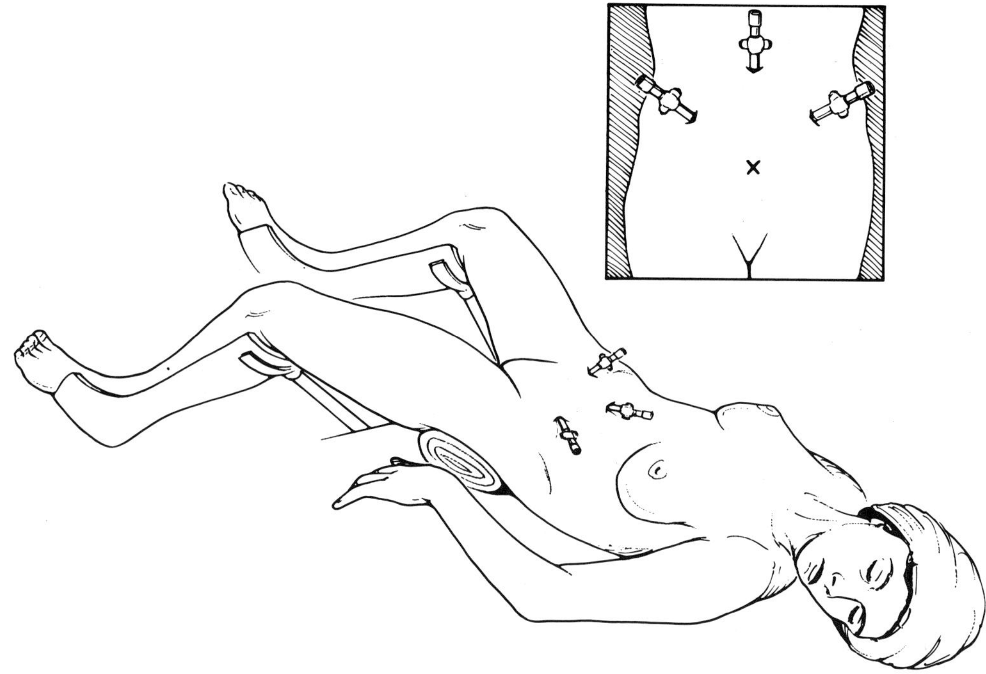

Figure 12-1 Patient positioning for laparoscopic bladder surgery. *Inset,* sites of trocar placement for laparoscopic bladder surgery.

oxygenation and avoid hypercarbia. Autonomic dysreflexia is a concern in paraplegics, and the anesthesiologist should be cognizant of the patient's premorbid status. Consideration to preoperative Nifedepine should be given in these circumstances.

Patient Positioning

We prefer positioning the patient in a modified lithotomy using Allen stirrups with the buttocks at the edge of the operating table (Fig. 12-1). A rolled sheet is placed below the hips to spread the pelvic girdle. This allows access to the rectum and perineum should cystourethroscopy or elevation of the anterior vaginal wall be necessary. An O'Connor sheath should be placed in either the rectum or the vagina. The patient's arms are tucked at the side to allow full movement by the operating team.

As effective retraction of bowel contents is not yet available for laparoscopy, considerable rotation of the patient occurs during the operation. Extreme lateral and Trendelenburg positions are common, and the patient needs to be secured to the table. Chest straps and shoulder braces are essential. Furthermore, as pressure points will change during the operation, all conceivable points need to be padded. Immediately prior to induction of the pneumoperitoneum the table is tilted to a Trendelenburg position of approximately 20 degrees. This will assist in displacing the bowels cephalad. Decompression of the continent pouch or management of an ileal conduit is accomplished by continuous catheter drainage. Gastric decompression by means of a nasogastric tube is also done.

Induction of Pneumoperitoneum

In our experience establishing a pneumoperitoneum in the virgin abdomen is simple if the Mitchell technique of Veress cannula placement is used.[30] However, the most innocuous and reliable way of establishing the pneumoperitoneum is by using a Hasson trocar via a minilaparotomy incision.[31] Once the trocar is in place it can be secured with sutures and rapid insufflation accomplished. The laparoscope with the video camera attached can then be passed and additional trocars placed under direct visual control.

Trocar Placement

The tendency for the neophyte endocavitary surgeon is to think that the more trocars used, the better. As experience is gained, though, the surgeon will find that less is superior. An excess of trocars and instruments in the abdomen resembles an overgrown jungle and more often impedes rather than augments the procedure. Fewer trocars also results in less pain for the patient postoperatively. We advocate starting with a three-port access for most pelvic procedures.

Our usual approach is to place a 10.5-mm trocar at the umbilical area through which the laparoscope

(a)

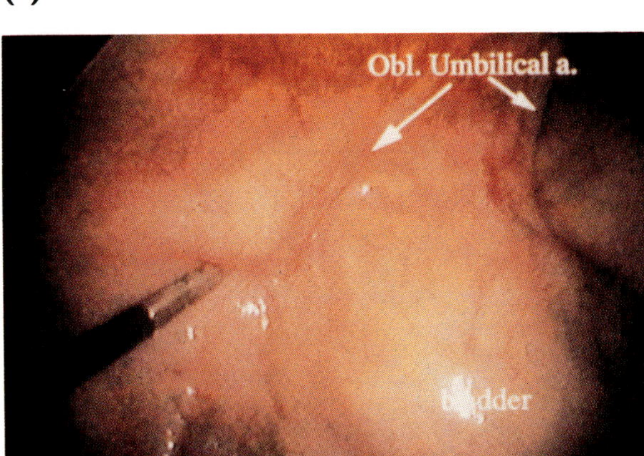

(b)

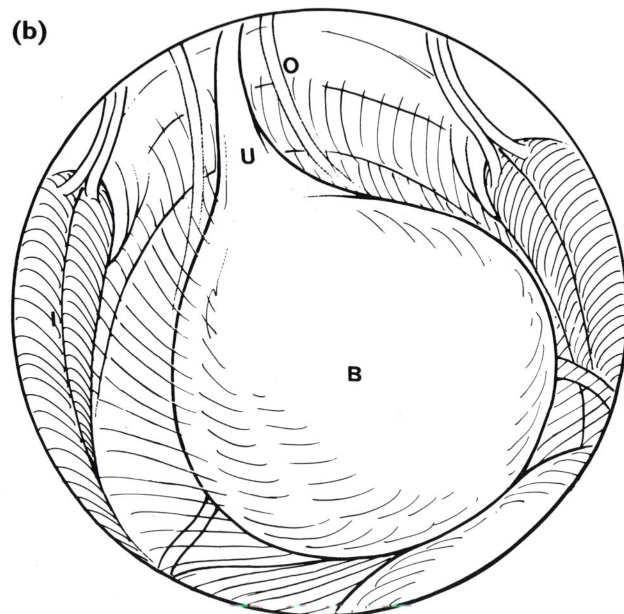

Figure 12-2 Pertinent anatomical surgical landmarks of laparoscopic bladder surgery. (a) Intraoperative photograph. (b) Line drawing.

and camera are used. An additional two ports, placed bilaterally approximately 2 cm below the navel along the mid-clavicular line, are all that is customarily needed. These are either 10.5 or 12 mm in diameter, depending upon the procedure planned, and whether or not the endo-GIA stapler is to be employed. Disruption of the epigastric vessels can occur with placement of the lateral ports. In addition to being aware of their usual course, the surgeon can often identify them by visualization through the laparoscope or by transillumination.[32] If an additional port is necessary for retraction, a 5- or 10.5-mm trocar can then be placed in the midline approximately 2 cm above the pubis (Fig. 12-1).

Surgical Technique

Pertinent Anatomy

Adhesiolysis is performed as needed. Quite often the sigmoid colon is adherent to the side wall at the internal ring and needs to be moved out of the operative field. Usually, the urine reservoir and/or conduit is displaced out of the operating field by the pneumoperitoneum. The essential anatomy should be clear after the adhesions are released (Fig. 12-2). Reference to the internal ring will assist the surgeon in his orientation. It is necessary to identify the obliterated umbilical arteries bilaterally. The laparoscope should be oriented such that the umbilical ligament is visualized on the monitor in a relatively constant course. The surgeon should work in line with the laparoscope to avoid mirror image effect. A Foley catheter balloon is usually visible in the bladder to assist in its identification. As far as possible without extensive dissection, the course of the external iliac vessels should also be identified. A transrectal or transvaginal probe is often useful in delineating the posterior anatomy. Such a probe will be helpful in the subsequent dissection.

Initial Dissection

Common practice in standard cystectomies is to develop the cul-de-sac or recto-vesical plane first. In laparoscopy, the pneumoperitoneum will tent the abdomen anteriorly. Dissection of the anterior plane will therefore greatly facilitate bladder mobilization and subsequent posterior dissection. The peritoneal reflection is sharply incised bilaterally extending from the bifurcation of the common iliac artery to the pubic rami (Fig. 12-3). The incision follows the lateral borders of the obliterated umbilical arteries, which are cauterized or clip ligated and divided.

With a combination of sharp and blunt dissection, the space between the lateral wall of the bladder and pelvis is developed as far as the endopelvic fascia. The dissection is continued until the prevesical space is entirely open (Fig. 12-4).

In the *male*, the anterior dissection of the prevesical space is continued to the level of the puboprostatic ligaments and endopelvic fascia (Fig. 12-5). If a

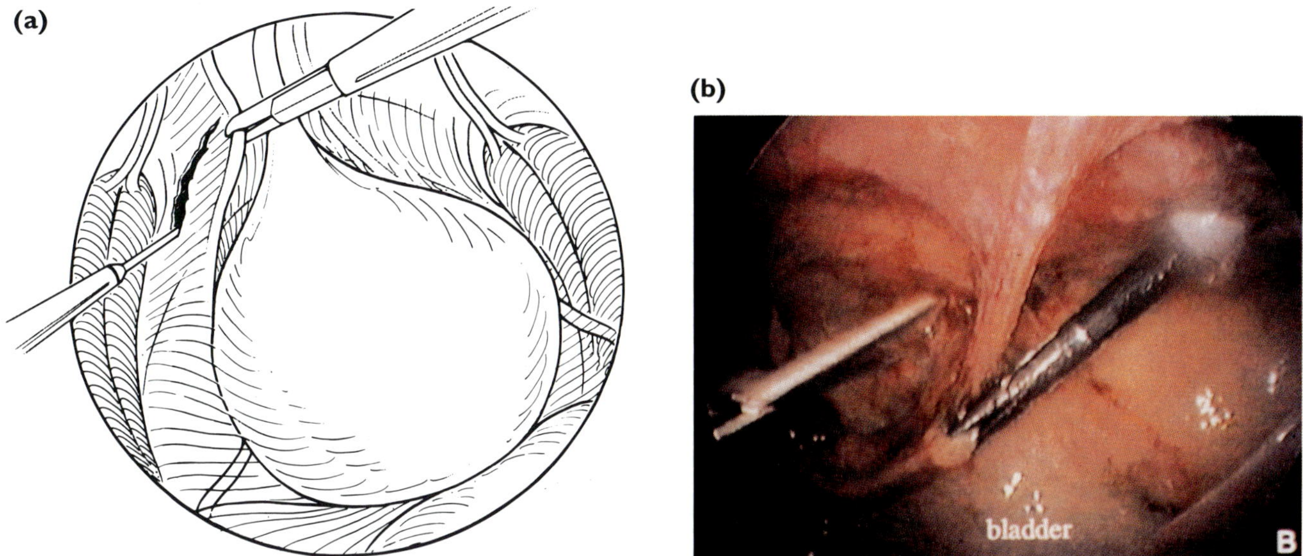

Figure 12-3 Initial step of laparoscopic cystectomy, incision of the peritoneal reflection from the bifurcation of the pubi rami to the common iliac artery. (a) Line drawing. (b) Intraoperative photograph.

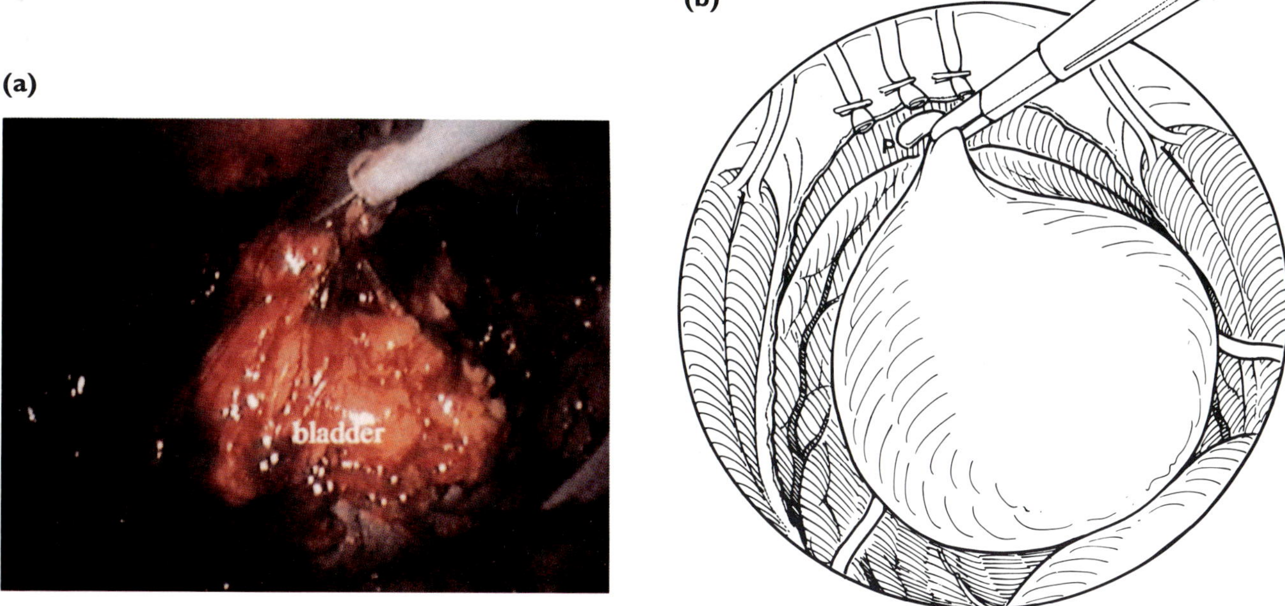

Figure 12-4 Completed bilateral anterior dissection of the prevesical space. (a) Intraoperative photograph. (b) Line drawing.

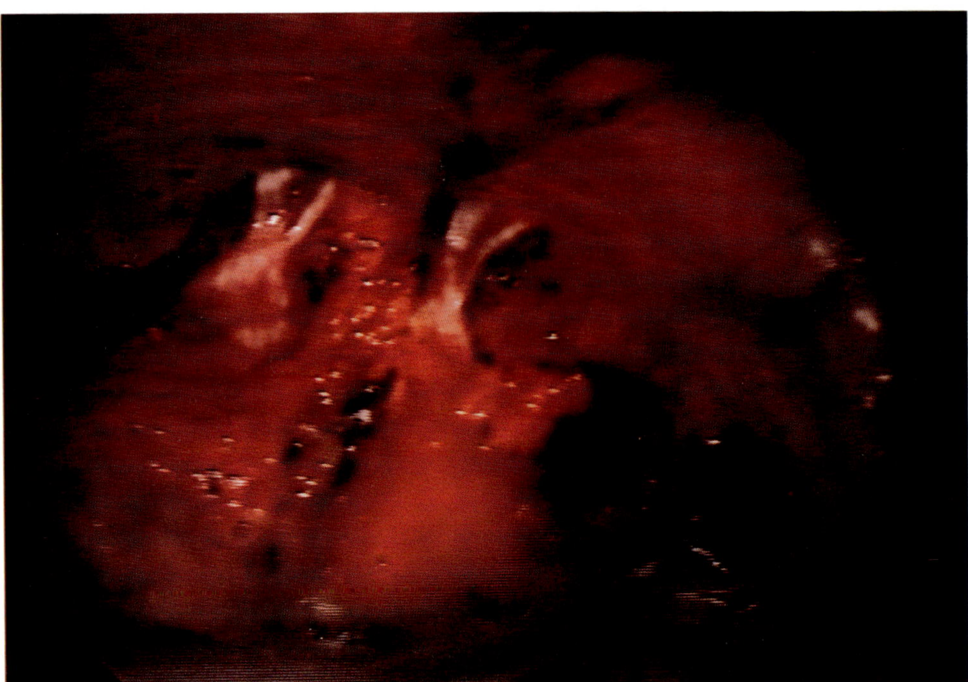

Figure 12-5 Completed anterior dissection of prevesical space in a male patient, note puboprostatic ligaments and endopelvic fascia.

prostatectomy is contemplated or further mobilization is needed, the endopelvic fascia can be opened bilaterally. At this point, it is useful to complete the posterior dissection before attempting transection of the prostatic urethra at the bladder neck.

In the *female*, the isolation and division of the urethra can often be accomplished before the posterior dissection is started. The vesicourethral junction is dissected clear using anterior/posterior traction and countertraction. A grasping forceps on the bladder is used to pull it posteriorly and a transurethral probe or cystoscope is used to force the bladder neck anteriorly. The multifire endo-GIA 30 stapler is passed through a 12-mm-diameter trocars and then placed across the urethrovesical angle to divide the urethra (Fig. 12-6).

Vascular Control

Using grasping forceps to exert cephalic traction on the bladder will assist in creating the posterior plane (Fig. 12-7). In the female the dissection is between the posterior vesical wall and the uterus to the level of the cervix. The application of electrocautery scissors is essential here. Lateral dissection is directed at isolation of the vascular pedicles. The endo-GIA stapler is used to ligate and divide the vascular pedicles (Fig. 12-8).

Final Dissection

Male. With cephalad traction on the bladder, the plane between the posterior vesical wall and the rectum to the level of the vesicoprostatic junction is developed. Complete detachment of the bladder from the rectum is performed by sequential staplings along the fascia plane. Finally, the vesicourethral junction is divided. A combination of electrocautery and stapling is used to transect the bladder and occlude the prostatic urethra. *Female*. Detachment of the bladder from the vagina is performed by sequential firing of the stapling instrument along the vesicovaginal angle (Fig. 12-9).

Specimen Retrieval

The specimen can usually be delivered in toto through one of the 12-mm trocars. If necessary, the trocar can be removed and the specimen retrieved through the wound, which is easily stretched. Irrigation and inspection of the pelvis is essential to evaluate for hemostasis and the integrity of the vagina or rectum, and to confirm that no residual bladder tissue remains. Usually no external drainage is needed.

Avoiding Complications

Trocar Injuries

Abdominal wall injuries to vessels are best managed by avoidance of the vessels. Transillumination or direct visualization will often reveal the epigastric artery and vein. Transected vessels can occasionally be controlled by the distention pressure from the trocar or traction on an inflated Foley catheter placed through the incision. Often they will require either

(a)

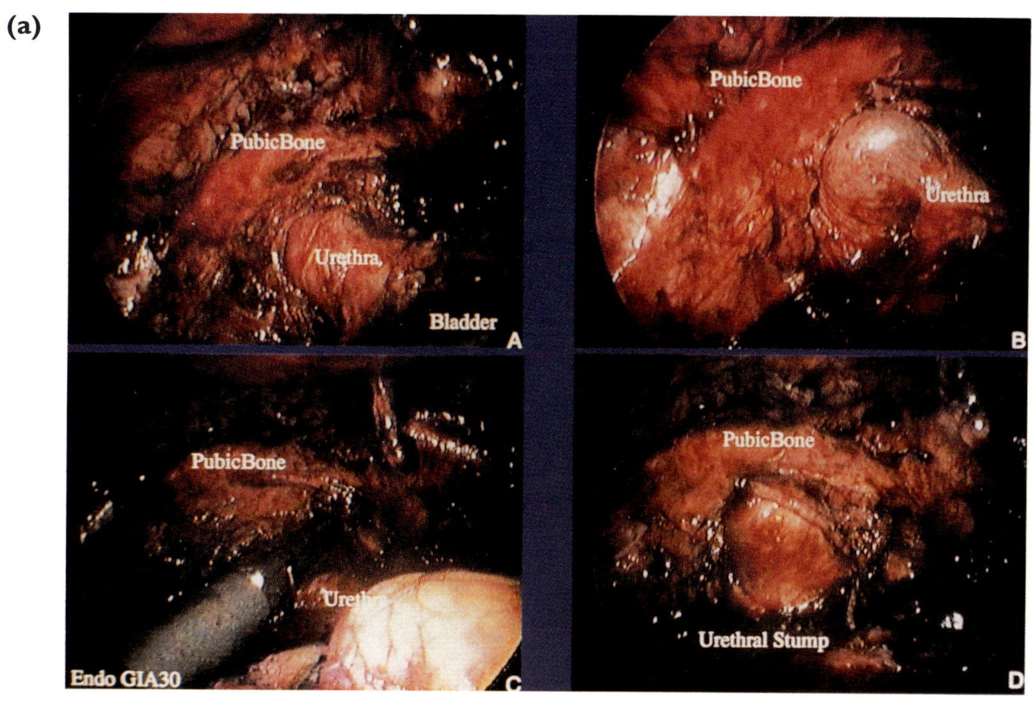

(b)

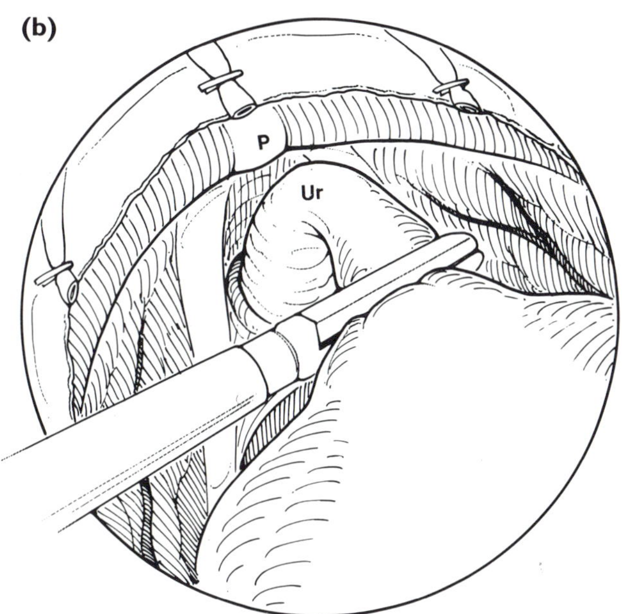

Figure 12-6 (a) Sequence of division of the urethra in a female patient with endo-GIA 30 stapler. (b) Depiction of endo-GIA 30 stapler across urethra.

cauterization or suture ligation. Cut-down and ligation is definitive, but often requires an extensive search for the vessel. A percutaneous technique using a figure-eight suture passed with a Stamey needle has been described by Green.[32]

Intra-abdominal vessel injury is considerably more serious. Preparation is essential to assist in the rapid identification and management of larger vessel injury. Before the first needle or trocar is passed, all instruments, including the laparoscope (for immediate visualization) and a scalpel (for emergent laparotomy), must be ready.[33] Aortic puncture has been reported. Large vessel injury is probably more likely in thin individuals and those having extensive adhesions. The use of a Hasson trocar and direct visualization of the placement of all tocars will minimize this risk. Avoidance of previous surgical scars will decrease the potential for injuring adherent underlying viscera.

Perforations of intestines or solid organ occurred in 8 of 500 cases in one series.[34] Unrecognized injury is likely to be much more common. Decom-

(a)

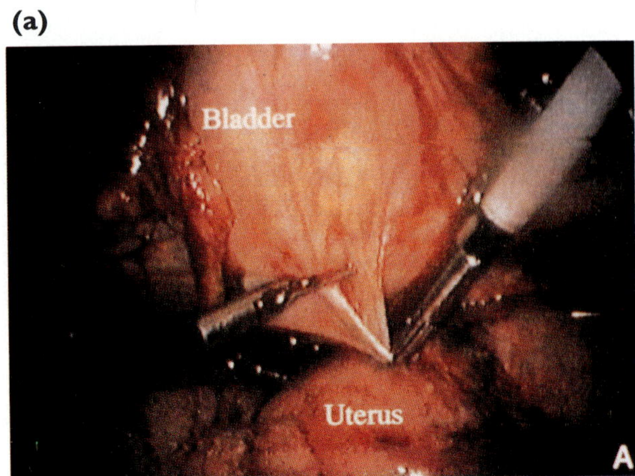

(b)

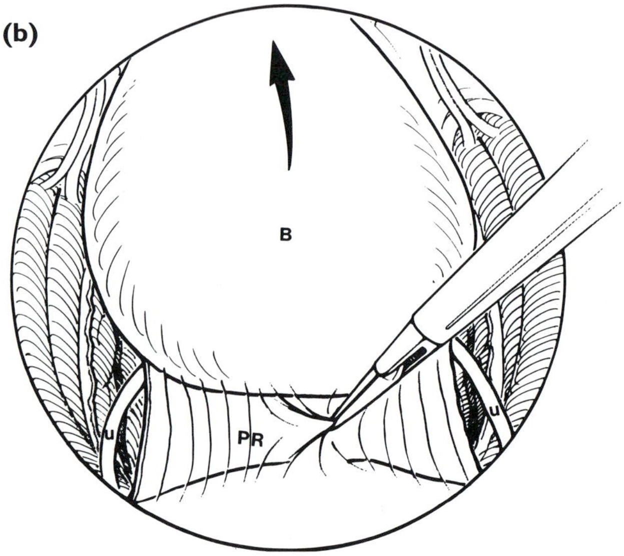

Figure 12-7 With cephalad traction on the bladder, dissection of the posterior plane is initiated (a) Intraoperative photograph. (b) Line drawing; B=bladder, U=ureter, PR=peritoneal reflection.

(a)

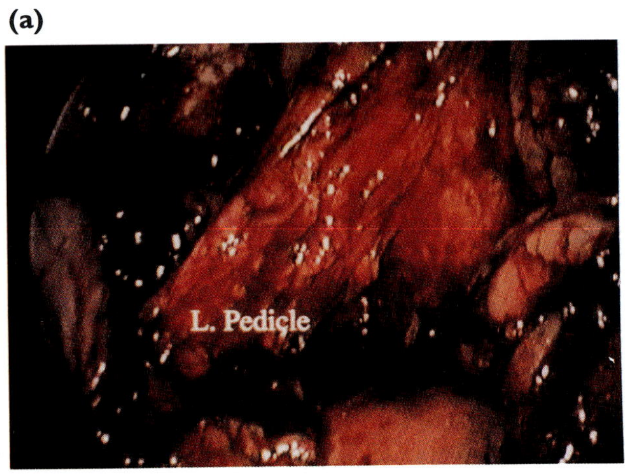

(b)

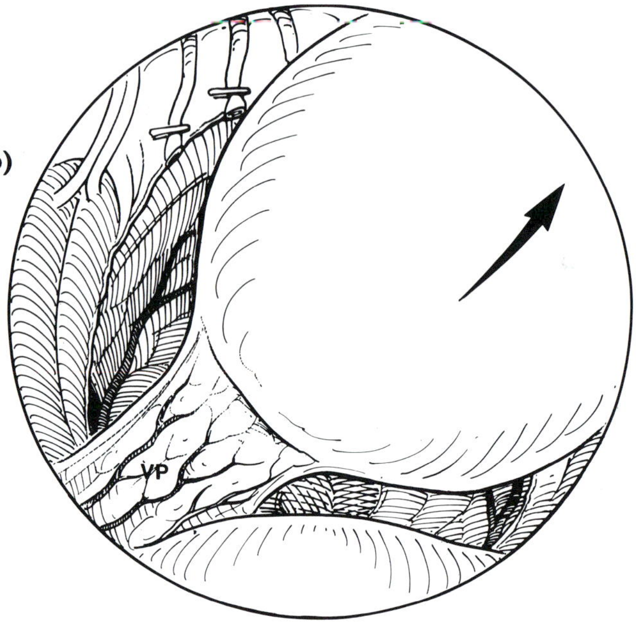

(c)

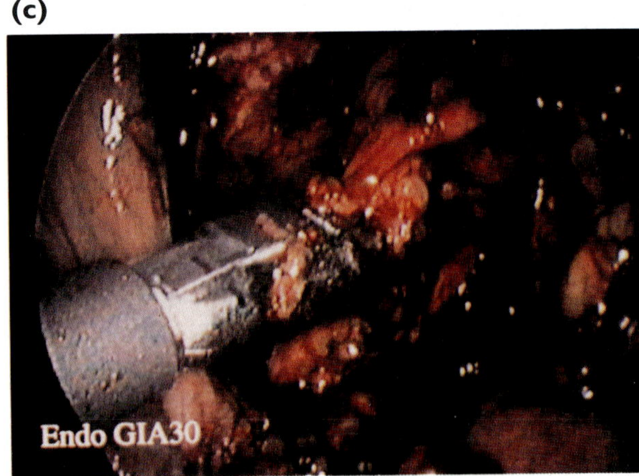

(d)

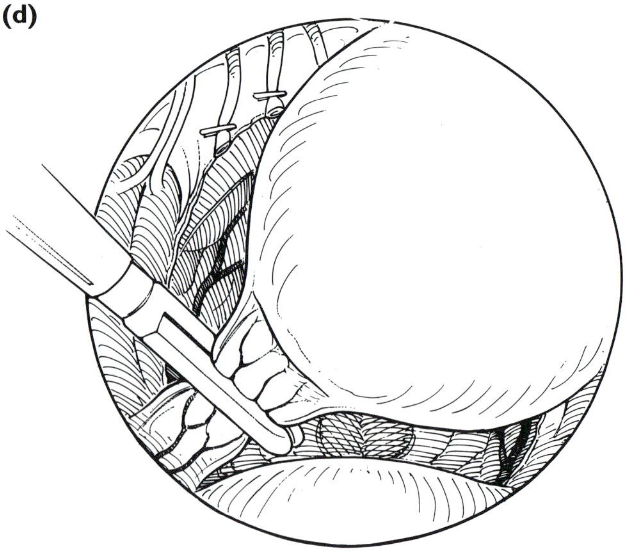

Figure 12-8 (a & b) Isolated left vascular pedicle. (c & d) Transection of left vascular pedicle with endo-GIA 30 stapler

(a)

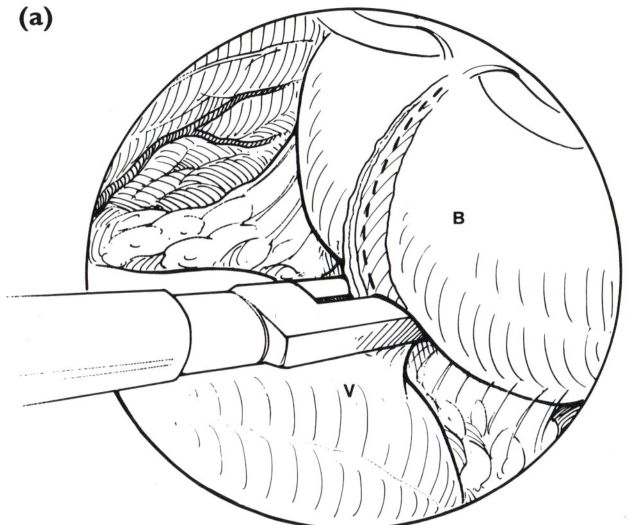

(b)

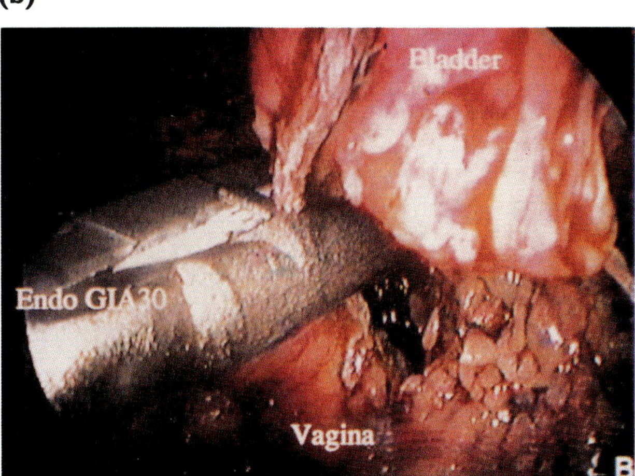

Figure 12-9 Detachment of the bladder from the vagina by sequential firing of the endo-GIA 30 stapler. (a) Line drawing; V=vagina, B=bladder. (b) Intraoperative photograph

pression of bowel with a bowel prep and a nasogastric tube may be useful. Often small holes can be closed primarily using laparoscopic suturing techniques. Gross contamination is probably best handled by laparotomy and irrigation.

Rectal Injury

As most cystectomy patients with the above indications have had numerous episodes of cystitis, significant perivesical fibrosis is to be expected. Careful sharp dissection is aided by the use of a probe or finger in the bladder and/or rectum. To limit the potential for a devastating mucosal thermal injury, the electrocautery should rarely if ever be used near the rectum. The liberal use of metal clips or an endostapler will limit the bleeding. A clean incision into the rectum can often be repaired primarily, although it may be wise to do so in an open fashion. Where a large vein or artery is encountered, the endo-GIA stapler can be used safely. Obviously preoperative bowel preparation is essential.

Vaginal Injury

The same principles apply to the posterior vaginal dissection as mentioned above for the avoidance of rectal injuries, although the use of electrocautery is not as strictly contraindicated. Traction and countertraction with a vaginal probe or a finger in the O'Connor sheath is useful in establishing the plane of dissection.

Vascular Injury

With the division of the obliterated umbilical ligaments the major landmarks for dissection are gone. Completing the anterior dissection to the pubis and identifying the external iliac vessels at their exit from the pelvis prior to division of the umbilical ligament is often the easiest method of maintaining the surgical perspective. Dissection above the bifurcation of the iliacs is not needed.

Frequent use of the endostapler along the vesical pedicle and anterior tributaries of the internal iliac artery is preferred to electrocautery. Prophylactic ligation of the hypogastric artery is seldom effective and can be hazardous to the lateral nerves and thin veins.

As noted above, the use of electrocautery should be limited above the rectum. As possible this dissection should be along Denonvilliers fascia.

In a few patients the obliterated umbilical ligament is misnamed. Profuse bleeding from a patent umbilical artery is impressive. We now use clips on all ligaments prior to division.

It should be noted that disruption of a large vein can lead to CO_2 pulmonary embolism. Prompt laparotomy to close the vein and decompress the pneumoperitoneum is the safest course in this event.

Bladder Neck Occlusion

Use of the endostapler makes for expedient closure of the bladder neck and limits the potential for intraabdominal contamination by vesical contents. An alternative method of bladder neck closure is intracorporeal suturing, although this is considerably more tedious and difficult to learn. Complete occlusion by whatever method is confirmed by gently probing the obliterated urethra with a soft red rubber catheter while inspecting the pelvis with the laparoscope. Intra-abdominal drainage is not necessary.

Bowel Obstruction/Hernia

Strict attention must be given to the precise closure of the fascial defects. Some suggest closure of all working trocar sites under direct vision with the laparoscope with the pneumoperitoneum intact.[35] Herniation of loops of bowel through trocar sites has been reported, and the surgeon should not be fooled by the apparent insignificance of the wounds.[36] At the very least, visual and manual inspection should be done to confirm that no viscera are trapped.

Deep Vein Thrombosis

There is no evidence to suggest that there is an increased risk of DVT in laparoscopy, but standard precautions with pneumatic compression stockings is fundamental.

Lymphoceles

We have seen an increased incidence of lymphocele formation when the peritoneum is reapproximated following lymphadenectomies. Although this is not observed in laparoscopic cystectomies, there is no utility in trying to staple the cut edges of the peritoneum.

Complications of Pneumoperitoneum

A rapid rise in pressure can lead to cardiovascular collapse. One patient in our series sustained a stroke when the automatic regulator failed and the pressure rose above 35 mm Hg in the abdomen.[33] The pressure monitor should be visible at all times to the surgeon and the operating nurses. Subcutaneous emphysema can be avoided by use of a Hasson trocar. Short of this, strict attention to the insufflation pressure will alert the surgeon of improper placement of the Veress needle.

Postoperative Considerations

Postoperative management begins with the closure of the fascia at each trocar location. As indicated above, bowel herniation is a real concern. We use interrupted figure-eight 0 polyglycolic acid (PGA) sutures on the fascia. The skin is closed with subcuticular 4-0 PGA. As the pneumoperitoneum is released it is helpful to decompress any pneumoscrotum. Usually no drains are required.

Standard surgical practices must be maintained in the care of the patient after laparoscopy. The practices of instituting full oral intake without assessment of the patient or discharging patients home at a predetermined time are ludicrous to the surgeon. Pressure to do just such things is increasing in the laparoscopic era and is to be decried.

As most patients have only minimal pain, severe pain should be considered the result of a surgical complication until proven otherwise. There are reports to suggest that delayed complications may be more common in laparoscopic procedures than traditional operations.[34] This may result from both a delayed mechanism of injury (for example from thermal injuries to bowel and ischemia from mesenteric vein thrombosis) as well as from delayed diagnosis. Late thermal bowel injuries usually present between 4 and 10 days after operation. Puncture wounds will usually manifest themselves within 48 h.[37] Unseen needle and trocar injuries in particular are probably much more common than traditionally acknowledged.

Results

In our experiece with three patients the total operative time averaged 155 min and the average estimated blood loss was 200 mL. All patients were discharged home within 5 days (range 3–5). In the one male paraplegic, the NG tube was removed on the first postoperative day (12 h) and he was able to tolerate a regular diet within 24 h. All patients resumed a regular diet within 48 h. Postoperative pain or use of analgesics was not required in one man. The average IM Meperidine used was 150 mg followed by less than 10 acetaminophen with codeine tablets.

Histologic exam of the bladder specimens showed clear margins with no evidence of bladder tissue left behind.

Diverticulectomy

Indications

Treatment for bladder diverticula may be considered under a variety of circumstances. Diverticula complicated by calculi, urinary retention, chronic infection, or carcinoma definitely require therapy.[38] Others have even recommended the prophylactic excision of diverticula because of the high incidence of associated neoplasia and the poor prognosis of such cancers.[39]

Excision of a bladder diverticulum by means of a laparoscope is a feasible alternative to open surgery.

This technique is particularly suitable for those diverticula with a narrow neck. Consideration for laparoscopic diverticulectomy may be given when the diverticulum is in an accessible position, has a narrow neck, and does not involve the ureter. In fact, we consider ureteral involvement to be an absolute contraindication to an endocavitary diverticulectomy.

The most difficult cases involve cancerous diverticula. The incidence of neoplasia in a vesical diverticulum ranges up to 13.5 percent.[39–42] Often these tumors are high grade and metastatic at presentation.[43–45] Many report a worse prognosis for these patients,[39,44] the few survivors having low-grade, superficial tumors.[38,39,41,44] A radical cystectomy is rarely a satisfactory solution, as it is often merely palliative. Conversely, a truly confined tumor can be readily treated with a less morbid diverticulectomy or partial cystectomy. As laparoscopy can effect complete resection and decrease the potential for tumor spillage, we believe this substantially improves the treatment options for these patients. It is also possible that a more accurate assessment of the tumor's extravesicle spread can be determined by laparoscopic inspection. In addition, a concomitant laparoscopic node dissection would improve staging.

Contraindications include all those listed for a cystectomy and a diverticulum that is intimately involved with a ureter.[1]

Preoperative Evaluation/Studies

The patient should be evaluated preoperatively with cystoscopy and cystography to carefully delineate the anatomy. Upper tract evaluation is essential to localize the position of the diverticulum with respect to the ureters.

Patient Preparation

Preoperative preparations are essentially the same as for a cystectomy, although a few special circumstances need consideration. Sterile urine must be assured, utilizing extended preoperative antibiotics when necessary. Stones in a bladder diverticulum are best managed via a transurethral approach.

Patient Positioning

To facilitate cystoscopy the patient is positioned in a modified lithotomy posture as for a cystectomy (Fig. 12-1). The use of a laparoscopic drape with a perineal breach is essential as well as a Connor rectal sheath.

Anesthesia

The same recommendations for the use of general endotracheal anesthesia exist as for cystectomy.

Induction of Pneumoperitoneum

In patients without previous abdominal surgery we place a Veress cannula subumbilically and create a pneumoperitoneum of 12 to 15 mm Hg with carbon dioxide. If a previous laparotomy has been performed, a blunt Hasson trocar is used to avoid injury to underlying viscera.

Trocar Placement

After the introduction of an adequate pneumoperitoneum, three or four operative ports are positioned as described for the cystectomy (Fig. 12-1). Cystoscopic examination is performed simultaneously, preferably with a rigid 21 French cystoscope. This not only assists in visualization of the diverticulum, but it is also essential to confirm total occlusion once the diverticulum has been excised. The placement of ureteral stents is also advised in most cases.

Surgical Technique

Pertinent Anatomy

The critical anatomy is seen after any adhesiolysis is accomplished. Identification of the ureters will be essential as the dissection proceeds, but they can only rarely be seen initially. The ipsilateral ureter will be inferior and often widely lateral or superior to the diverticulum. If doubt about their location exists at any time, ureteral stenting should be done.

Initial Dissection

In most bladder surgery we have found it preferable to proceed from the anterior first, then retract the bladder or diverticulum anteriorly for the more complex posterior dissection. The diverticulum is identified with the assistance of transillumination from the cystoscope, and the peritoneum is opened directly over it using a combination of blunt and sharp dissection (Fig. 12-10).

Vascular Control

Bleeding is controlled using cautery and clip ligation. Vigorous dissection of the ureter and periureteral tissue is to be avoided to minimize both direct trauma and devascularizing injury. Staying

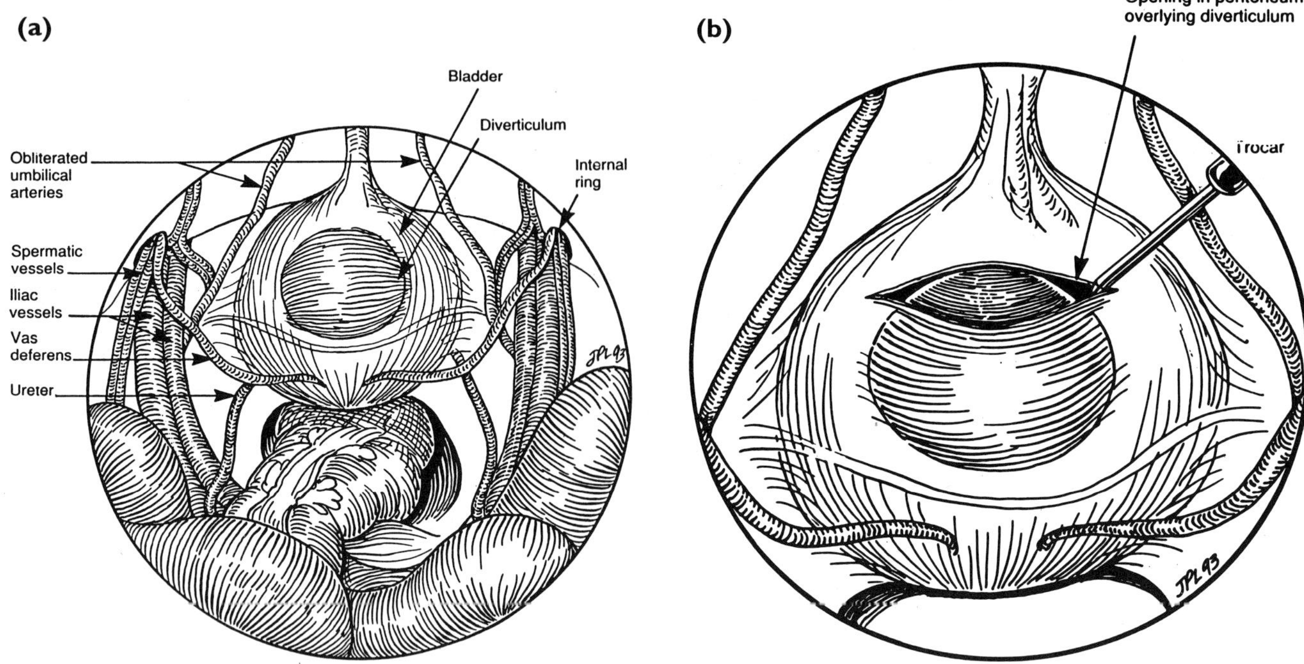

Figure 12-10 (a) Laparoscopic perspective of pertinent anatomy depicting relative position of diverticulum in relation to other pelvic structures. (b) Opening of parietal peritoneum directly over the diverticulum.

medial to the umbilical ligaments will limit the potential for major vascular trauma. While the vascular pedicle of the bladder will often be inferior to the diverticulum, rarely if ever is it necessary to dissect through the pedicle itself. The use of the endo-GIA is therefore limited here.

Final Dissection

The diverticulum is dissected free of the peritoneum and bladder until the neck is completely circumscribed (Fig. 12-11) The inferior limit of the neck is occasionally difficult to discern. Obviously, this is where trauma to the ureter and vascular pedicle is most likely to occur. Repeated filling of the bladder and diverticulum is helpful in this regard. The cystoscope can also be used to transilluminate and exert countertraction at the neck.

Finally, the endostapler is introduced through one of the 12-mm ports and used to clamp across the bladder wall at the diverticular neck (Fig. 12-12). The ureter should be visualized at all times during this procedure. Firing the stapler automatically divides and hermetically approximates the tissue. This portion of the operation is simultaneously visualized cystoscopically, confirming the total occlusion of the diverticular neck. Overdistention of the bladder is to be avoided, as it complicates the closure and may predispose to leaking of the staple line. Depending on the size of the diverticulum, two or three successive staplings should accomplish the complete division of tissue. Hydrodilation of the bladder is then done to assure that the closure is watertight. An alternative method of bladder closure is intracorporeal suturing.[46]

Specimen Removal

The diverticular tissue is removed with gall bladder grasping forceps through a 12-mm port. It may on rare occasions be necessary to remove the trocar as the specimen is retrieved. In instances where diverticulectomy has been performed for malignancy, it is preferable to place the specimen in an organ retrieval bag prior to removal.

Avoiding Complications

Transection of Ureter

Injury to the ureter is the most probable adverse consequence of this procedure. Identification of the ureter proximal to the iliac vessels can be helpful in avoiding this problem. The ureter is then traced distally, and if it terminates at the diverticular neck, open intervention is indicated. Constant reference to the ureter with hydrodilation and cystoscopic tran-

(a)

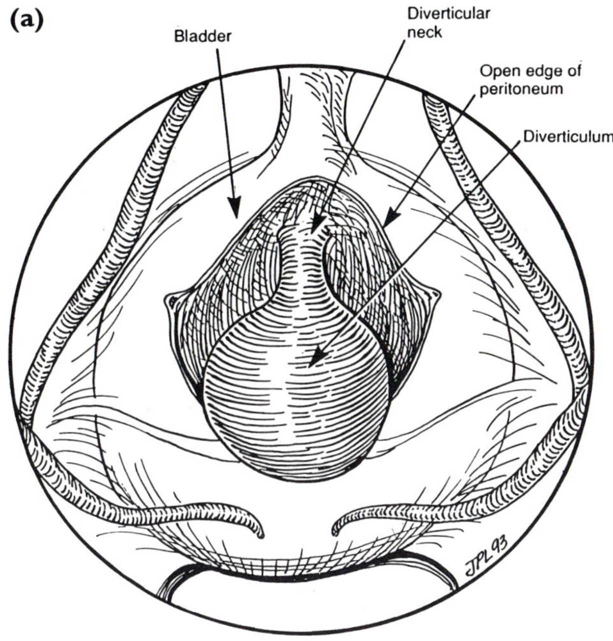

(b)

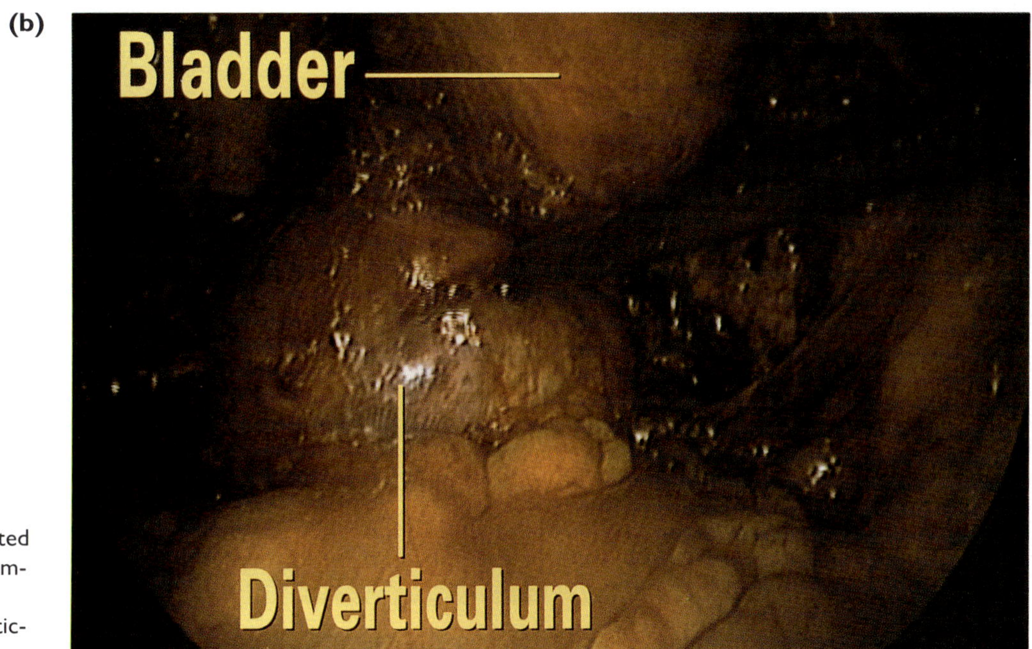

Figure 12-11 (a) Dissected diverticulum with neck completely circumscribed. (b) Actual dissection of diverticulum.

sillumination during the procedure is helpful. Aggressive periureteral dissection and devascularization should be avoided.

Diverticular Stones

Although we have yet to encounter this situation, it is conceivable that the entire dissection and removal can be accomplished with a stone in situ. Obviously, an intraperitoneal cystostomy should be avoided in this situation.

Inadvertent Cystostomy and Spill of Bladder Contents

An alternative method of bladder closure is intracorporeal suturing. This has been described by others for diverticulectomies.[46] Its main advantage is that absorbable suture can be used. It does require considerably more time and involves an intraperitoneal cystostomy.

From a preventive standpoint, the use of the endostapler allows expedient closure of the divertic-

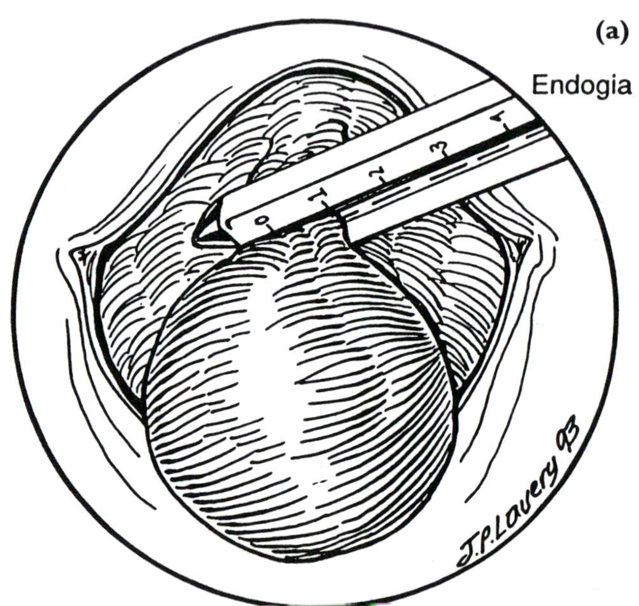

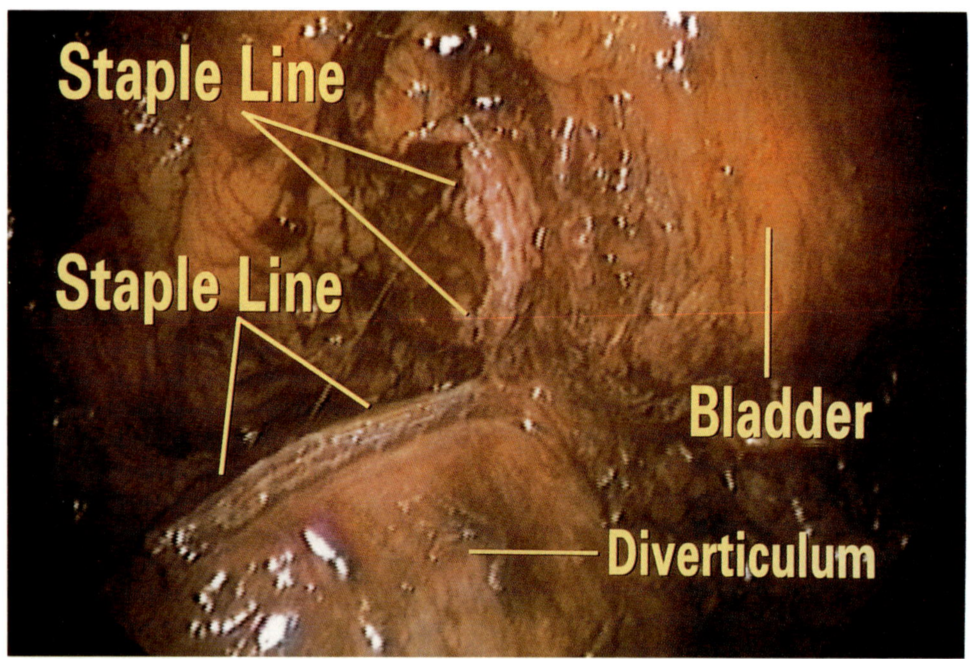

(b)

Figure 12-12 (a) Dissection of diverticular neck with endo-GIA 30 stapler. (b) Partially transected diverticular neck.

ular neck without an intraperitoneal cystotomy. Although the presence of staples in the urinary tract is thought to predispose to stone formation, the use of titanium staples may obviate this possible complication, as has been demonstrated in other areas where this metal has been used within the urinary tract.[47] Clayman has done extensive work with staples and the bladder, and has yet to see encrustations present a problem.[48] Stapling techniques are potentially most useful when excising diverticula with carcinoma present, as this would preclude tumor spillage. Should tumor or other grossly contaminated bladder contents be spilled, conversion to a laparotomy may be prudent. Laparoscopic irrigation systems may be sufficient, but caution is advised.

If following complete transection of the diverticular neck a leak is identified, the cystostomy can be closed one of two ways. If it is small, a laparoscopic hernia needle can be used to close the defect with one or two figure-eight polygalactin sutures. Larger defects can be occasionally closed by grasping both edges of the bladder wall and using the endo-GIA stapler. This requires a fourth port if one is not in place already.

Postoperative Considerations

After inspection for hemostasis, the pneumoperitoneum is expelled and the trocars removed. The fascial defects are closed with 0 polygalactin sutures and the skin closed with 4-0 polygalactin subcuticular sutures. No peritoneal drains are needed. Foley catheter drainage is maintained for 7 days. Cystography is then performed to confirm absence of extravasation, and the catheter is removed.

Repair of Bladder

We have recently closed a bladder rupture via the laparoscope.[49] A man undergoing transurethral bladder biopsies sustained an intraperitoneal bladder perforation, which was diagnosed immediately.

A three-port laparoscopic approach readily revealed the rupture in the anterior, lateral bladder. The bladder was filled with a dilute solution of methylene blue and saline, augmenting the identification of the edges of the wound (Fig. 12-13). The abdomen was inspected carefully for bladder tissue, then copiously irrigated with normal saline through the laparoscope.

The bladder defect was closed with three passes of an absorbable suture (2-0 polyglycolic acid) in running fashion, followed by a serosal layer of interrupted sutures (Fig. 12-14). Simultaneous cystoscopy assisted in identifying the safe position of the ureter, and hydrodilation of the bladder confirmed complete closure. The man was discharged home the next day and returned for urethral catheter removal in 7 days.

Cystoprostatectomy and Urinary Diversion

For pathologies other than a retained bladder, concomitant urinary diversion is necessary. The general indications for cystectomy with diversion are well described for open procedures and a discussion is not germane to this chapter. We will briefly discuss the specific comparative advantages and disadvantages of laparoscopic cystectomy (simple and radical) with urinary diversion. It should be noted that laparoscopic surgeons are just beginning to attempt such procedures.

A laparoscopic prostatectomy[50] and a laparoscopic radical cystectomy and ileal conduit have been performed.[51] Urinary diversion with laparoscopic assistance had been previously reported by Kozminski.[11] The arduous task of performing the bowel anastomosis and ureteroileal anastomosis was done with the bowel pulled extracorporeally through a trocar site in both instances. Many researchers are reporting ureteral surgery (ureterolysis,[52] ureteroureterostomies,[53] and extravesical vesicoureteroplasties[54]) that suggests the practical application of intracorporeal anastomosis of ureter to ileal con-

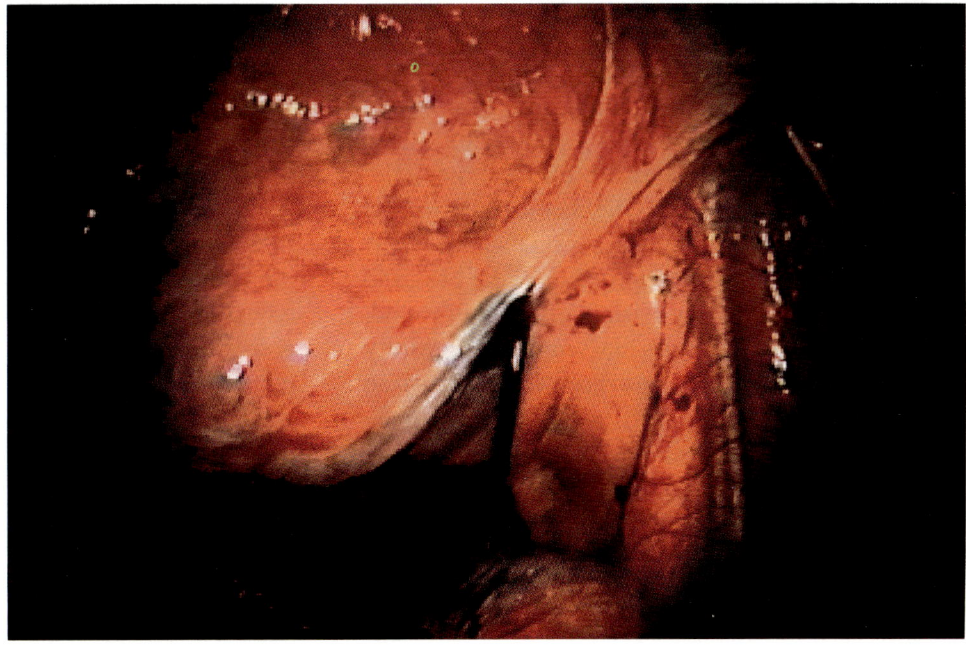

Figure 12-13 Injection of indigo carmine through catheter confirms location of injury.

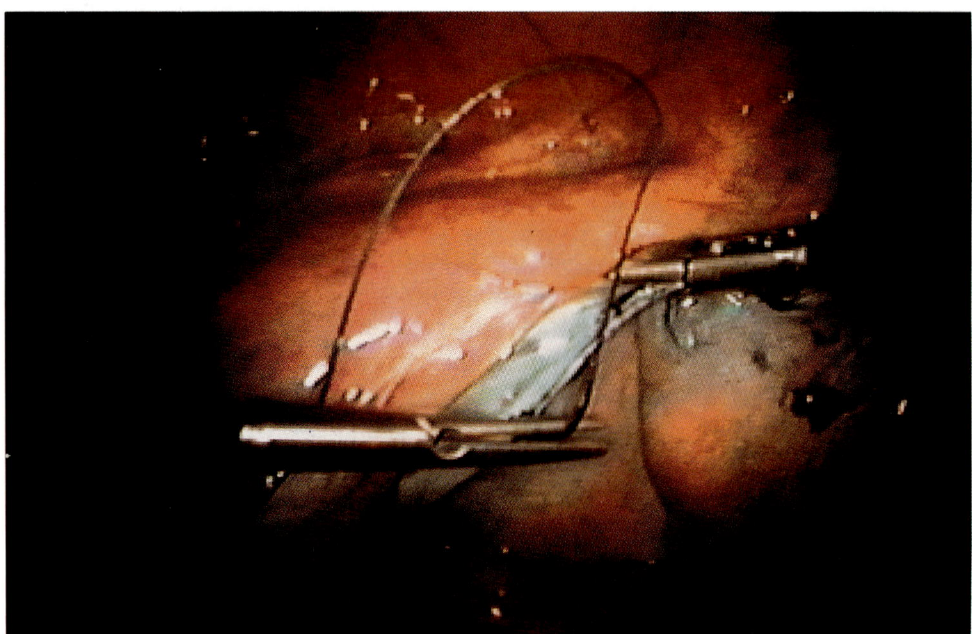

Figure 12-14 Rupture was closed with intracorporeal suturing techniques. Closure of peritoneal layer is demonstrated.

duits. Laparoscopic bowel techniques are also improving rapidly.[55] Recently, totally incorporeal bowel resections with ureteral anastomosis have been accomplished.[56] Jordon has performed a laparoscopic Mitronoff procedure, with the majority of the bowel work done extracorporeally.[57] Obviously, laparoscopic cystectomy and cystoprostatectomy with ileal conduits may soon be reasonably considered. Despite the report from Jordon, a continent urinary diversion with nonrefluxing ureteral anastomosis via the laparoscope still presents considerable problems. An inadequate bowel prep will compromise a traditional open diversion procedure. In a closed abdomen, gross spillage of bowel contents would probably necessitate conversion to an open procedure.[34] The most pressing technical problems are providing adequate exposure for the bowel and ureteral resection, and the bowel reconstruction.[28] At this point the surgeons are waiting on technology.

When considering a new procedure, the pros and cons must be compared on relatively equal ground. First, it is hard to justify a decrease in morbidity when compared with the increased mortality of an unsatisfactory cancer operation. Entrapment systems for tissue removal are in use to limit the intraperitoneal spread of cancer or contagion, but at present their ability to guarantee tissue isolation is not assured. Furthermore, such endo-bags generally require tissue morcellization, which effectively eliminates comprehensive pathological assessment.[28] For most patients, a standard continent diversion, although presenting more initial morbidity, is more satisfactory in the long run. At this time, the laparoscope has not proven itself equal to standard surgical oncologic techniques, and the minor savings in terms of morbidity should be viewed with a modicum of circumspection.

Conclusion

Delayed cystectomy is a major operative procedure that can be associated with serious complications and prolonged hospitalization. In the five patients in our series requiring bladder removal for recurrent pyocystis the average hospital stay was over 20 days. Reduction of the morbidity of this cystectomy is a legitimate goal.

Three obstacles to the laparoscopic approach included the anticipated presence of adhesions, the risks of bleeding from the vascular pedicles, and the possibility of intraperitoneal spillage of infected material from an open bladder. The first concern was addressed by use of the Hasson trocar through a minilaparotomy incision. The excision of the bladder from its vascular attachments was made possible by the employment of the multifire endo-GIA stapler. This instrument also allowed for the expedient detachment of the bladder from its urethral, vaginal, and/or rectal connections in a watertight fashion, thereby averting spillage of vesical contents into the peritoneal cavity.

We believe there are multiple potential advantages to laparoscopic cystectomy. There is no need for a large abdominal incision, which is more cosmetically appealing while decreasing the probability of wound dehiscence and incisional hernia formation. Postoperative pain is also reduced, and hospital stay can be markedly shortened, allowing the individual to return to normal activities sooner.

Since Czerny in 1897 first reported a diverticulectomy,[44] a variety of approaches have been described, including intravesical,[58] extravesical,[59] and transurethral techniques.[60,61] Disadvantages of the open methods include the morbidity of a large incision into the abdominal cavity with resultant pain and added convalescence time. Although the transurethral approach eliminates this morbidity, not all diverticula are amenable to correction via this route. Our experience with the laparoscopic excision of diverticulum demonstrates its feasibility, although considerably more needs to be done to define appropriate indications for this procedure.

The efficient laparoscopic closure of a traumatic rupture of a bladder perforation significantly reduced the morbidity that a laparotomy would have produced. In our case the procedure added little to the patient's pain, burden, or length of hospitalization. Given these circumstances, laparoscopic management of such ruptures is highly recommended.

Considerable experimental evidence supports the prospect of total laparoscopic management of other bladder pathologies, including those that require radical extirpation and urinary diversion. As technologies are developed for improved retraction of viscera, more complex procedures will be possible. The potential for tumor spillage and specimen procurement needs to be more firmly settled. The surgical efficacy in terms of cancer-free margins and nerve preservation (where indicated) also needs to be critically examined.

Finally, one conceivable disadvantage, inherently common to laparoscopy in general, is that significant operator experience is required. However, with appropriate training and guidance, together with the rapid development of improved instruments for urologic laparoscopy, this can be overcome. The addition of laparoscopy to the urologic armamentarium has given considerable breadth to the management of diverse bladder and other pelvic procedures. The depth of practicality of this tool may prove equally impressive as appropriate trials are conducted.

References

1. Parra RO, Jones JP, Andrus CH, Hagood PG: Laparoscopic diverticulectomy: Preliminary report of a new approach for the treatment of bladder diverticulum. *J Urol* 148:869, 1992.
2. Parra RO, Andrus CH, Jones JP, Boullier JA: Laparoscopic cystectomy: Initial report on a new treatment for the retained bladder. *J Urol* 148:1140, 1992.
3. Lowe BA, Novy MJ, Strang E: Laparoscopic segmental cystectomy. *J Urol* 147:408A, 1992.
4. Albala DM , Schuessler WW, Vancaillie TG: Laparoscopic bladder neck suspension. *J Endourol* 6(2):137, 1992.
5. Chiu AW, Chen MT, Huang WJS, Juang GD, Lu SH, Chang LS: Case report: Laparoscopic nephroureterectomy and endoscopic excision of bladder cuff. *Min Inv Ther* 1:299, 1992.
6. Neufang T, Ludtke FE, Lepsien G: Laparoscopic excision of an urachal fistula: A new therapy for a rare disorder. *Min Inv Ther* 1:245, 1992.
7. Hagood PG, Mehan DJ, Worischeck JH, Andrus CH, Parra R0: Laparoscopic varicocelectomy: Preliminary report of a new technique. *J Urol* 147:73,1992.
8. Clayman RV, Kavoussi LR, Soper NJ, et al: Laparoscopic nephrectomy: Initial case report. *J Urol* 146:278, 1991.
9. Parra RO, Jones JP, Hagood PG: Laparoscopic intraperitoneal marsupialization: Report on a new technique for lymphoceles. *Surg Laparosc Endosc* 2:306, 1992.
10. Parra RO, Andrus CH, Boullier JA: Staging laparoscopic pelvic lymph node dissection: Comparison of results with open pelvic lymphadenectomy. *J Urol* 147:857, 1992.
11. Kozminski M, Partamian K0: Case report of laparoscopic ileal loop conduit. *J Endourol* 6:147, 1992.
12. Burney SW, Graves RC, Friedell GH: Multiple malignancies in the urinary bladder following a bypass procedure. Report of a case. *Urol Int* 25:69, 1970.

13. Silber SJ: Carcinoma in the bladder left behind. *J Urol* 110:675, 1973.

14. Rege PR, Evans AT: Carcinoma in isolated bladder after ileoconduit diversion. *Urology* 5:652, 1975.

15. O'Flynn JD, Mullaney J: Vesical leukoplakia progressing to carcinoma. *Br J Urol* 46:31, 1974.

16. Garvin DD, Weber CH Jr, Polsky MS: Carcinoma in the defunctionalized bladder: Report of a case and review of literature. *J Urol* 117:669, 1977.

17. Melzak J: The incidence of bladder cancer in paraplegia. *Paraplegia* 4:85, 1966.

18. Moloney PJ, Fenster HN, McLoughlin MC: Carcinoma in the defunctionalized urinary tract. *J Urol* 126:260, 1981.

19. Eigner EB, Freiha FS: The fate of the remaining bladder following supravesical diversion. *J Urol* 144:31, 1990.

20. Retik AB, Perlmutter AD, Gross RE: Cutaneous ureteroileostomy in children. *N Engl J Med* 277:217, 1967.

21. Holland JM, Schirmer HKA, King LR, Gibbons RP, Scott WW: Pyeloileal urinary conduit: An 8-year experience in 37 patients. *J Urol* 99:427, 1968.

22. Engel RN: Complications of bilateral uretero-ileo cutaneous urinary diversion: A review of 208 cases. *J Urol* 101:508, 1969.

23. Schmidt JD, Hawtrey CE, Flocks RH, Culp DA: Complications, results and problems of ileal conduit diversions. *J Urol* 109:210, 1973.

24. Guerrier K, Albert DJ, Persky L: Experiences with pyocystis. *Arch Surg* 103:63, 1971.

25. Stewart WW, Alexander SC, Ireland GW: Experience with pyocystis following intestinal conduit urinary diversion. *J Urol* 109:375, 1973.

26. Richie JP: Intestinal loop urinary diversion in children. *J Urol* 111:687, 1974.

27. Stevens PS, Eckstein HB: The management of pyocystis following ileal conduit diversion in children. *Br J Urol* 47:631, 1975.

28. Coptcoat MJ, Wickham JEA: Laparoscopy in urology. *Min Inv Ther* 1:337, 1992.

29. Matsuda T, Horii Y, Higashi S, Oishi K, Takeuchi H, Yoshida O: Laparoscopic varicocelectomy: A simple technique for clip ligation of the spermatic vessels. *J Urol* 147:636, 1992.

30. Mitchell MB, Stiegmann GV, Mansour A: Improved technique for establishing pneumoperitoneum for laparoscopy. *Surg Laparosc Endosc* 1(3):198, 1992.

31. Hasson HM: Open Laparoscopy: A report of 150 cases. *J Reprod Med* 12:234, 1974.

32. Green LS, Loughlin KR, Kavoussi LR: Management of epigastric vessel injury during laparoscopy. *J Endourol* 6:99, 1992.

33. Parra RO, Hagood PG, Boullier JA, Cummings JM, Mehan DJ: Complications of laparoscopic urologic laparoscopy: Experience at St. Louis University. *J Urol* 151:681, 1994.

34. Reich H: Laparoscopic bowel injury. *Surg Laparosc Endosc* 2:74, 1992.

35. Winfield HN, Donovan JF: Laparoscopic varicocelectomy in. *Semin Urol* 10:152, 1992.

36. Kavoussi LR, Sosa E, Capelouto, CC: Complications of laparoscopic surgery. *J Endourol* 6:95, 1992.

37. Penfield AJ: How to prevent complications of open laparoscopy. *J Reprod Med* 30:660, 1985.

38. Das S, Amar AD: Vesical diverticulum associated with bladder carcinoma: Therapeutic implication. *J Urol* 136:1013, 1986.

39. Kelalis PP, McLean P: The treatment of diverticulum of the bladder. *J Urol* 98:349, 1967.

40. Kutzmann AA: Diverticulum of the urinary bladder: An analysis of 100 cases. *Surg Gynecol Obstet* 56:898, 1933.

41. Gerridzen GR, Futter GN: Ten year review of vesical diverticula. *Urology* 20:33, 1982.

42. Peterson LJ, Paulson DF, Glenn JF: The histopathology of vesical diverticula. *J Urol* 110:62, 1973.

43. Knapperberger ST, Uson AC, Melicow MM: Primary neoplasms occurring in vesical diverticula: A report of 18 cases. *J Urol* 83:153, 1960.

44. Ostroff EB, Alperstein JB, Young JD Jr: Neoplasm in vesical diverticula. *J Urol* 110:62, 1973.

45. Micic S, Ilic V: Incidence of neoplasm in vesical diverticula. *J Urol* 129:734, 1983.

46. Das S: Laparoscopic bladder diverticulectomy. *J Urol* 147:407A, 1992.

47. Parra, RO: Treatment of posterior urethral strictures with a titanium urethral stent. *J Urol* 146:997, 1991.

48. Clayman RV: The use of staples in the urinary bladder. Personal communication.

49. Parra RO: Laparoscopic repair of intraperitoneal bladder perforation. *J Urol* 151:1003, 1994.

50. Schuessler WW, Kavoussi LR, Clayman RV, Vancaille THE: Laparoscopic radical prostatectomy: Initial case report. *J Urol* 147:246A, 1992.

51. Sanchez de Badajoz E, Gallego Perales JL, Reche Rosado A, Gutierrez de la Cruz JM, Jimenez Garrido A: Laparoscopic radical cystectomy and ileal conduit. *Arch Esp Urol* 46:621, 1993.
52. Kavoussi LR, Clayman RV, Burnt LM, Soper NJ: Laparoscopic ureterolysis. *J Urol* 147:426, 1992.
53. Nezhat C, Nezhat F, Green B, Gonzalez G: Laparoscopic ureteroureterostomy. *J Endourol* 6:143, 1992.
54. Erlich RM, Gershman A, Fuchs G: Laparoscopic vesicoureteroplasty in children: initial case reports. *Urology* 43:255, 1994.
55. Cooperman AV, Zucker KA: Laparoscopic guided bowel resection. In: *Surgical Laparoscopy* edited by Zucker KA. St. Louis: Quality Medical Publishing, p 344, 1991.
56. Kozminski M: Laparoscopic urinary diversion. In: *Laparoscopy: Surgical Learning Center*. AUA Office of Education. p 97, 1992.
57. Jordon GH, Winslow BH: Laparoscopically assisted continent catheterizable cutaneous appendicovesicostomy. *J Endourol* 7:517, 1993.
58. Young HH: The operative treatment of vesical diverticulum with report of four cases. *Johns Hopkins Hosp Rep* 13:411, 1906.
59. Jarow JP, Brendler CB: Urinary retention caused by a large bladder diverticulum: A simple method of diverticulectomy *J Urol* 139:1260, 1988.
60. Vitale PJ, Woodside JR: Management of bladder diverticula by transurethral resection: Re-evaluation of an old technique. *J Urol* 122:744, 1979.
61. Orandi A: Transurethral fulguration of bladder diverticulum. New Procedure. *Urology* 10:30, 1977.

13

Laparoscopic Intraperitoneal Drainage of Lymphoceles

Raul O. Parra
John A. Boullier

Introduction

Lymphocele formation occurs in 1 percent to 49 percent of patients who have undergone pelvic lymphadenectomy, renal transplant, or other radical pelvic procedures.[1,2] Their formation is believed to result from inadequate closure of the lymph channels and the inability of the peritoneal surface to accommodate the increased fluid load.[2,3] Studies have demonstrated the ability of lymph fluid to clot and occlude open lymphatic vessels, but at a rate considerably slower than that of serum.[4] Furthermore, the lymph channels do not spasm to assist in closure.[5] Other factors that could contribute to the formation of lymphoceles include perioperative use of heparin, diuretics, infection, lack of drains, use of drains, presence of metastatic tumor, radiation, extensive nodal dissection, and transplant rejection.[2-7]

Most lymphoceles are small and asymptomatic and can be treated expectantly, as spontaneous regression is common.[2] Symptoms are usually related to infection or to the compression of adjacent organs, namely, the ureter, uterus, iliac vessels, bladder, sigmoid colon, or an allograft kidney.[2,8]

When treatment is necessary, a number of methods are available, all equally effective, but each attended by significant disadvantages. External drainage, either percutaneous or open, is widely used, but treatment can be prolonged and secondary infection is common.[1,8] Sclerotherapy can be used as an adjunct, but it also subjects the patient to prolonged treatment. In addition, vital structures directly adjacent to the cavity may be inadvertently sclerosed.[9,10] Internal marsupialization via laparotomy is considered definitive therapy but subjects the patient to considerable morbidity and prolonged convalescence.[10] For these reasons, many physicians are not inclined to administer active treatment.

A recent report on the laparoscopic drainage of a post-transplant lymphocele presented a reasonable and attractive alternative to the management of symptomatic lymphoceles.[10]

In this chapter the basic technique required for drainage of lymphoceles intraperitoneally will be described.

Indications

The basic indications for laparoscopic intraperitoneal drainage are the same as for an open procedure; a symptomatic lymphocele following a radical pelvic surgical procedure or renal transplant.

Contraindications

The most important consideration when deciding how to treat a symptomatic fluid collection suspected of being a lymphocele is to be absolutely certain that the fluid is of lymphatic origin and not a urinoma or hematoma. Equally important is to ascertain that one is not dealing with an infected lymphocele or abscess. Therefore, appropriate attention to the clinical history, symptoms, and appropriate use of imaging studies is imperative. If any doubt exists, percutaneous aspiration of the fluid with chemical analysis and or culture will establish the diagnosis.

Patient Preparation

Parenteral broad spectrum antibiotics should be administered to prevent introducing external pathogens into the rich culture medium that the lymphocele fluid represents.

If the lymphocelectomy is being carried out on a renal transplant recipient, judicious adjustments of the immunosuppressive agents must be carried out prior to the procedure. Likewise a careful review of the operative report is essential in order to anticipate the location of the transplanted ureter and vessels in respect to the lymphocele.

Surgical Technique

Induction of the Pneumoperitoneum and Trocar Location

Since virtually all patients developing a lymphocele have had a previous surgical procedure, most likely an extraperitoneal operation, we advise the use of the open minilaparotomy technique for gaining access. If the surgeon desires to use the Veress cannula, however, then a site other than the umbilicus should be considered in order to avoid the potential bowel loop adherent to the umbilical area.

The number and location of the trocars are basically identical to that employed in a varicocelectomy: three ports arranged in a triangular array (a supraumbilical 10-mm trocar for introduction of the laparoscope, and a 5- and 10-mm trocar at the midclavicular lines placed approximately 5 cm below the navel).

Dissection and Creating the Peritoneal Window

Once access has been obtained and the laparoscope introduced, the lymphocele is readily apparent as a translucent, well-circumscribed bulge immediately over the iliac vessels (Fig. 13-1). Difficulty can arise in discerning the lymphocele mass from the adjacent anatomic structures, as may be the case with those forming after renal transplantation. Identification of the bladder can be facilitated by filling it with 200 to 400 mL of fluid. The lymphocele can usually be seen medial to the fluid-filled bladder and somewhat superomedial to the graft. Another way of confirming the nature of the structure in question is by placing the laparoscope directly against the wall of the mass. A lymphocele should readily transilluminate the light.

Drainage is accomplished by opening the wall of the lymphocele with the electrocautery scissors. After draining the lymph fluid it is important to completely break and evacuate any loculations or coagulated lymph present (Fig. 13-2).

Marsupialization is completed by excising as much of the lymphocele wall as possible (Fig. 13-3). Too small a window can lead to lymph reaccumulation and clinical recurrence.

If the lymphocele is recurrent or the window created is felt to be inadequate—as may be the case in chronic lymphoceles, where the wall becomes quite thick and difficult to resect—then harvesting a vascularized omental patch and placing it inside the lymphocele cavity may help prevent reaccumulation.

Conclusion

The judicious treatment of symptomatic lymphoceles is compromised by the limited number of patients reported on and the considerable divergence of opinion in these reports. In our recent review of the literature it was evident that each proposed therapy has significant disadvantages.[11]

Aspiration is generally unsuccessful, with recurrence rates of up to 90 percent. Repeat aspiration has led to infection of the lymphocele in 10 percent of cases. Two deaths have been reported: One patient died of sepsis,[12] the other from infection and hemorrhage.[8] The duration of therapy and number of aspirations necessary can be considerable but are not routinely reported. One patient with a symptomatic lymphocele was followed for 17 months,[13] and therapy extending to months is not uncommon.

Overall, percutaneous drainage was effective in 73 percent of the cases, but it subjects the patient to a lengthy treatment course (a mean of 30 days) and carries a risk of infection of up to 26 percent. Occasionally percutaneous drainage is not feasible, or is hazardous, when the lymphocele is located posterior to an allograft kidney. Furthermore, fistula formation can be a complication.[8]

Sclerosing of the cavity was effective in 19 of 24 patients; as with other percutaneous methods, the

(a)

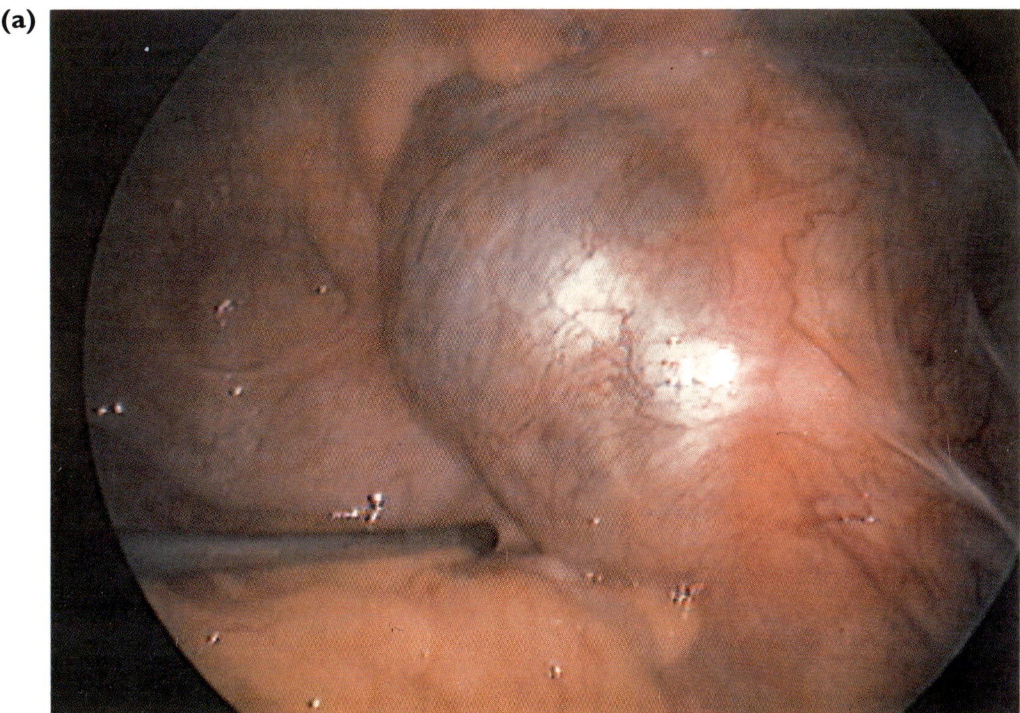

(b)

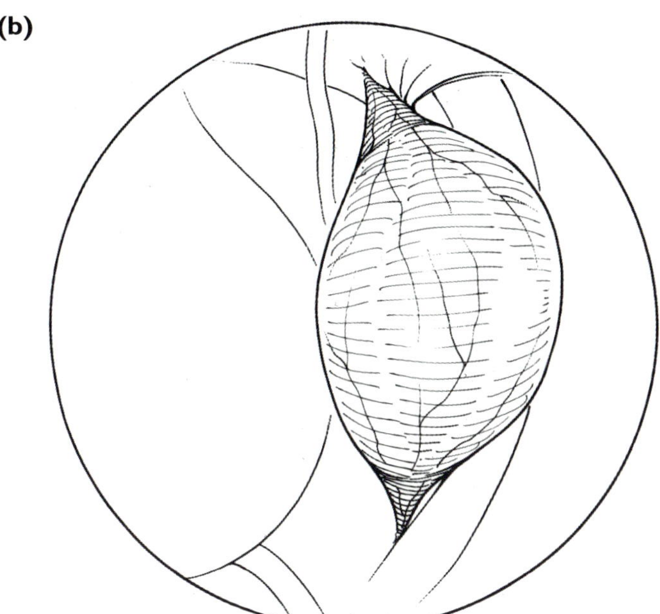

Figure 13-1 (a) Intraoperative view of a right lymphocele overlying the iliac vessels. (b) Line drawing depicting typical appearance of lymphocele.

duration of treatment can be prolonged to several weeks, with a mean of 20 days overall. Also, the distribution of the sclerosing agent cannot be completely controlled, and collateral damage is a considerable hazard. Sclerosing therapy is therefore not recommended when nerves, blood vessels, or vital organs transverse the immediate area.[9,10] Gilliland's report on nine patients is one of the largest and most detailed series. In the eight patients successfully treated, the catheter was left in place an average of 25 days (range, 15 to 37 days), and multiple treatments were the norm.[14]

External drainage is as effective as percutaneous catheterization, but it offers no advantage over the other methods and adds the burden of prolonged wound care. In the cases we reviewed, 18% of patients developed an infection secondary to treatment. Fistula formation is another reported compli-

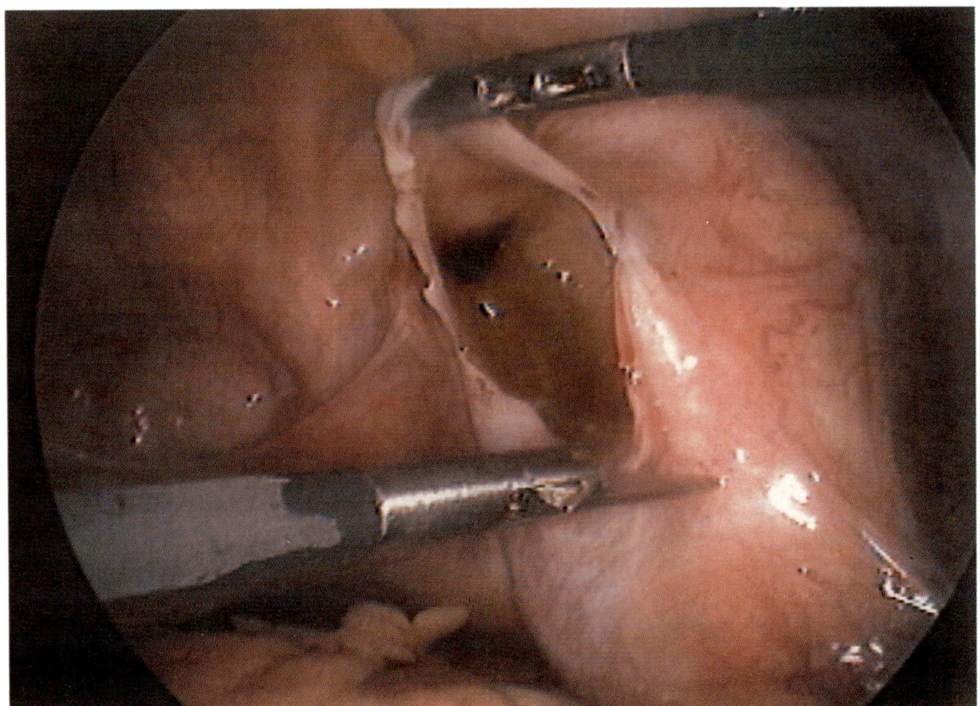

(a)

Figure 13-2 (a) and (b) Opening of the lymphocele wall (note the gelatinous nature of the coagulated lymph). (c) The coagulated lymph must be evacuated from the lymphocele cavity.

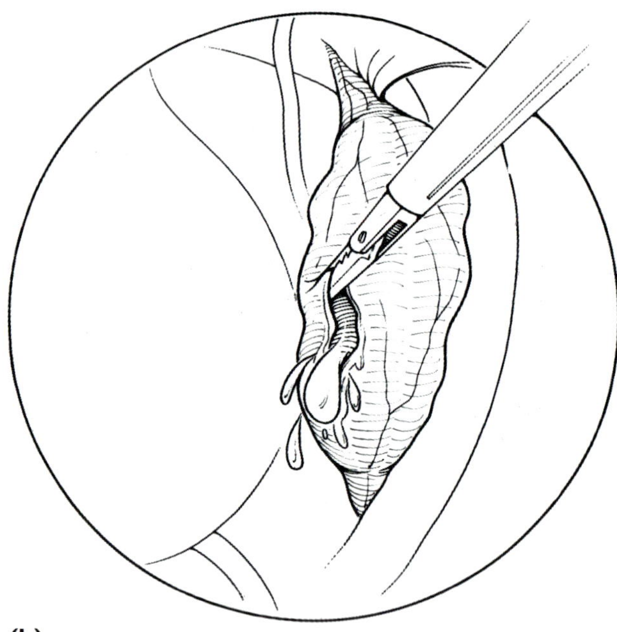

(b)

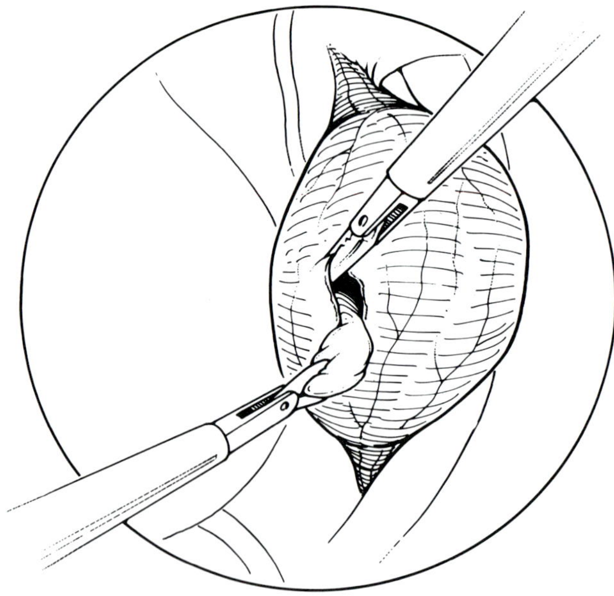

(c)

cation.[15] Two deaths were attributed to this therapy or its failure, one from sepsis[15] and one from pulmonary embolism.[16]

Internal marsupialization is quite effective, but success is not certain.[7] Of 14 failed internal marsupializations, 7 required repeat laparotomy,[9,12,17,18] 3 underwent external drainage,[7,18] 1 had sclerotherapy,[14] and 3 were observed.[19-21] A second consideration is the prolonged recovery secondary to laparotomy. The duration of hospitalization and convalescence is not routinely reported in the published cases. In our experience, having treated 3 patients by internal drainage via laparotomy, all patients left the hospital within a week, but none were able to resume regular activity in less than 3 weeks.

Finally, conservative treatment can occasionally be recommended, especially with incidentally discovered, asymptomatic collections. Although Mori showed that most lymphoceles are small and will resolve spontaneously,[2] conservative treatment can

17. Bear RA, McCallum RW, Cant J, Goldstein MB, Johnson M: Perirenal lymphocyst formation in renal transplant recipients. *Urology* 7:581, 1976.

18. Brockis JG, Hulbert JC, Patel AS, et al: The diagnosis and treatment of lymphoceles associated with renal transplantation. A report of 6 cases and a review in the literature. *Br J Urol* 50:307, 1978.

19. Greenberg BM, Perloff LJ, Grossman RA, Naji A, Barker CF: Treatment of lymphocele in renal allograft recipients. *Arch Surg* 120:501,1985.

20. Lerut T, Lerut J, Broos P, Gruwez JA, Michielsen P: Lymphatic complications in renal transplantation. *Eur Urol* 6:83, 1980.

21. McLoughlin MG, Williams GM: Late perirenal lymphocele causing ureteral and arterial obstruction in renal transplant patients. *J Urol* 114:527, 1975.

22. Basinger GT, Gittes RF: Lymphocyst: Ultrasound diagnosis and urologic management. *J Urol* 114:740, 1975.

23. Spring DB, Schroeder D, Sankaran B, Agee R, Gooding GAW: Ultrasonic evaluation of lymphocele formation after staging lymphadenectomy for prostatic carcinoma. *Radiology* 141:479, 1981.

24. Gray MJ, Plentl AA, Taylor HC Jr: The lymphocyst: a complication of pelvic lymph node dissections. *Am J Obstet Gynecol* 45:1059, 1958.

14

Laparoscopic Renal and Ureteral Surgery

J. G. Valdivia-Uria

Introduction

Until recently the application of laparoscopy in urology was limited to the localization of intra-abdominal nonpalpable testes and the investigation of intersexual states.[1,2,3,4] Over the last several years, however, laparoscopic surgery has materialized as an alternative surgical modality for many urological diseases. Hitherto, transperitoneal monitoring of percutaneous kidney surgery in pelvic ectopia,[5] laparoscopic corrections of varicoceles,[6] orchiectomies for intra-abdominal testes,[7] nephrectomies,[8] nephroureterectomies,[9] ureterolysis,[10] ureterolithotomy,[11] ureterorrhaphies,[12] cystorrhaphies,[13] cervicourethropexies,[14] laparoscopic excision of bladder diverticula,[15] lymphadenectomies,[16,17] cutaneous ureteroileostomies,[18] drainage of lymphoceles,[19,20,21] renal biopsies,[22] marsupialization of renal cysts,[23] and even cystectomies[24] have been performed.

In this chapter the basic laparoscopic techniques applied to the kidney and ureter will be described.

Laparoscopic Approach to the Kidney

In spite of the retroperitoneal location of the kidney its laparoscopic approach can readily be accomplished transperitoneally. The retroperitoneal route (retroperitoneoscopy) nevertheless represents another valuable adjunct to the laparoscopic surgeon as illustrated in Chap. 17. We will limit our discussion in this chapter to the classic transperitoneal technique.

Access to the Abdominal Cavity

When dealing with kidney and upper-ureteral laparoscopic surgery, there is no need to modify the periumbilical access of the first trocar (10 to 12 mm). To introduce the laparoscope a cutaneous (semilunar) incision is usually performed in the upper or lower aspect of the umbilicus. Alternatively, a short vertical incision 2 or 3 cm above the navel may be utilized.

When dealing with a patient who has had a previous laparotomy via a midline incision, and is therefore, suspected of adhesions in this area, we would utilize a Hasson trocar (Chap. 5). If a Hasson trocar is not available, we insufflate the abdomen with approximately 5 L of CO_2 via an upper-quadrant stick, followed by the placement of a 5-mm trocar through the insufflation site. Then either a 5-mm laparoscope or, if that is not available, a 12-degree cystoscope lens is passed to allow the placement of a 10- to 12-mm trocar under direct vision, eliminating the potential risk of bowel injury.

The pneumoperitoneum can also be induced with the patient already in the lateral decubitus position by simply inserting the Veress needle lateral to the corresponding rectus muscle at the level of the umbilicus. Inserting the first trocar through this site instead of employing the usual umbilical location avoids repositioning of the patient. Lately, we have avoided patient repositioning and blind Veress needle insertion by introducing a 10- to 12-mm trocar directly via a minilaparotomy with the patient in the lateral decubitus position.

Trocar Placement and Location

When the patient is supine a 10- to 12-mm trocar is placed via the umbilical incision. Once the initial umbilical trocar is in place, two additional ports are placed under visual control, one located subcostally along the corresponding midclavicular line and the other following the same direction at the level of the iliac fossa near McBurney's point (Fig. 14-1). We prefer to use 10- to 12-mm sizes for all trocars because it allows more flexibility in terms of passage of instruments and tissue retractors. Renal cyst marsupialization or ureteral lithotomies can be readily performed with this trocar configuration. For a nephrectomy two additional access ports are usually necessary, and prior to their placement the patient is turned into the lateral decubitus position. Following repositioning, two 5- to 12-mm trocars are then inserted along the mid-axillary line, one subcostally and the other at the level of the umbilicus (Fig. 14-2). Alternatively, as described above, all trocars may be placed with the patient in the lateral decubitus position from the onset.

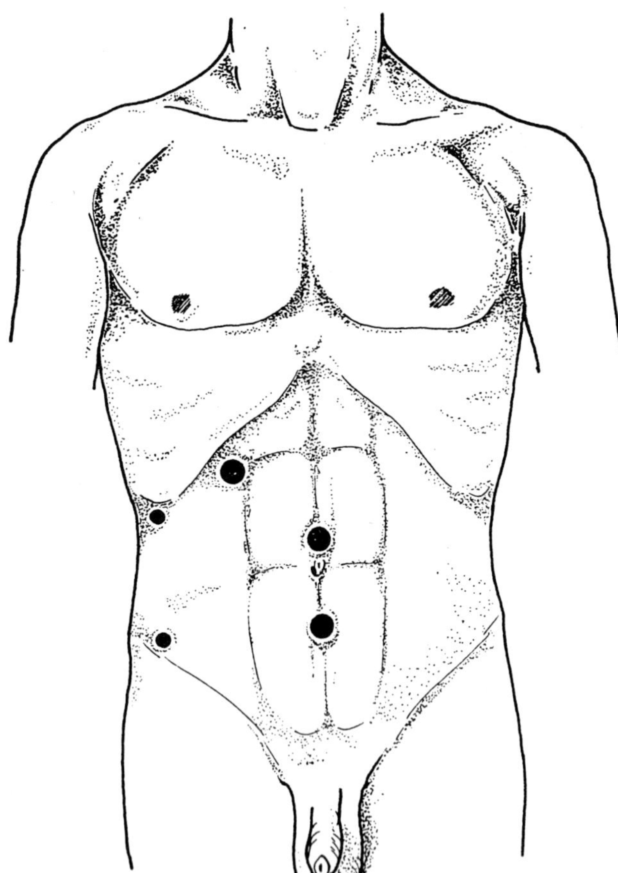

Figure 14-2 Portals for laparoscopic nephrectomy.

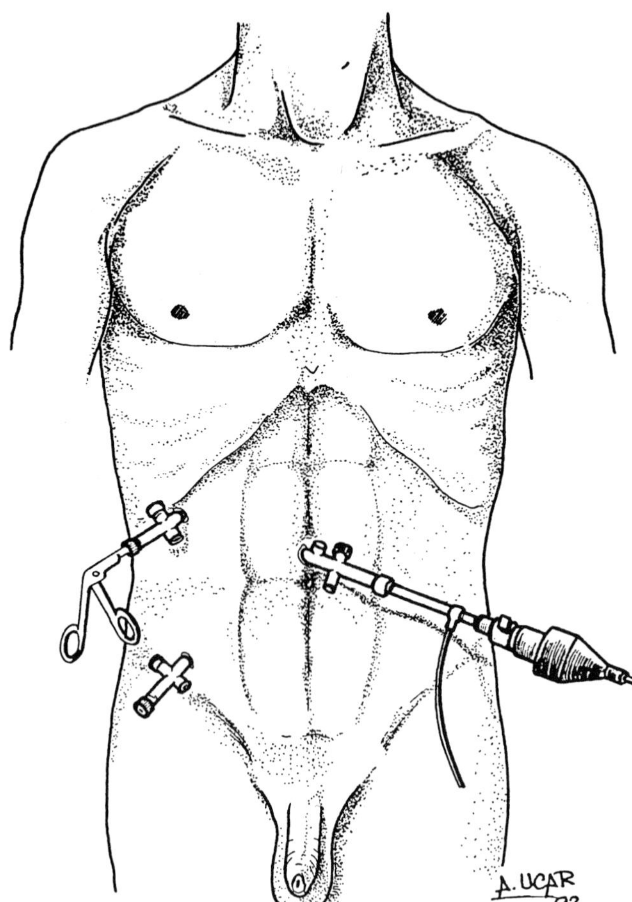

Figure 14-1 Initial portal placements for a simple kidney operation.

Renal Exposure

The transperitoneal laparoscopic access to the renal area does not differ from that carried out through an open laparotomy. In order to enter the renal cell it is necessary to separate the colon of the corresponding side from its attachment to the lateral body wall. The following steps are usually followed in exposing the kidney endocavitarily.

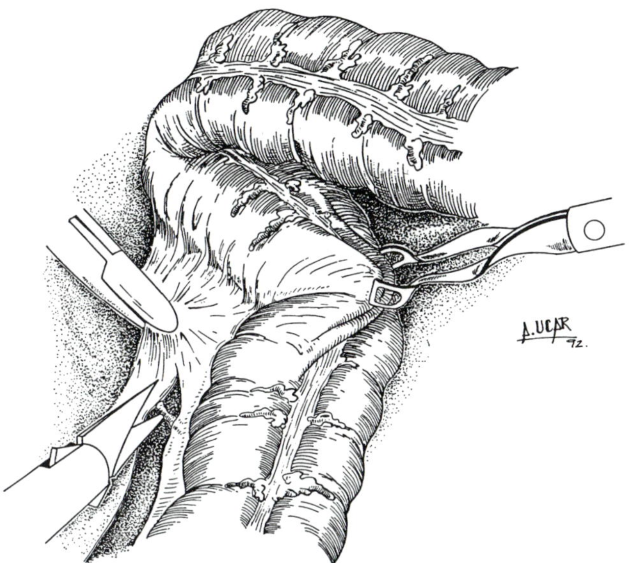

Figure 14-3 Opening of the line of Toldt. The endo-Babcock forceps retracts the colon towards the midline.

Opening of the Parietal Colic Space (Incision of the Line of Toldt)

Using the principles of traction and countertraction, an assistant grasps the lateral parietal peritoneum with tooth forceps while the surgeon retracts the colon itself with atraumatic forceps or an endo-Babcock (Fig. 14-3). This places the lateral peritoneal reflection under tension, facilitating its incision with the electric scissors. The incision extends from the aortic bifurcation caudally to past the hepatic or splenic flexure cranially depending upon the side being operated upon. The hepato or spleno-renal ligaments are then divided to facilitate the exposure of the upper pole of the kidney. A combination of blunt and sharp dissection assisted by medial retraction of the colon results in the development of the corresponding retroperitoneal space. On the right side, exposure of the medial aspect of the kidney is accomplished by the performance of a Kocher maneuver. We have found the use of the endo-Kitner dissector quite useful for this step. Following completion of these steps the vena cava on the right and lateral aorta on the left should be easily identified. The kidney(s) covered by Gerota's fascia are then approached. Special care must be taken with regard to exposure and liberation of the upper renal poles, especially on the right. The superior half of the right kidney is covered by the subhepatic peritoneal reflection. In order to obtain optimum mobilization, this segment of parietal peritoneum must be divided. This can be made easier by cephalad retraction of the liver with a fan retractor passed through a upper anterior mid-clavicular-line port (Fig. 14-4). The peritoneal reflection is then divided in a medial to lateral fashion. During this maneuver one sometimes encounters small vessels, which must be either cauterized or clipped.

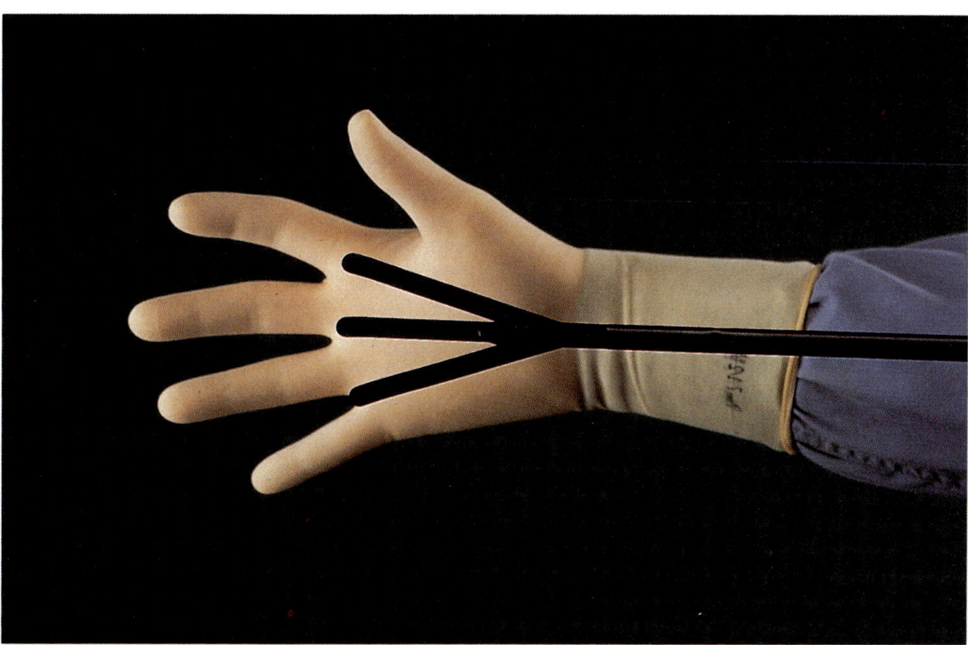

Figure 14-4 Endo-fan retractor.

Dissection of the Retroperitoneal Structures

The degree of dissection carried out depends upon the intent of the procedure. When a simple biopsy or lower pole renal cyst marsupialization is the sole purpose of the operation, one only needs to expose the renal capsule over the area of interest. This is accomplished by grasping Gerota's fascia and dissecting with cautery scissors until the plane between the renal capsule and perirenal fat is developed. Once the capsule is visualized, sharp and blunt dissection is then used to separate the kidney from the rest of the contents of the renal cell.

Ureteral Dissection and Securement

If the upper pole or posterior aspect of the kidney needs to be accessed or if the planned procedure is a nephrectomy, the next step must be the dissection and securement of the ureter. Placement of a 7 or 8 French ureteral catheter prior to the surgery has been recommended to aid this dissection. We have found that the easiest way to identify the ureter is to go directly to the iliac bifurcation. Once the ureter is identified it is grasped with atraumatic forceps or an endo-Babcock. Alternatively, securement of the ureter may be accomplished by encircling it with an umbilical tape brought out through a trocar port. A combination of sharp and blunt dissection is then employed to detach the ureter from the surrounding retroperitoneal tissues (Fig. 14-5). The ureter can then be followed as high as the renal pelvis. During the dissection, one commonly encounters the gonadal veins coursing parallel and medial to the ureter. These veins are best clipped and divided to avoid their inadvertent avulsion. In cases where the ureter is difficult to identify, (because of anatomical variance, inflammation, or fibrosis) the previously placed ureteral catheter can be useful. Movement of the stent from below is transmitted to the retroperitoneal structures overlying the ureter, thereby facilitating its identification.

Renal Dissection

The dissection starts at the lower pole and proceeds along its internal border to the upper pole. By sequentially grasping the perirenal tissues and dissecting with endoscissors between the renal capsule and perirenal fat, the plane between these structures is developed just as one would do in an open procedure. The upper pole is handled as previously explained. If the operation is to be a radical nephrectomy, then the dissection must be carried out extrafascially.

Hilar Dissection

Three maneuvers facilitate the exposure and dissection of the renal vascular pedicle; liberation of the upper pole, caudal traction on the ureter, and lateral displacement of the upper pole with an endo-Kitner dissector or similar instrument. This latter maneuver

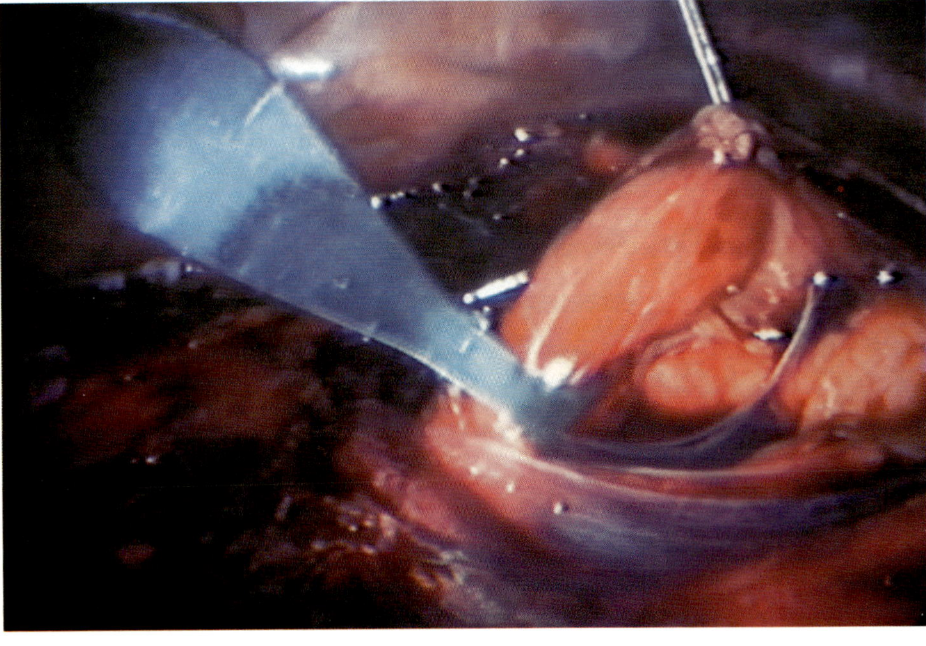

Figure 14-5 Ureter exposed and grasped by endo-Babcock.

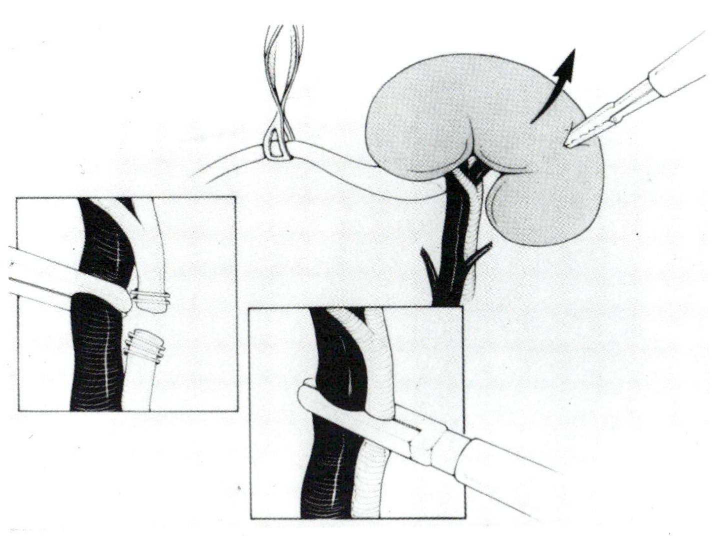

Figure 14-6 *Right*, Traction on upper pole and ureter which facilitates exposure of renal pedicle. *Left*, Demonstration of transection techniques of the renal pedicle with the GIA endostaple.

places the renal pedicle under stretch, which facilitates its dissection with a combination of sharp and blunt maneuvers (Fig. 14-6). The renal vein is first exposed and dissected free of its perivascular attachments. Once this is done it can be retracted superiorly and the artery dissected by progressively dividing the overlying tissues with the aid of the electrocautery scissors. Once isolated, the renal artery is clip ligated with 9-mm titanium clips. If possible, 2 or 3 clips are placed proximally and 2 distally (Fig. 14-6, Box). Then the artery can be safely transected. The vein can be similarly handled. However, it is not unusual to find a renal vein, especially on the right, whose diameter is such that it cannot be safely handled with existing endoclips. In this situation, it is better to use the endo-GIA linear stapler, which not only divides but simultaneously places three rows of staples on each side of the cut vessel (Fig. 14-6, Box). Once the pedicle is safely transected, any remaining attachments are either cut or cauterized (Fig. 14-7).

Division of the Ureter

The final step consists of dividing the ureter at the level of the iliac bifurcation by simply double clip ligating its proximal and distal ends and transecting it.

Removal of Specimen

Removal of the kidney can be accomplished in several ways.

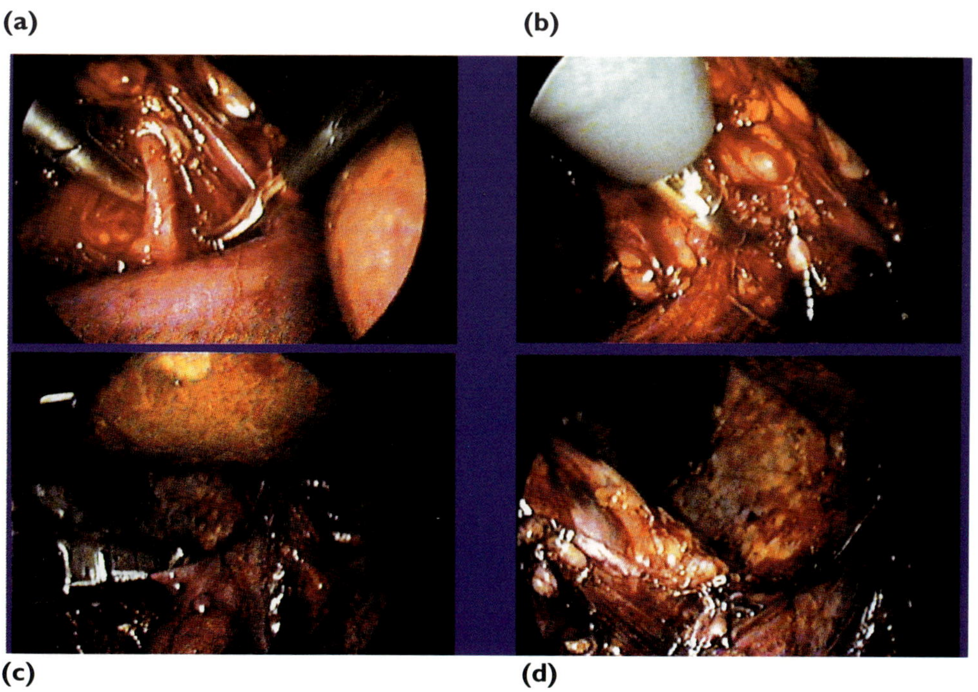

Figure 14-7 Typical sequence of the most commonly utilized technique for division of the renal pedicle. (a) Dissection of the renal artery. (b) Clipping and transection of the renal artery. (c) Endo-GIA division of renal vein. (d) Transected renal pedicle

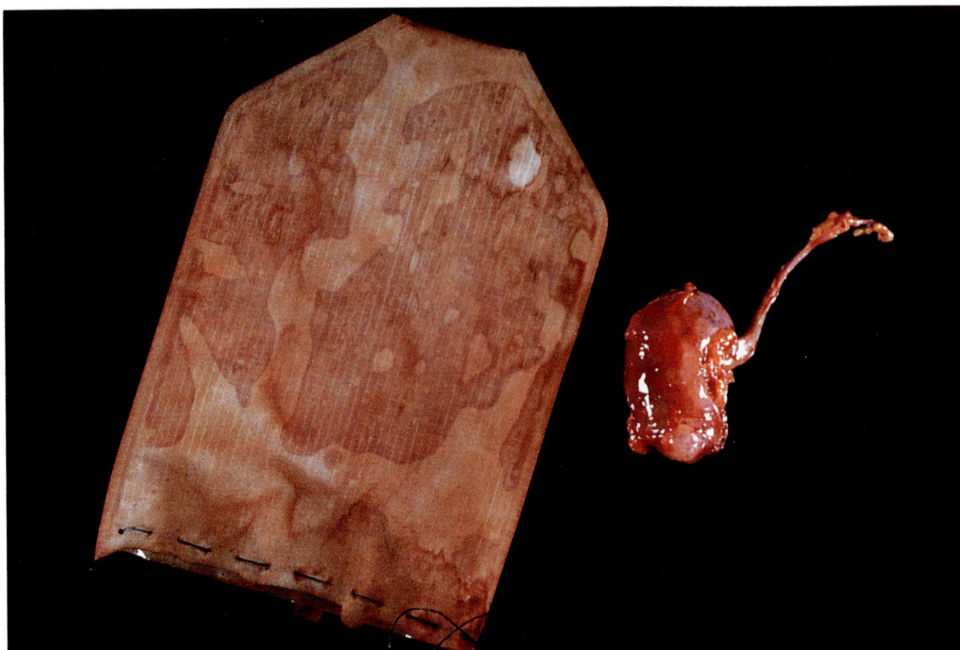

Figure 14-8 Relationship of small intact kidney and commonly employed endo-retrieval bag.

Intact without an Entrapment Bag

If the renal unit is small, it may be grasped by the ureter with either a 10-mm cup biopsy or a large tooth gall bladder grasping forceps and removed via the 12-mm umbilical port. This can be facilitated by withdrawing the trocar sheath while applying continuous traction on the kidney. Occasionally the incision must be slightly enlarged to deliver the specimen. Alternatively, in the female patient the kidney can be retrieved transvaginally after making an incision through the cul-de-sac.

Intact with an Entrapment Bag

Several organ retrieval bags are commercially available. They are usually introduced via a 12-mm port. Once inside the peritoneal cavity they must be opened by grasping the edges with traumatic grasping forceps. The kidney is then placed inside the bag, the bag closed and its neck drawn as far as possible into the trocar sheath of a 12-mm trocar. The sheath and the sac can then be removed in toto as mentioned above (Fig. 14-8).

Removal with Tissue Fragmentation

If the kidney is of such volume that it does not allow intact removal it must be fragmented. Although the use of the endo-tissue morcellator has been advocated, it is not universally available. We have found the following alternative technique efficacious and inexpensive. Once the organ retrieval bag has been pulled through the trocar site, its mouth is opened and with close endoscopic control a pair of long heavy scissors is introduced and the kidney is cut into pieces. The bag and its contents can then be delivered out of the body (Fig. 14-9).

Other Laparoscopic Operations upon the Kidney

Laparoscopic Excision of Renal Cysts

The steps to obtain renal exposure are the same as that described for a nephrectomy. The exeresis of the cyst wall is simple once the contents are evacuated with an endoscopic needle. When removing the cyst fluid it is advisable to transfix or grasp the edges of the wall of the cyst in the area near the renal parenchyma, since there is a tendency for the cyst to disappear into the depth of the operating field after the fluid is removed. The cyst wall is totally excised and any loculations broken up (Fig. 14-10). Careful inspection of the cyst wall must be performed so that the rare neoplasm is not missed. Following excision of the cyst it is desirable to cover the resulting defect with any remaining perirenal fat. This tissue approximation can be readily accomplished with an automatic hernia stapler.

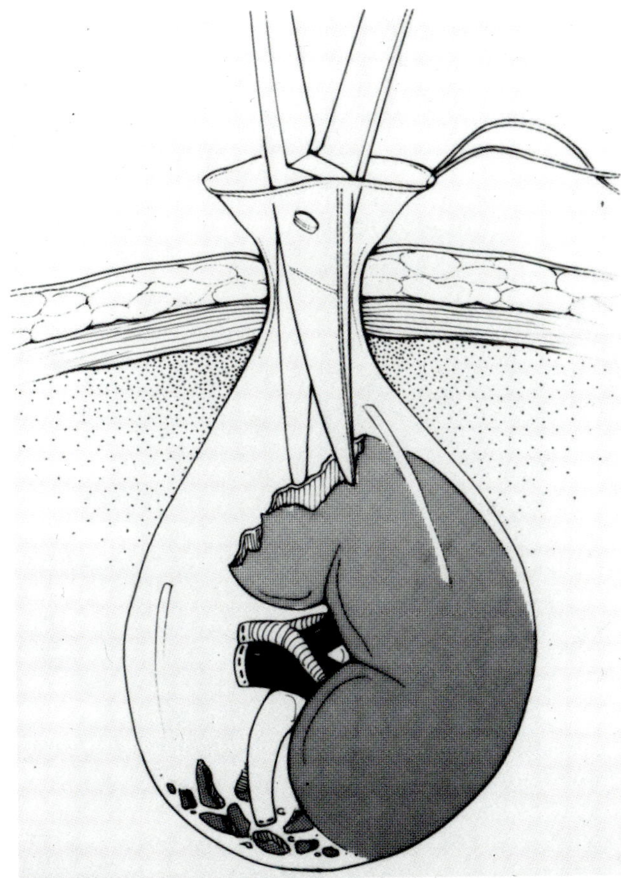

Figure 14-9 Morcellation of kidney with scissors.

Renal Tumorectomy

At present no indication exists for this technique if malignancy exists. However, in the rare instance of a known benign renal mass such as an angiomyolipoma this procedure may represent an alternative to open enucleation. After renal exposure the parenchyma near the tumor mass is circumscribed with the electrocautery scissors and the tumor enucleated (Fig. 14-11). Recent technological advances such as the coagulating Argon laser can prove useful in obtaining hemostasis. If necessary, superselective embolization of the arteries feeding the mass can be undertaken. Following excision the defect can be covered with remaining perirenal fat or Gerota's fascia as previously described.

Renal Biopsy

Laparoscopic guided percutaneous renal biopsy is an alternative in those individuals who because of medical contraindication or body habitus are candidates for an open renal biopsy. At this moment we advocate a retroperitoneoscopic approach rather than a transperitoneal access for this procedure (Chap. 17).

Laparoscopic Monitoring of Percutaneous Access to Pelvic Kidneys

This procedure has been described by Eshghi and colleagues in patients with pelvic kidneys and a

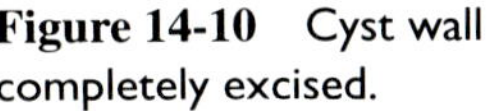

Figure 14-10 Cyst wall completely excised.

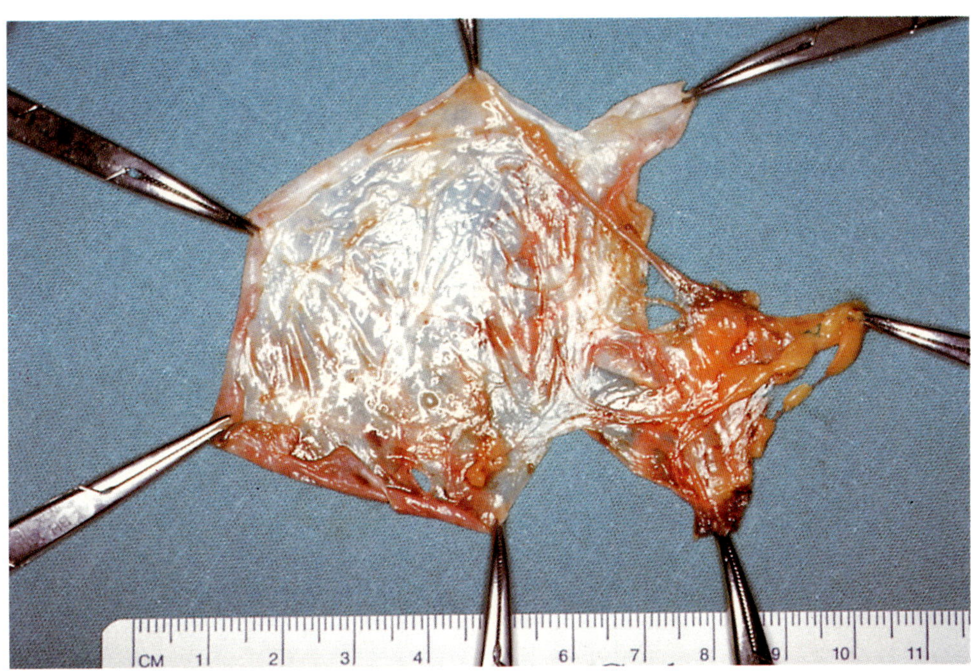

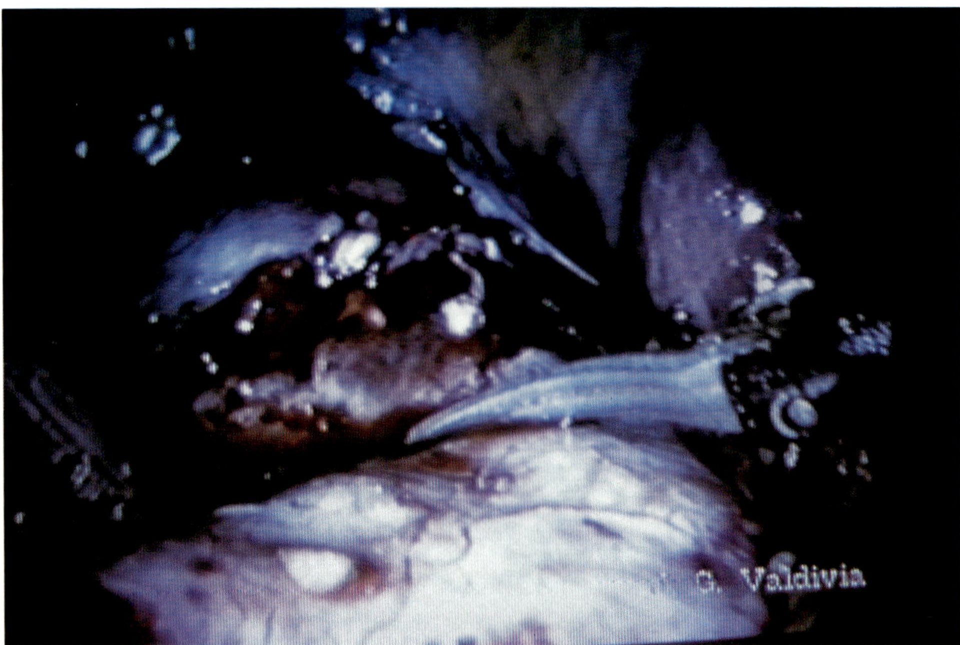

Figure 14-11 Renal tumorectomy. The electrocautery scissors separate the tumor from the renal parenchyma.

staghorn calculus as a means of obtaining safe and accurate percutaneous access.[5]

Laparoscopic Pyelo-Ureterolithotomy in Cases of Complex Lithiasis

This is a feasible alternative which we have employed in a case involving stones located in an anomalous kidney. The same technique can be applied to patients with horseshoe kidneys (Fig. 14-12).

Partial Nephrectomy

Laparoscopic partial nephrectomy is a feasible procedure which has been performed in patients with lower pole calculi beneath a thin layer of renal tissue.[25] The technical principles outlined in the section on tumorectomy apply here as well.

Pyeloplasty

The Anderson Hine technique of dismembered pyeloplasty has been successfully performed in selected patients by Schuessler and Kavousi.[26] It should be noted, however, that the intracorporeal suture techniques currently used to accomplish the procedure are tedious and time-consuming. A more practical approach may be that of tissue welding with biological glues activated with a laser. Given the multiple alternative minimally invasive techniques for the treatment of UPJ obstruction, it is unlikely that this procedure will find widespread acceptance.

Nephroureterectomy

The technique for the nephrectomy is the same. The ureterectomy, however, requires dissection of the ureter to the vesical junction and in the male may require division of the vas deferens for adequate mobilization of the distal ureteral segment. Excision of the entire ureter may be accomplished by either of the following two methods. Prior to the laparoscopic procedure, a transurethral resection of the hemitrigone and intramural ureter may be performed allowing intracavitary removal of the entire ureter (Fig. 14-13). Alternatively, the hemitrigone may be partially resected followed by the laparoscopic excision of the bladder cuff with the endo-GIA stapler.[27]

Laparoscopic Ureteral Surgery

At present the best indications for laparoscopic ureteral surgery are retroperitoneal fibrosis and impacted ureteral calculi not amenable to other treatments. Ureteral repair and ureteral reimplantation, although anecdotally performed, must at pre-

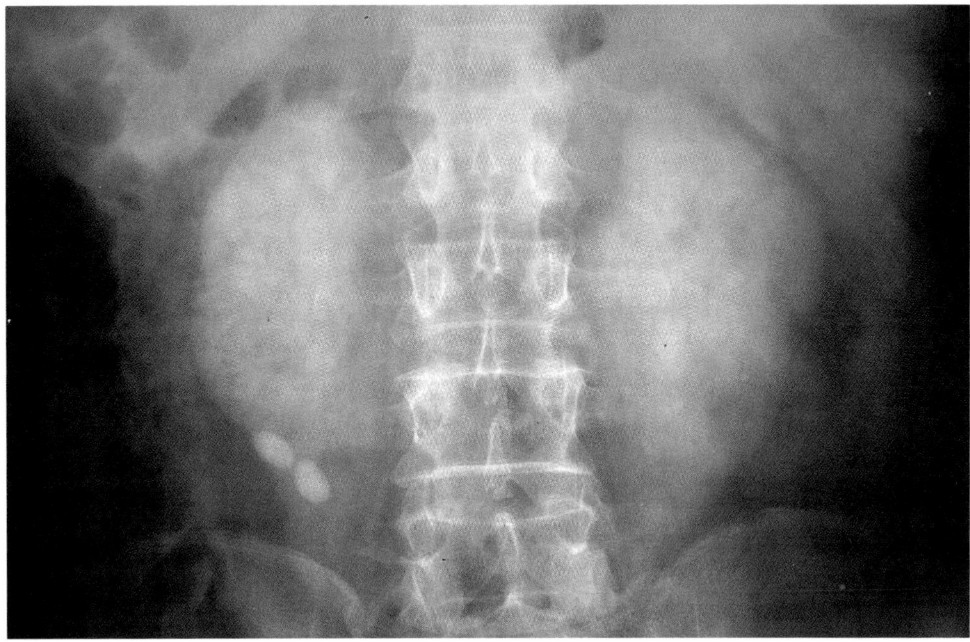

(a)

(b)

Figure 14-12 (a) Lithiasis in pelvis of horseshoe kidney. Patient who failed previous PCNL and ESWL.
(b) Urographic study of the same case.

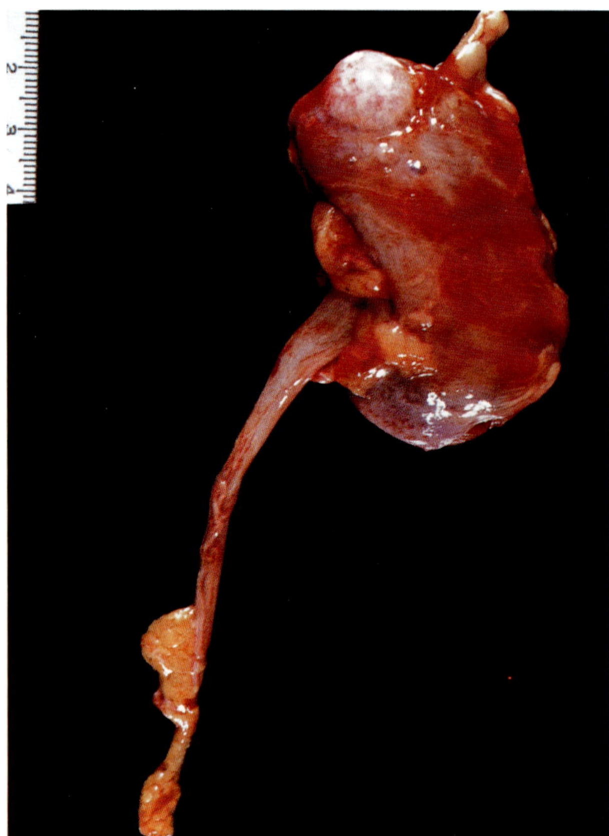

Figure 14-13 Nephroureterectomy specimen after transurethral ureteral detachment.

sent be considered experimental techniques. Patient preparation and positioning, establishment of the pneumoperitoneum, and trocar placement are virtually identical to that previously described for laparoscopic renal surgery.

Ureterolysis

The main reason to perform ureterolysis is obstruction. Every effort should be made preoperatively to establish not only the diagnosis and significance of the hydronephrosis but also the length of ureter involved. Minimum preoperative studies include a CT scan of the abdomen and pelvis and retrograde pyelogram of the involved ureter. If renal function is in question, a renal scan with DTPA and Lasix washout should be obtained. When dealing with an azotemic patient, temporary drainage by either ureteral stenting or percutaneous nephrostomy is imperative until the clinical picture stabilizes.

As in renal surgery, a 7 or 8 French ureteral catheter is passed to the renal pelvis over a guidewire. The guidewire should be left in so that after the ureterolysis is completed an internal double J stent can be exchanged with the external stent. The steps for exposure are exactly as those for a nephrectomy or nephroureterectomy.

In cases of retroperitoneal fibrosis it is best to first locate, free, and secure the upper ureter in an area close to the renal pelvis that is not involved by the fibrotic process. This is easily accomplished by grasping the ureter with atraumatic forceps, pulling it upward and then with the tips of the scissors creating a window through which one side of the endo-Babcock can be passed to grasp the ureter in a secure fashion. The ureter can then be placed under tension, allowing the plane between the ureter and the retroperitoneum to be established to the level of the obstruction. At this point, a biopsy of the fibrotic plaque must be performed to rule out a possible malignancy. If the frozen section returns with a positive result, we recommend a formal laparotomy. If no cancer is found, sharp and blunt dissection is used to completely free the ureter. If necessary the vas deferens in the male or the round ligament in the female can be divided between hemoclips to allow access to the pelvic ureter. Once the ureter has been freed, the external stent is extracted and a 6 or 8 French double J catheter is exchanged with the external stent over a guidewire. The ureter is then intraperitonealized by approximating the edges of the peritoneal reflection with the endo-hernia stapler posterior to the ureter.

Ureteral Lithotomy

Obviously only those large impacted ureteral stones in which all other forms of therapy have failed are considered candidates for this approach. Identification of the ureter may be aided by the previously described techniques. In instances where the size of the calculus does not allow the passage of a stent or guidewire, or when the often present reactive periureteral inflammation makes visualization of the ureter difficult, the availability of intraoperative fluoroscopy is essential .

Under fluoroscopic guidance the tips of an instrument may be placed at the level of the calculus, facilitating the dissection of the involved ureteral segment. Once the segment of ureter containing the impacted stone has been isolated, an endo-Babcock is used to secure the ureter above the calculus to avoid its possible cephalad migration. If possible, we place a stay suture of 4-0 Vicryl through half the thickness of the ureteral wall immediately proximal and distal to the stone. These sutures are not tied; instead, they are pulled through one of the trocars, placing the ureteral wall on stretch and away from the calculus. Using a hook electrode, the ureter is incised directly over the stone. Once the calculus is visualized it may be necessary to dislodge it with the tips of atraumatic forceps. After the stone is extracted, a stent is passed over the previously placed guidewire and the edges of the ureteral wall approximated with 4-0 polyglycolic sutures. The procedure is terminated by approximating the edges of the peritoneal reflection with the endo-hernia stapler to retroperitonealize the ureter.

Exiting the Abdomen

Exiting the abdomen is the same as for any endocavitary procedure. The intra-abdominal pressure is lowered to about 5 mm of mercury, and the area of dissection is inspected with special attention, in the instance of nephrectomies, to the transected renal pedicle. Irrigation is carried out, and each trocar is removed individually under direct vision. The fascia of every trocar site is closed with 2-0 Vicryl sutures and the skin approximated with a running subcuticular 4-0 Vicryl.

References

1. Silver SJ, Cohen R: Laparoscopy for cryptorchidism. *J Urol* 124:928–929, 1980.
2. G. Páramo P: Utilidad de la laparoscopia en el diagnóstico del testículo intra-abdominal. In: Jornadas Internacionales de Actualización Urológica, Madrid, pp 23–30, 1983.
3. Lowe DH, Brock WA, Kaplan GW: Laparoscopy for localization of non-palpable testis. *J Urol* 131:728–729, 1984.
4. Manson AL, Terhune D, Jordan G, Aumar JR, Peterson N, MacDonald G: Preoperative laparoscopic localization of non-palpable testis. *J Urol* 134:919–920, 1985.
5. Eshghi AM, Roth JS, Smith AD: Percutaneous transperitoneal approach to a pelvic kidney for endourological removal of staghorn calculus. *J Urol* 134:525–527, 1985.
6. Sánchez de Badajoz E, Diaz F, Marín J: Tratamiento endoscópico del varicocele. *Arch Esp Urol* 41:15–16, 1988.
7. Nogueira-Castilho L, Ferreira U, Rodrigues-Netto N Jr, et al: Laparoscopic pediatric orchiectomy. *J Urol* 6:155–157, 1992.
8. Clayman RV, Kavoussi LR, Soper NJ, Albala DM, Figenshau RS, Chandhoke PS. Laparoscopic nephrectomy: Review of the initial 10 cases. *J Endourol* 6:127–132, 1992.
9. Coptcoat MJ: Laparoscopy in Urology: Perspectives and practice. *Br J Urol* 69:561–567, 1992.
10. Kavoussi LR, Clayman RV, Brunt LM, Soper NJ: Laparoscopic ureterolysis. *J Urol* 147:426–429, 1992.
11. Escovar P, Rey M, López JR, Rodriguez M, La Riva F, González RD: Ureterolitotomía Laparosc.*Urol Panamericana* 4:29–34, 1992.
12. Nezhat C, Nezhat F, Green B, Gonzalez G: Laparoscopic Ureteroureterostomy. *J Endourol* 6:143–145, 1992.
13. Reich H, McGlynn F: Laparoscopic repair of bladder injury. *Obstet Gyencol* 76:909–910, 1990.
14. Albala DM, Schuessler WW, Vancaillie TG: Laparoscopic bladder neck suspension. *J Endourol* 6:137–141, 1992.
15. Parra RO, Jones JP, Andrus CH, Hagood PG: Laparoscopic diverticulectomy: Preliminary report of a new approach for the treatment of bladder diverticulum. *J Urol* 148:869–871, 1992.
16. Schuessler WW, Vancaille TG, Reich H, Griffith DP: Transperitoneal endosurgical lymphadenectomy in patients with localized prostate cancer. *J Urol* 145:988–991, 1991.
17. Parra RO, Andrus C, Boullier J: Staging laparoscopic pelvic lymph node dissection: Comparison of results with open pelvic lymphadenectomy. *J Urol* 147(3):875–878, 1992.
18. Kozminski M, Partamian K: Case report of laparoscopic ileal loop conduit. *J Endourol* 6:147–150, 1992.
19. Mulganonkar S, Jacobs MG, Viscuso R, et al: Laparoscopic internal drainage of lymphocele in renal transplant. *Am J Kidney Dis* 19:490–492, 1992.
20. Voeller G, Butts A, Vera S: Kidney transplant lymphocele: Treatment with laparoscopic drainage and omental packing. *J Laparoendosc Surg* 2:53–55, 1992.
21. Khauli RB, Mosenthal AC, Caushaj PF: Treatment of lymphocele and lymphatic fistula following renal transplantation by laparoscopic peritoneal window. *J Urol* 147:1353–1355, 1992.
22. Squadrito JF Jr, Coletta AV: Laparoscopic renal exploration and biopsy. *J Laparoendosc Surg* 1:235–239, 1991.

23. Winfield HN, Farage Y, Godet A, Loening SA: Laparoscopic renal cyst marsupialization. *J Urol* 147:204A, 1992.

24. Parra RO, Andrus CH, Jones JP, Boullier JA: Laparoscopic cystectomy: Initial report on a new treatment for the retained bladder. *J Urol* 148:1140–1144, 1992.

25. Chandhoke S, Clayman RV, Stone AM, McDougal EM, Figenshau RS, Kavoussi LR: Laparoscopic partial nephrectomy (LPN). *J Urol* 147:206A, 1992.

26. Brooks JD, Preminger GM, Kavoussi LR, Schuessler WW, Moore RG: Comparison of endourologic approaches to the ureteropelvic junction obstruction. *J Urol* 151:394A, 1994.

27. Clayman RV, Kavoussi LR, Figenshau RS, Chandhoke PS, Albala DM: Laparoscopic nephroureterectomy: Initial clinical case report. *J Laparoendosc Surg* 1:343–349, 1991.

15

Laparoscopic Adrenalectomy

Raul O. Parra

Introduction

Surgical approaches to the adrenal glands can be classified as either intraperitoneal or extraperitoneal. The intraperitoneal incisions most commonly utilized include anterior accesses via a midline or chevron incision or a thoracoabdominal approach. Extraperitoneal procedures are generally through posterior incisions such as the flank or supracostal. Selection of one operation over the other is dependent on the size and nature of the tumor as well as the surgeon's preference or experience.[1] Regardless of which of the above is performed, postoperative pain and a lengthy convalescence is usually the result experienced by most patients.[2]

The standard postoperative sequelae of the classic surgical approaches described above prompted the performance of laparoscopic adrenalectomies in an effort to provide the patient with those advantages unique to laparoscopic surgery.[3–5] The relative success of these initial cases encouraged others to approach adrenal pathology laparoscopically.[6–12] Currently the adrenals can be endoscopically accessed by either the classic intraperitoneal laparoscopic approach or by retroperitoneoscopy. This chapter will exclusively address the former while the retroperitoneal technique is amply described in Chap. 17.

Contraindications

At present, we do not advocate a laparoscopic adrenalectomy in any patient suspected of harboring an adrenocortical carcinoma. Most malignant adrenal tumors are larger than 6 cm and their capsule is quite thin. The large size of the mass, together with its friability, not only makes their excision difficult but potentially predisposes to intraoperative tumor rupture and dissemination of malignant cells intraperitoneally. Moreover, the surgical approach to a malignant adrenal tumor must be radical, which is difficult to adequately accomplish laparoscopically.

Although functional pheochromocytomas have been successfully removed endocavitarily,[4,6,7,10,12] the simple process of inducing the pneumoperitoneum as well as the manipulation necessary during the dissection can stimulate the tumor and create a hypertensive emergency. Consequently, it has been our policy to abstain from performing laparoscopic surgery in tumors secreting catecholamine.

Other contraindications are identical to those for laparoscopy in general.

Indications

The best indications at the present time for a laparoscopic adrenalectomy include cortical adenomas with hypercorticoid production and tumors inducing hyperaldosteronism. Patients with incidentalomas greater than 3 cm or that demonstrate an increase in

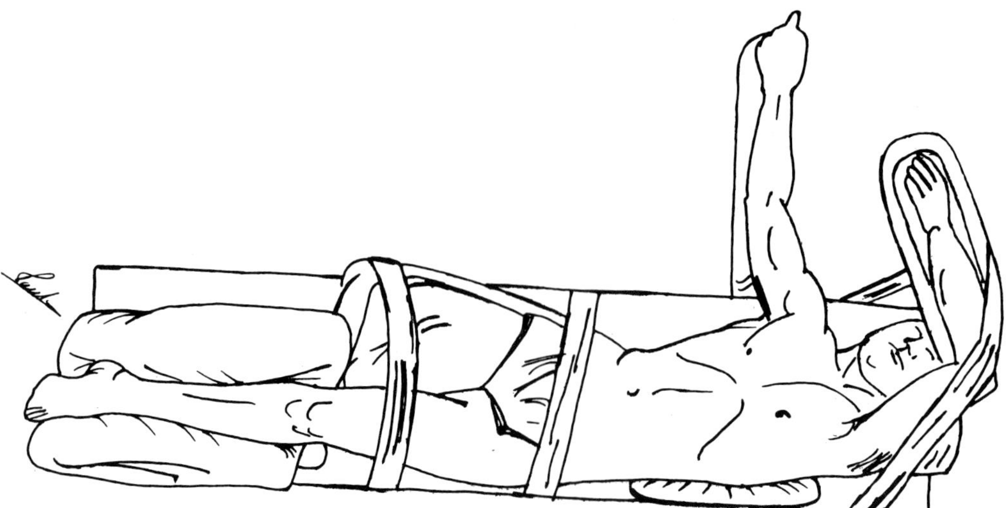

Figure 15-1 Patient positioning for a left laparoscopic adrenalectomy, modified flank position similar to that employed for a thoracoabdominal operation.

growth during follow up also represent candidates for an endocavitary approach.

Preoperative Preparation

Other than the special precautions necessary in any form of adrenal surgery, adequate corticoid or mineral corticoid replacement in the pre- and postoperative period, the preparation is quite similar to that for laparoscopic nephrectomy (Chap. 14). Appropriate imaging studies must be obtained so that the exact size, location, and vascularization of the mass in question can be clearly delineated prior to surgery. Particular attention must be paid in cases being performed for Cushing's syndrome. Not only must special steps be taken with regard to the altered metabolic derangements and possible pulmonary impairment frequently present in these patients, but the body habitus of each individual patient should be carefully evaluated. Indeed, in a morbidly obese patient, strong consideration should be given to an open procedure in order to prevent possible complications.

Patient Positioning and Trocar Placement

Positioning

We place the patient in a modified flank position similar to that employed for a thoracoabdominal operation. With the body at approximately 45 degrees, the ipsilateral arm is brought across the chest and supported on a Krauss stand while the hips are maintained nearly flat (Fig. 15-1).

Pneumoperitoneum and Trocar Location

Since we initiate the procedure with the patient in a modified flank position, it is our preference to utilize an open technique via a minilaparotomy incision to establish the pneumoperitoneum. The incision is made supraumbilically and a Hasson trocar introduced through which prompt insufflation is accomplished. The rest of the trocars are then placed under direct visual control.

Three or four additional ports are necessary. All trocars are 10 to 12 mm and located as depicted in Fig. 15-2. If supplemental trocars become necessary

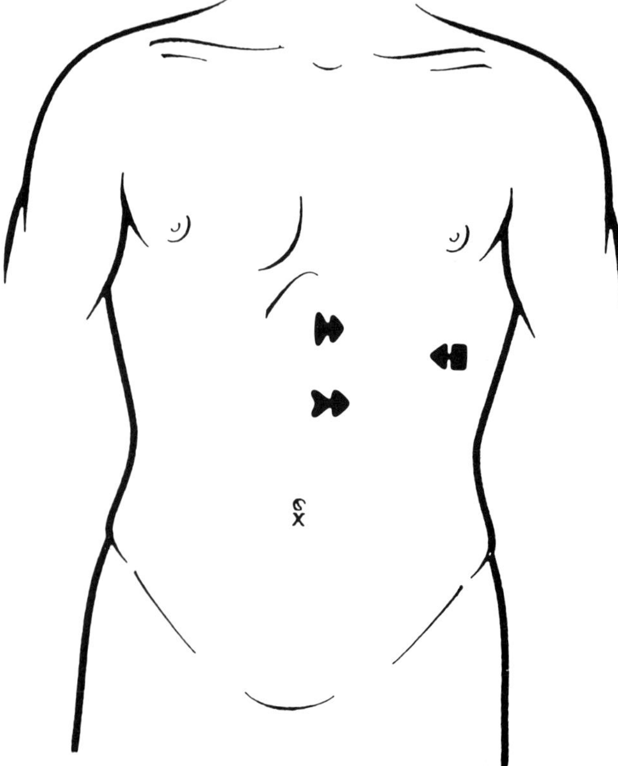

Figure 15-2 Preferred trocar locations for a left adrenalectomy. Conversely, if a right adrenalectomy is to be performed trocar placement mirrors that demonstrated.

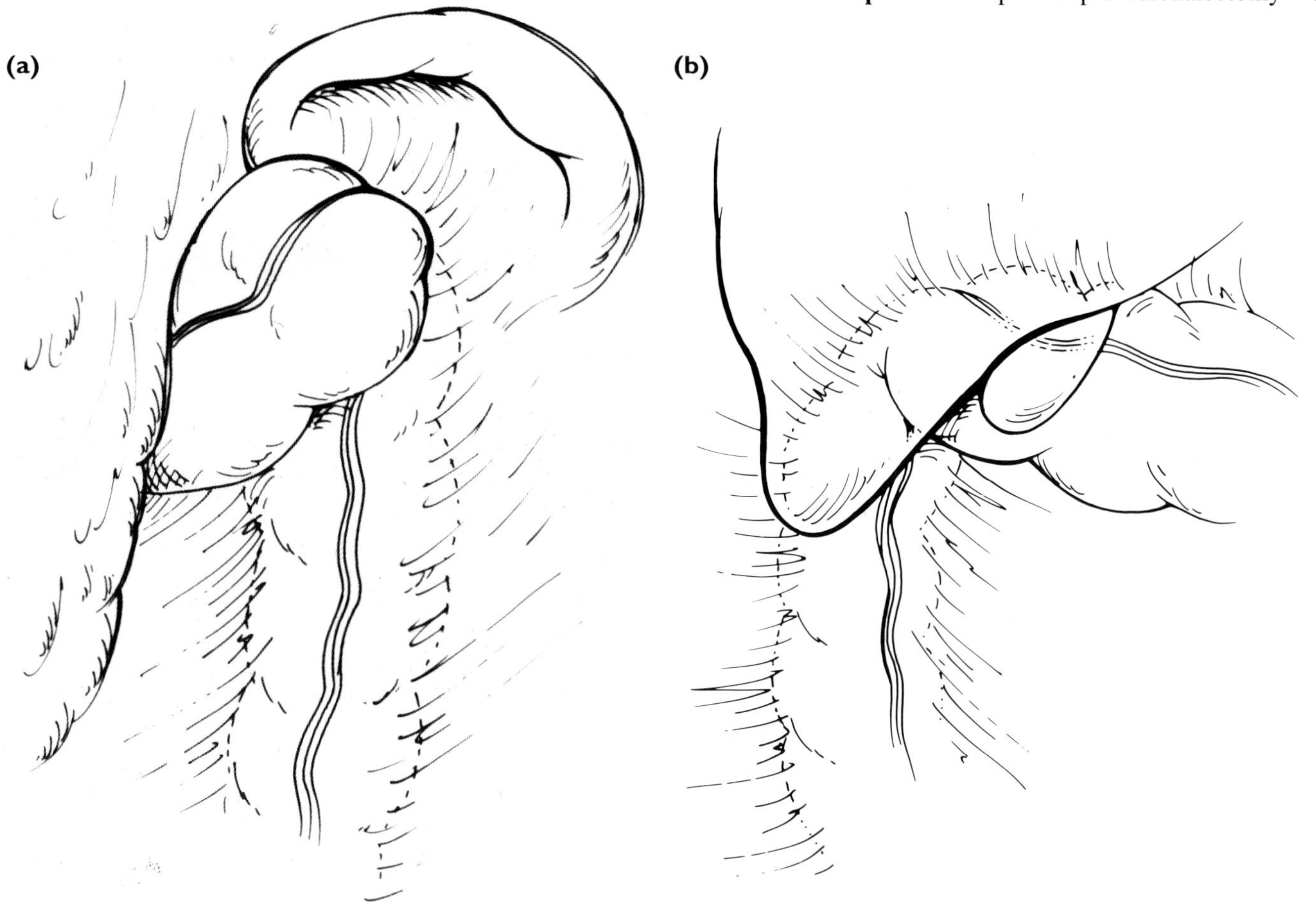

Figure 15-3 (a) Left retroperitoneal exposure is obtained by division of line of Toldt past splenic angle. The spleno-renal and spleno-colic ligaments must be divided for adequate exposure. (b) Exposure for a right adrenalectomy requires opening of the parieto-colic gutter and division of the hepato-colic and hepato-renal ligaments.

as the procedure progresses, these can be arranged in positions dictated by their intended purpose.

Surgical Dissection

Exposure of the adrenal is achieved by incising the line of Toldt all the way past the hepatic or splenic flexure, depending upon which side of the patient is explored (Fig. 15-3). The colon is retracted medially to expose the renal area. Additional bowel displacement can be obtained by rotating the operating table to the contralateral side. An endoscopic fan retractor is quite helpful in retracting the right lobe of the liver or the spleen as the case may be (Fig.15-4).

If a left adrenalectomy is being performed, the dissection is now focused on localizing the left adrenal vein. This is achieved by exposing the left renal vein. The adrenal vein usually drains into the middle or proximal third of the renal vein. Once identified and dissected, the adrenal vein is clip ligated and divided (Fig. 15-5). The perirenal fat attached to the tumor is then dissected from the upper pole of the kidney. I have found this maneuver facilitates manipulation of the adrenal gland with decreased risk of fracture. Once dissected, the upper renal pole is distracted laterally and inferiorly by a blunt instrument and held there by an assistant. A combination of sharp and blunt dissection is then used to separate the diseased adrenal from attachments to the posterior body wall and aorta. Any adrenal vessels encountered are sequentially clip ligated and divided or electrocauterized. When free, the specimen is placed into an endo-bag and extracted through the corresponding trocar site.

The technique for a right adrenalectomy is similar to that described above except that special care must be exercised in controlling the right adrenal vein, which usually enters the inferior vena cava in a posterior and cephalad location. Once the peritoneal

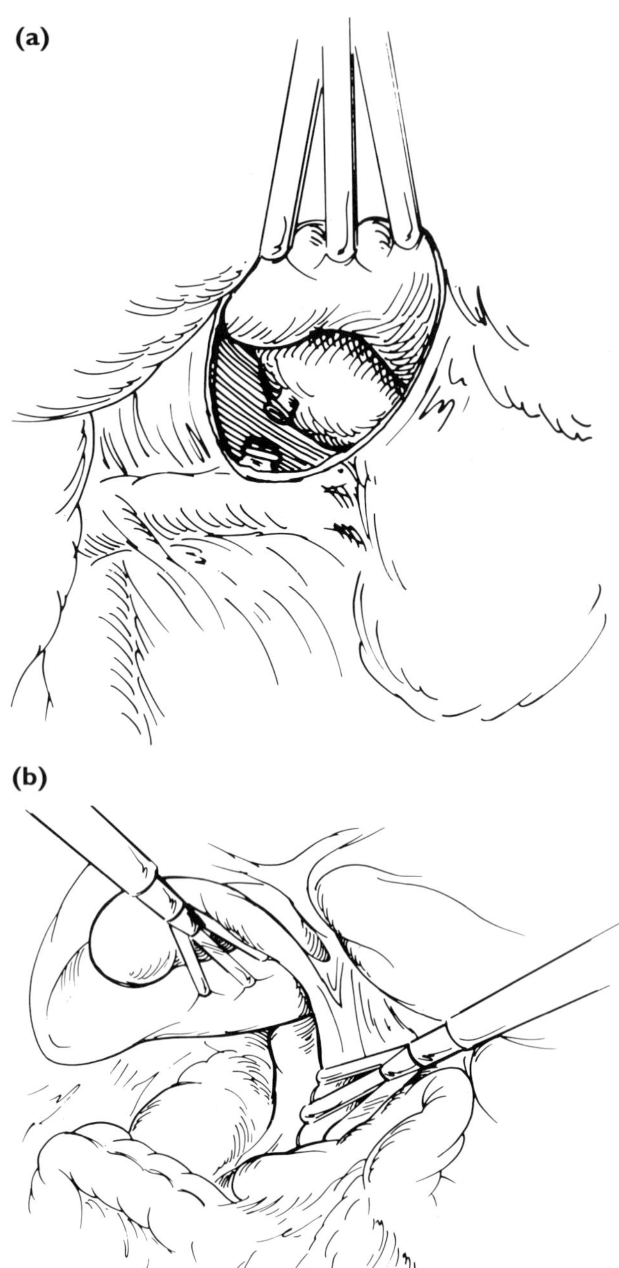

Figure 15-4 (a) Left suprarenal area is exposed. The left renal vein is clearly visible as well as the left adrenal vein. (b) Exposure of the right suprarenal area, (note the fan retractor displacing the liver cephalad).

reflection has been incised, a fan retractor is used to retract the right lobe of the liver superiorly. The posterior peritoneum overlying the inferior vena cava is then incised. This maneuver facilitates exposure of the right renal vein. The dissection then proceeds along the lateral border of the vena cava in a cephalad direction to the level where the adrenal gland and the undersurface of the liver join. The plane between the upper pole of the kidney and adrenal gland is established by sharply dissecting the pararenal fat and Gerota's fascia from the upper renal region. The adrenal is carefully grasped and retracted laterally. This step together with continued dissection along the lateral margin of the vena cava will expose the right adrenal vein (Fig. 15-6). The vein is double clip ligated on the caval side, once on the adrenal side, and divided carefully between the clips. The remaining attachments as well as vascular supply to the gland are then sequentially cauterized or clipped as needed, and the specimen removed as previously described.

Potential complications

Although care must be taken to anticipate and avoid the obvious vascular mishap, the avulsion or slippage of a clip from the adrenal vein, one must also be aware of other potential vascular complications. If the renal vein is not clearly identified, an injury to it can occur during the dissection. If the adrenal mass is large or encroaching upon the renal pedicle, an injury to the renal artery may occur if the dissection is carried out too hastily. A firm knowledge of the regional anatomy is mandatory, particularly in

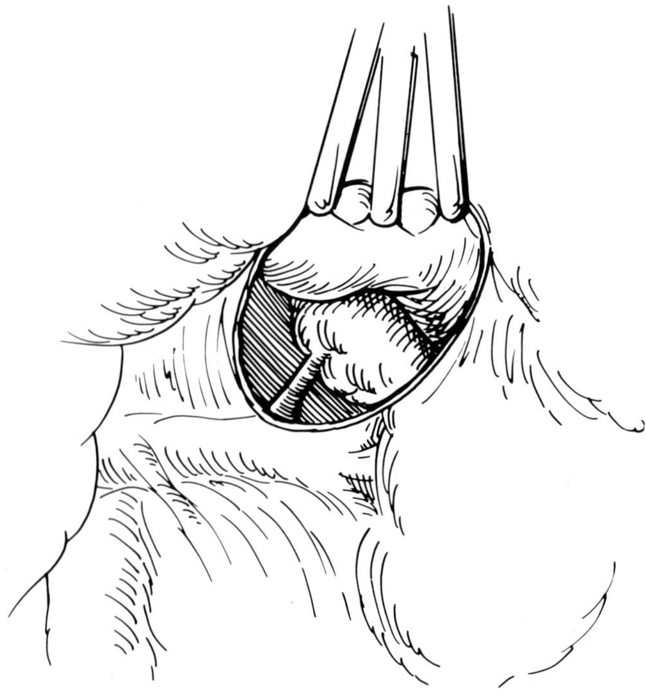

Figure 15-5 Division of the left adrenal vein with clips. This maneuver greatly facilitates the remainder of the dissection.

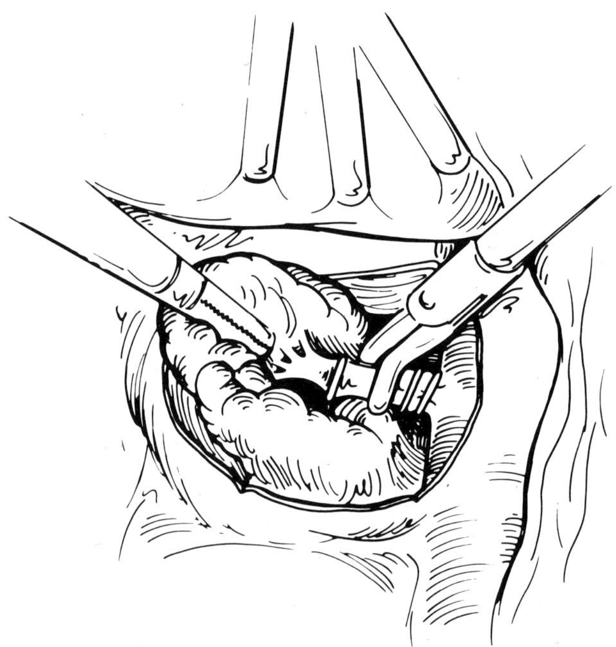

Figure 15-6 Exposure of the right adrenal vein. This is facilitated by lateral traction on the adrenal gland with simultaneous dissection along the vena cava.

view of the different perspective that laparoscopy gives the surgeon.

Other potential sources of problems often encountered are the small adrenal veins and arteries draining to the vena cava or emanating from the aorta and the phrenic, and even lumbar, vessels. Some laparoscopic surgeons advocate the use of the ultrasonic aspirator to perform the dissection.[11] This device, which vibrates at a very high speed, disrupts the connective tissues while sparing the vascular structures, which can then be visualized and handled appropriately.

The spleen on the left or the liver on right may be inadvertently injured during adrenal procedures. Most of the visceral injuries to these organs are caused by retractors. Every attempt to adequately control the bleeding must be employed, since once the pneumoperitoneum is released its tamponading effect will be lost and severe bleeding may ensue in the postoperative period. In such circumstances, the application of hemostatic agents alone or in combination with the coagulating argon laser may save the patient a laparotomy. Failure to satisfactorily control the bleeding is an indication for immediate open exploration.

Conclusions

Laparoscopic adrenalectomy is a novel procedure; nevertheless, more and more reports of its successful application with seemingly excellent results continue to appear in the literature. It seems likely that with experience, improved technique, and a refinement of indications, this laparoscopic technique will find a place in the surgical armamentarium of the urologic surgeon.

References

1. Vaughn ED Jr: Adrenal surgery. In: *Atlas of Urologic Surgery*. Edited by Marshall FF. Philadelphia, WB Saunders, 1991.
2. Scott HW Jr: Anatomy of the adrenal gland and bilateral adrenalectomy. In: *Surgery*. Edited by Nyhus LM, Baker RJ. 2nd ed., vol II, Boston: Little, Brown & Co., p 1373, 1992.
3. Higashihara E, Tanaka Y, Horie S: Laparoscopic adrenalectomy: The initial 3 cases. *J Urol* 149:973, 1993.
4. Gagner M, Lacroix A, Bolte E: Laparoscopic adrenalectomy in Cushing's syndrome and pheochromocytoma [letter]. *N Engl J Med* 327:1033, 1992.
5. Sardi A, McKinnon W: Laparoscopic adrenalectomy for primary aldosteronism [letter]. *JAMA* 269:989, 1993.
6. Suzuki K, Kageyama S, Ueda D: Laparoscopic adrenalectomy: Clinical experience with 12 cases. *J Urol* 150:1099, 1993.
7. Fernandez-Cruz L, Benarroch G, Torres E, Astudillo E, Saenz A, Taura P: Laparoscopic approach to

the adrenal tumors. *J Laparoendosc Surg* 3:541, 1993.

8. Sardi A, McKinnon WMP: Laparoscopic adrenalectomy in patients with primary aldosteronism. *Surg Laparosc Endosc* 4:86, 1994.

9. Naito S, Uozumi J, Ichimiya H, et al: Laparoscopic adrenalectomy: Comparison with open adrenalectomy. *Eur Urol* 26:253, 1994.

10. Gagner M, Lacroix A, Bolte E, Pomp A: Laparoscopic adrenalectomy. The importance of a flank approach in the lateral decubitus position. *Surg Endosc* 8:135, 1994.

11. Takeda M, Go H, Imai T, Komeyana T: Experience with 17 cases of laparoscopic adrenalectomy: Use of ultrasonic aspirator and argon beam coagulator. *J Urol* 152:902, 1994.

12. Albala DM, Prinz RA: Laparoscopic adrenalectomy: Results of eight patients. Société Internationale D'Urologie 23rd Congress Abstracts, #790, p 286, 1994.

SECTION THREE

Other Applications

16

Laparoscopic Techniques in Pediatric Urology

Sakti Das

Historical Introduction

At the beginning of this century, Kelling and Jacobaeus separately reported their techniques of laparoscopy. These primeval developments of laparoscopy necessitated the use of the urologic cystoscope, yet for nearly half a century the gynecologists virtually monopolized the art and practice of laparoscopy. The urologic utility of laparoscopy was initially limited to the field of pediatric urology. In 1976 Cortesi et al. from the Department of Surgery and Endocrinology at the University of Modena in Italy pioneered the first urologic use of laparoscopy. They localized bilateral intraabdominal testes in an 18-year-old male and commended this diagnostic approach as a prelude to surgical exploration in the management of nonpalpable testes.[1] During the same period, Paramo in Madrid utilized laparoscopy in six males with cryptorchidism, though this was belatedly communicated by Dr. Uson in a letter to the editor of the *Journal of Urology*.[2] Thereafter, until recently, the only serious involvement of the urologist with the laparoscope has been for the diagnostic localization and evaluation of the nonpalpable testes.

Human ingenuity aided by technologic advancements has allowed us to extend the use of the laparoscope beyond the realm of diagnostic exploration. Developments in laparoscopic dissection emanating initially from our gynecologic colleagues have led our endeavors toward more complex urologic surgeries through the laparoscope. As the techniques and our expertise have matured, the indications have been extended to the extremes of ages. Laparoscopic urology carries special significance in the pediatric population. Reduced trauma of access and rapid recovery has led to less psychological burden and easier acceptance of surgery by this select group of patients and their parents. The following pages elaborate the existing indications and techniques of specific laparoscopic procedures in children, with special emphasis on laparoscopic techniques for cryptorchidism.

The Nonpalpable Testes

Since the original works of Cortesi and Paramo, many authors have substantiated the usefulness of laparoscopy in the diagnostic localization as well as other definitive surgical procedures upon cryptorchid children.[3–12] In a patient with nonpalpable testes, a laparoscope can aid in (1) the localization and evaluation of the missing gonad, (2) two-step orchiopexy, (3) laparoendoscopic orchiopexy, and (4) orchiectomy.

Laparoscopic Localization and Evaluation

Various diagnostic methods have been implemented in an effort to properly localize and assess the anatomic status of nonpalpable testes prior to surgical exploration so that one can rationally plan for the surgical approach. If an orchiopexy is deemed suitable, one planned with special attention to the vascular anatomy can be expected to yield better testicular salvage. Localization procedures for cryptorchid testes include spermatic venography, spermatic arteriography, herniography, radionuclide scanning, abdominal ultrasound, computed tomography (CT), and magnetic resonance imaging (MRI). Spermatic venography and arteriography are invasive procedures, often requiring a separate general anesthesia with its attendant morbidity. Abdominal ultrasound, radionuclide scanning, and CT yield inconsistent results. The hazards of ionizing radiation exposure to young boys with several of these procedures is of added concern. MRI is poorly tolerated by infants because of the claustrophobia aggravated by the long scanning time. Moreover, it is an expensive test, and imaging of small intraabdominal testes is often obscure. In contrast, laparoscopy immediately prior to exploration under the same anesthetic has proven successful in localizing cryptorchid testes in nearly all instances.

Laparoscopic anatomy of nonpalpable testes are classified into three types:

1. *Abdominal testes* are visible inside the abdomen proximal to the deep inguinal ring (Fig. 16-1). One can more critically gauge the extent of testicular atrophy by direct visual assessment through the laparoscope. Laparoscopy provides a more precise estimation of the location of the intraabdominal testis, thereby aiding in the determination of the preferred surgical technique to bring the testis toward the scrotum.

2. In the case of *Canalicular testes* the vas deferens and spermatic vessels are observed to converge and exit at the deep inguinal ring. This is often associated with an indirect inguinal hernia, and milking the inguinal canal may cause the testicle to emerge into the neck of the hernia at the deep ring (Fig. 16-2). It is often possible to negotiate the laparoscope through the large hernial opening at the deep ring and visualize a more distal inguinal testis. Presence of a substantial inguinal hernia does not automatically imply the association of a canalicular testicle. We have encountered a child who underwent an inguinal hernia repair and on subsequent laparoscopy two years later was proven to have a high intraabdominal testis.

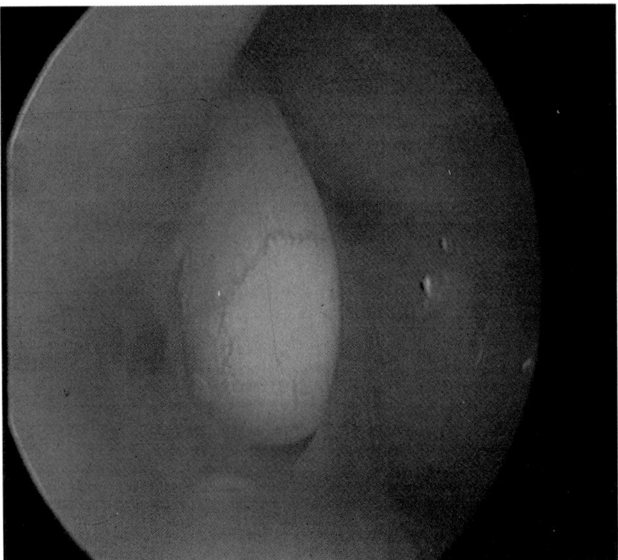

Figure 16-1 Intraabdominal testis just inside the deep inguinal ring,

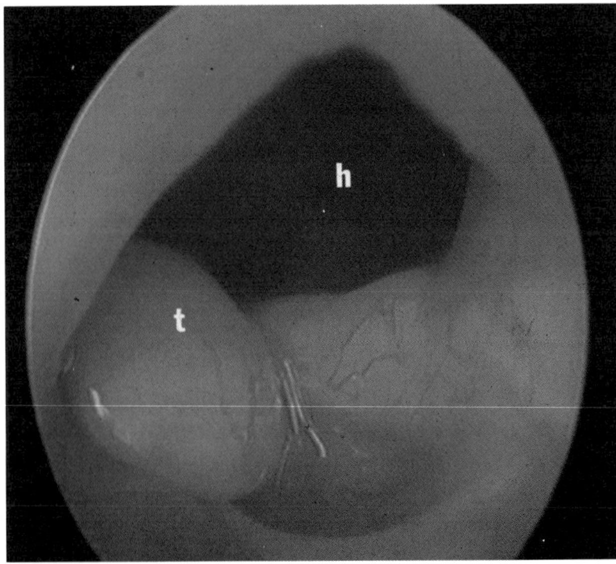

Figure 16-2 Indirect inguinal hernia with canalicular testes (h = hernia, t = testis).

3. Infrequently the vas deferens and spermatic vessels will be seen to terminate blindly proximal to the deep inguinal ring, thereby establishing the diagnostic entity of *unilateral or bilateral anorchia or vanishing testes* (Fig. 16-3a). Laparoscopic observation of the vas and gonadal vessels ending blindly proximal to the deep inguinal ring is convincing enough evidence of a vanishing testis that no further surgical exploration is necessary (Fig. 16-3b and c). In the literature there has never been a report of a testicle located geographically away from the termination of its gonadal vessels. One must see the blind-ending gonadal vessels before a diagnosis of anorchia can be entertained. On rare occasions when the vas deferens is seen to end blindly with no testes or spermatic vessels in the near vicinity, one should explore for the testes or spermatic vessels because they may be lying high and disjunct from the vas deferens. However, a testis whenever present cannot be separate from the termination of its vessels. One patient in our series and another in the series by Weiss and Seashore affirm the therapeutic axiom that whether one is working through the laparoscope or by open exploration, if the termination of the gonadal vessels is not identified, a meticulous intraperitoneal search should be undertaken to locate or exclude the possibility of a proximal high-lying testis.[8]

With the accumulation of our laparoscopic experience we are convinced that inguinal exploration alone for nonpalpable testes often is deceivingly inadequate. Boddy, Corkery, and Gornal reported on 13 boys declared to have no testes after extensive inguinal exploration and found 5 salvageable intraabdominal testes on subsequent laparoscopy.[7] The danger of developing malignancy in missed supracanalicular testes cannot be overemphasized.

Compared to other available localizing procedures, laparoscopy provides more direct visual evidence of the location and anatomic condition of the nonpalpable testes. Laparoscopy has only rare false negative and no false positive interpretations.

Two-Step Orchiopexy

Following the laparoscopic localization of a salvageable albeit high-lying intraabdominal testis, it may be worthwhile to attempt preservation and scrotal relocation. Such a procedure is particularly

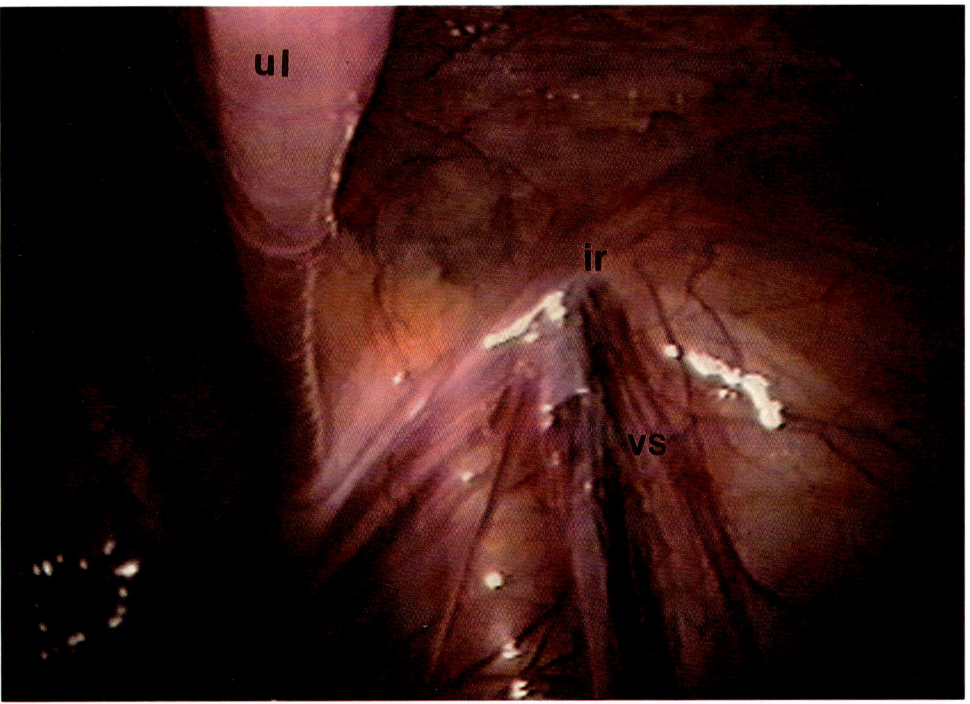

(a)

Figure 16-3 (a) Normal anatomy, right side (ir = internal ring, vs = spermatic vessels, ul = umbilical ligament.

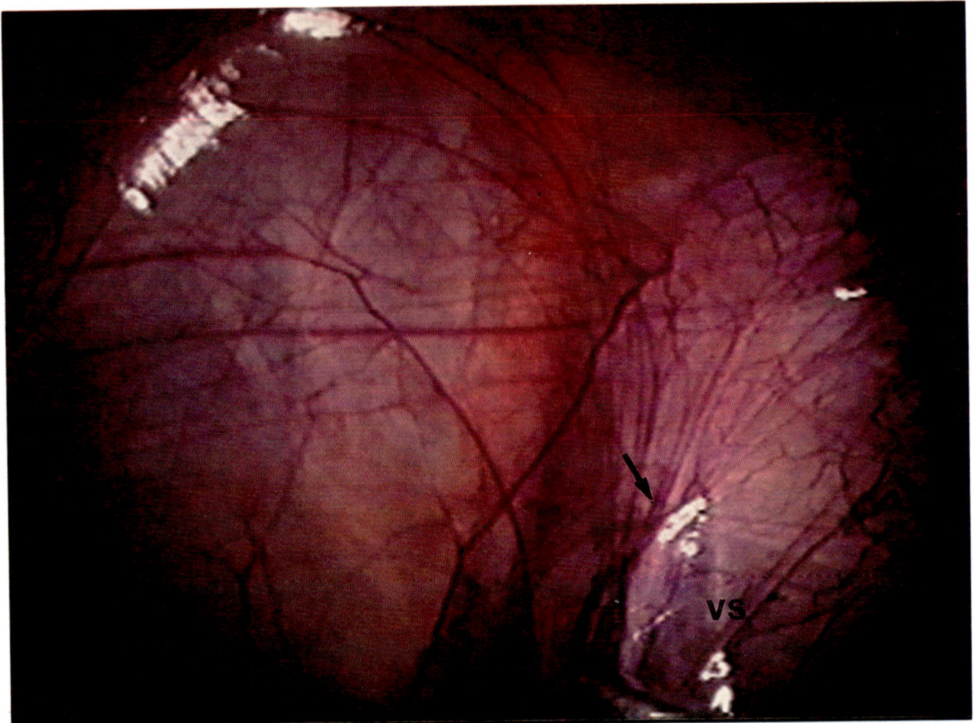

(b)

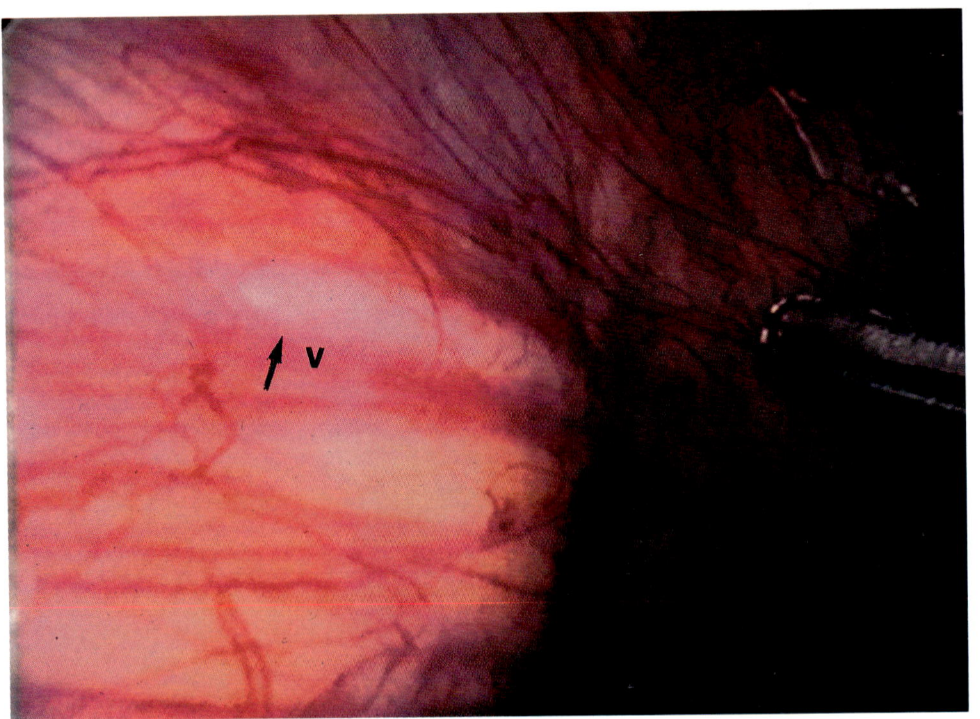

(c)

Figure 16-3 (*cont.*) (b & c) Anorchia as evidenced by spermatic vessels (vs) and vas deferens ending (v) blindly in a scarred area proximal to the deep inguinal ring.

desirable in the specific circumstances of a patient with an imperfect contralateral testicle. Testicular autotransplantation and staged orchiopexy are difficult, although they are possible surgical options in the management of abdominal testes. The preferred approach has been the Fowler-Stephens orchiopexy, whereby the spermatic vessels are divided and the testis is mobilized on the vas deferens with the hope that the vasal collateral circulation will sustain the vascular needs of the organ. The prerequisite anatomic criteria for success of the Fowler-Stephens orchiopexy include a long loop vas deferens, short spermatic vascular bundles, and Prune Belly Syndrome.[13] Unfortunately, a long loop vas, which is the most important criterion, is not a common form of vasal anatomy with intraabdominal testes. The success of the Fowler-Stephens procedure therefore ranges from 50 percent to 86 percent in highly selected patients. Duckett in 1982 proposed preliminary in situ ligation of the spermatic vessels with the intent that vasal collaterals would be enhanced and that subsequent late division of the spermatic vessels and vas-based orchiopexy would have improved chance for success.[14] Pascual et al. noted in the laboratory that following spermatic vascular interruption, the blood flow to the testes was reduced to 80 percent within 1 h but returned to normal by 30 days.[15] Ransley et al. in 1984 reported favorable results in their series of boys subjected to this staged Fowler-Stephens procedure.[16]

Laparoscopy permitted a new twist to these approaches, endocavitary application of hemostatic clips to interrupt the internal spermatic vessels away from the testes. Bloom continues to report his pioneering technique of applying clips to the spermatic vessels as a prelude to staged Fowler-Stephens orchiopexy.[14] At least 6 months after the laparoscopic clipping of the vessels, the patient is explored for the stage-II orchiopexy. The spermatic vessels are ligated and divided cephalad to the clip. After inscribing a wide peritoneal cuff around the testis and vas deferens, the latter structures are carefully mobilized to gain sufficient length for placement in the scrotum. Early results of two-step orchiopexy in the series reported by Bloom are encouraging. Six of the seven testes showed normal size and growth comparable to that of the contralateral gonad at 6 months to 3½ years of follow-up. The singular failure in the whole series was in a boy who already had significant testicular atrophy following two prior inguinal explorations.

There are several distinct advantages of laparoscopic two-step orchiopexy for high-lying supracanalicular testes over the orthodox Fowler-Stephens procedure. It is applicable for any salvageable abdominal gonad whether or not associated with a long loop vas deferens. Hemostatic clip ligation interrupts the internal spermatic vessels with virtually no dissection or disturbance of the testes or the vasal arcades of circulation. Although requiring two separate anesthetics and operative interventions, the laparoscopic first stage is rapid and minimally invasive. The second stage is of known quantity and is executed with no uncertainty of exploration. A precisely contrived dissection thereby optimizes the success of a vasal pedicled orchiopexy.

Laparoendoscopic Orchiopexy

Jordan and associates have reported their technique of laparoscopic orchiopexy whereby a high-lying intraabdominal testis was mobilized by laparoscopic dissection of the spermatic vessels, the vas deferens, and the associated inguinal hernia.[17] A 10-mm trocar was introduced through the scrotal dartos pouch into the peritoneal cavity. The mobilized testis was grasped through the scrotal trocar into the dartos pouch and anchored there (Fig. 16-4).

Bogaert et al. have recently reported dissection of the testicle during the second stage of Fowler-

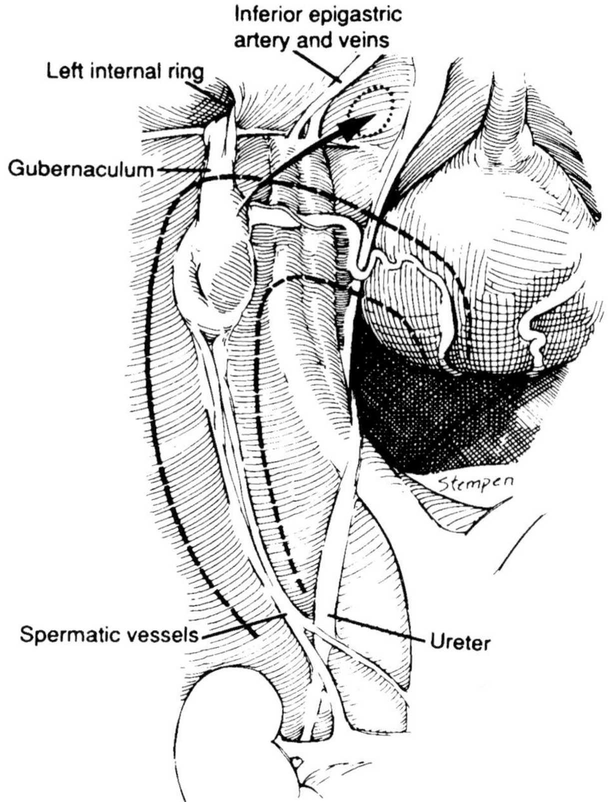

Figure 16-4 Laparoscopic approach for a laparoscopy-assisted orchiopexy.

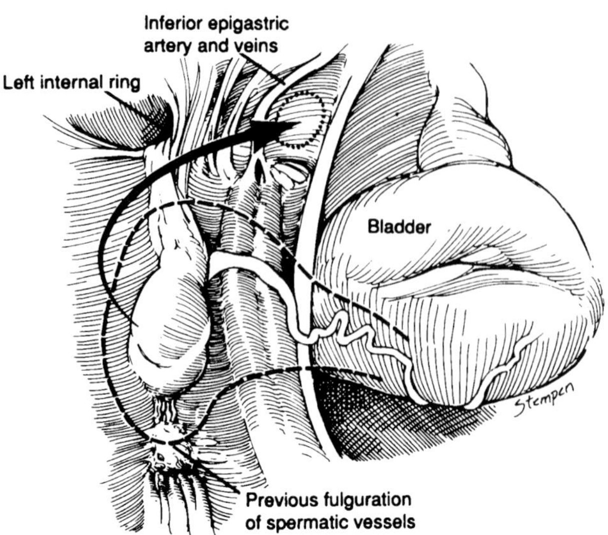

Figure 16-5 Laparoscopic approach for a second-stage Fowler-Stephens orchiopexy.

Stephens orchiopexies laparoscopically in 5 patients (6 testicles).[18] In 3 patients the entire procedure was performed through a laparoscopic approach (Fig. 16-5).

Orchiectomy

Small atrophic intraabdominal testes in postpubertal patients are often better removed. Unilateral high-lying testes with a normal contralateral gonad also constitute a relative indication for orchiectomy at any age. Carcinoma in situ and obvious malignancies have been reported in as many as 8 percent of these abnormally descended testes.[19] With the available instrumentation for laparoscopic dissection, orchiectomy can be carried out at the time of laparoscopy. Castilho et al. first described the removal of a prepubertal testis in a patient with ambiguous genitalia.[20] The spermatic vessels and vas deferens are clipped and divided in sequence. The distal peritoneal and gubernacular attachments are then dissected. The testis, freed from its vessels and attachments, is then removed through a port (Fig. 16-6).

Intersex States

Laparoscopy provides the most definitive as well as minimally invasive procedure for the inspection, necessary biopsy, or removal of intraabdominal gonadal structures in suspected intersex patients with ambiguous genitalia. Even during laparoscopy for nonpalpable testes, one must entertain the possibility of finding Mullerian structures. In a series of 33 patients with nonpalpable testes Lowe, Brock, and Kaplan detected 1 patient with gonadal dysgenesis by laparoscopy.[5] Wolfman and Kreutner reported their laparoscopic experience in 13 adolescents with gonadal dysgenesis, 3 with vaginal agenesis, and 2 with gonadal agenesis.[21] The spectrum of laparoscopic findings in intersex states in the several studies included absent, streak, and normal-looking gonads with various abnormal Mullerian derivatives. With the available laparoscopic expertise, a diagnostic open laparotomy in these children can no longer be recommended.

Varicoceles in Adolescents

Adolescent varicoceles are unique conditions of unknown etiology and natural history. There is no consensus regarding the timing and type of therapy. Not observed in childhood, the prevalence of varicocele is between 14.7 percent and 16.2 percent in the 10- to 14-year old male.[22,23] More than one third of these varicoceles are pronounced. Twenty-five percent are grade II and 11 percent are grade III. Increased scrotal temperature and an altered hormonal milieu secondary to varicocele often leads to progressive testicular atrophy. Okuyama et al. studied 40 adolescents with varicoceles, including 24 subjected to varicocelectomy and 16 on observation alone.[24] Significant improvement of testicular atrophy and normal seminal patterns were more commonly observed in the males subjected to varicocelectomy. The patients followed with no surgical venous interruption continued to have deterioration of their testicular size and seminal patterns. In adolescents with varicoceles, I therefore recommend internal spermatic vein ligation whenever there is 20 percent or more reduction in testicular volume compared to the normal contralateral testicle.

There are distinct advantages of laparoscopic internal spermatic vein interruption over open vein ligation in this age group. The small incisions for access are more cosmetically appealing. Significantly less pain allows quicker recovery and early resumption of activities such as sports and eduction. Open internal spermatic vein ligation has been associated with a 5 to 16 percent recurrence rate. The

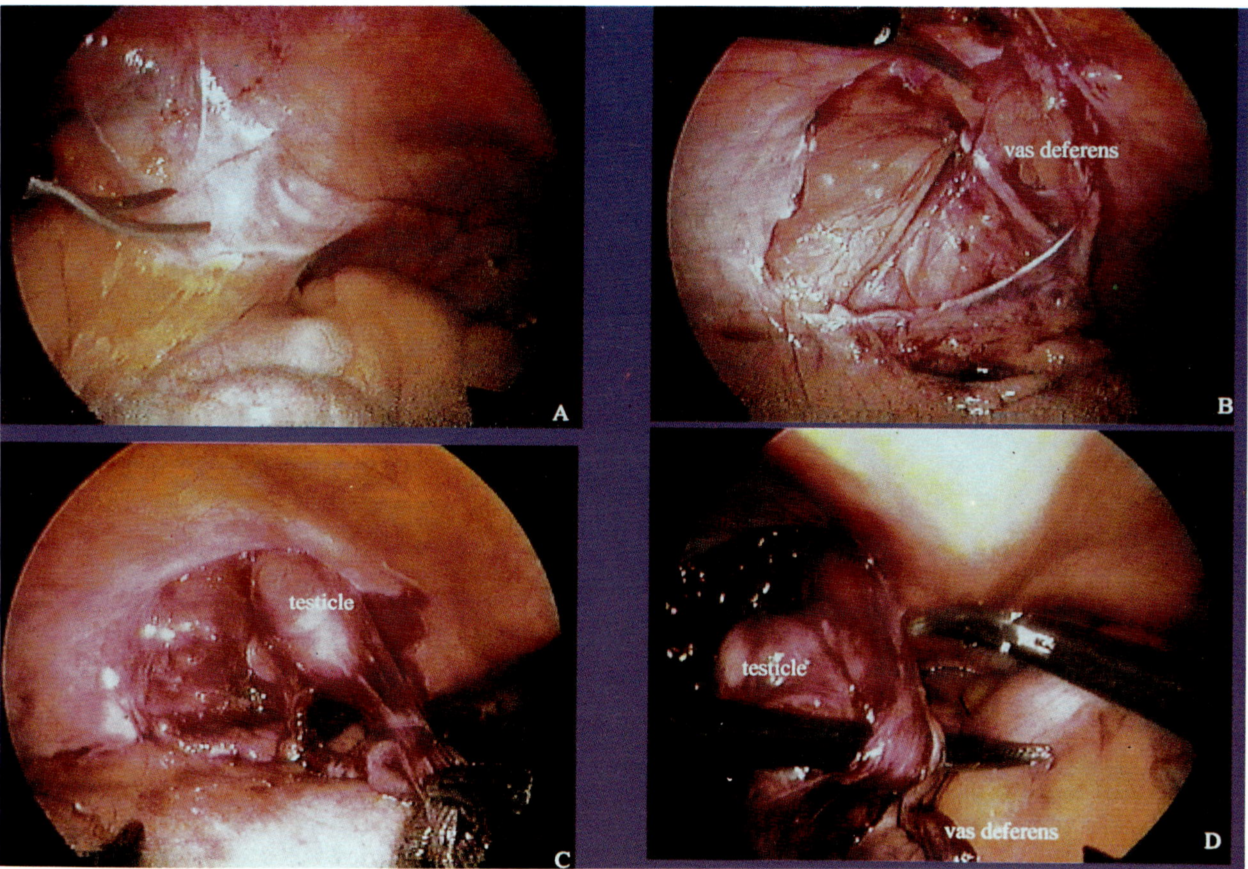

Figure 16-6 (a) Sequence demonstrates a left orchiectomy performed laparoscopically: The vas deferens and spermatic vessels are dissected. Traction is applied on the vessels which delivers the gonad to the field.

majority of these recurrences are attributable to missed accessory internal spermatic veins or aberrant tributaries communicating with cremasteric, vasal, and presacral venous trunks.[25,26] The retroperitoneal anatomy at and above the deep inguinal ring is more clearly observed by laparoscopy and allows better identification of these venous trunks. Therefore a more thorough venous interruption can be accomplished with less chance of recurrence.

The main indication for internal spermatic vein interruption in adolescent varicocele is to prevent and often reverse testicular atrophy. Every effort must be made to identify and preserve the integrity of the testicular artery during the interruption of the venous channels. During laparoscopic varicocelectomy one should try to avoid electrocautery to prevent inadvertent arterial injury or spasm. Identification of a testicular artery in spasm is often facilitated by sprinkling Papaverine solution in the area of laparoscopic dissection.

Other Surgeries upon the Urinary Tract

As a logical extension of our adult experience, laparoscopic nephrectomy, partial nephrectomy, and nephroureterectomy become more feasible in the pediatric population, since most commonly the indications involve small atrophic kidneys. We have successfully carried out a nephroureterectomy in an 11-year-old girl to remove an end-stage shrunken kidney secondary to vesicoureteric reflux. Similarly, removal of multicystic kidneys, congenital hypoplastic kidneys causing hypertension, and partial nephrectomy in duplex kidneys with obstruction, ectopia, or reflux can be accomplished by laparoscopic dissection.

With increasing experience and refinements of our technical finesse, especially in laparoscopic endosuturing, many more potential laparoscopic

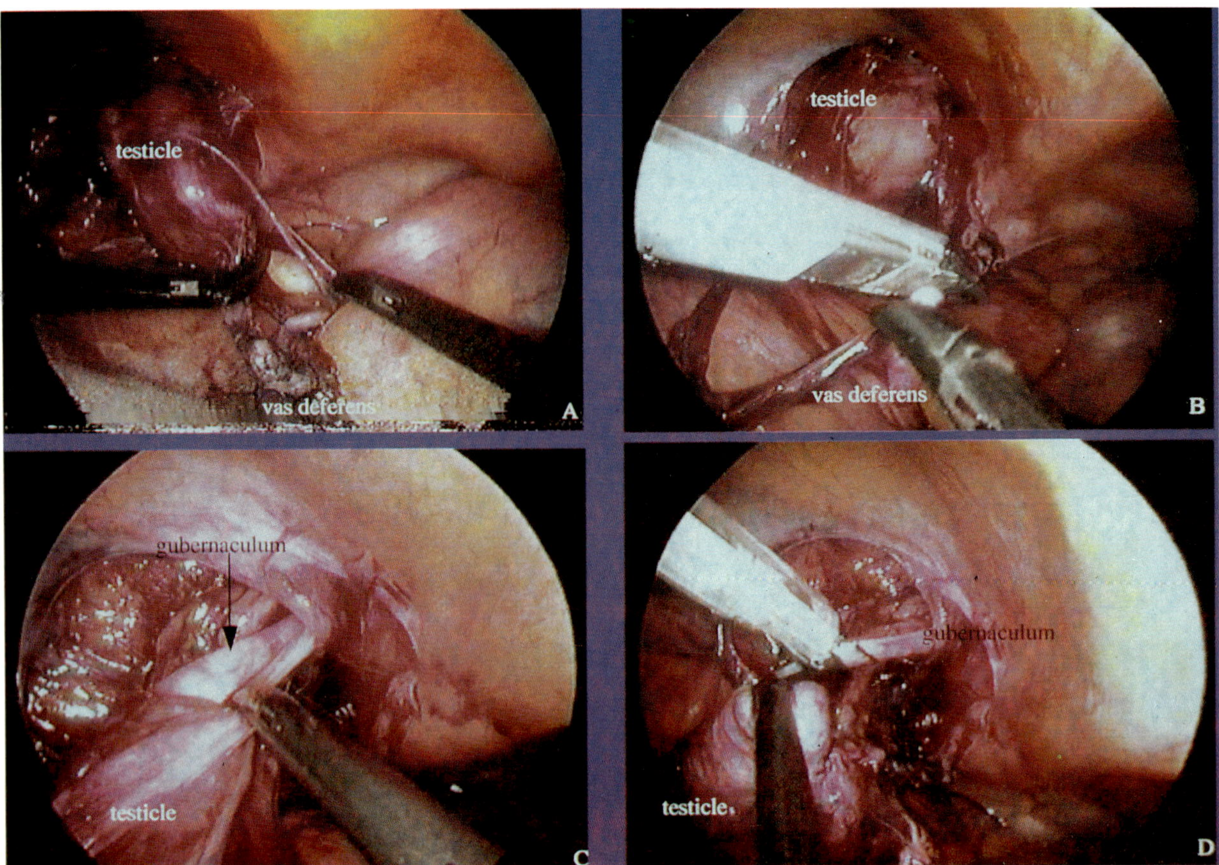

Figure 16-6 (*cont.*) (b) The testicular attachments—vessels, vas deferens, and gubernaculum—are serially clipped and divided.

procedures in pediatric urology continue to evolve. Examples of such procedures are (1) anti-reflux surgeries, especially the extravesical ureterovesicoplasty, (2) repair of ureteropelvic junction obstruction, either by intubated ureterotomy or by dismembered pyeloplasty, (3) ureteroureterostomy or pyeloureterostomy in duplicated ureters, (4) repair of inguinal hernia, (5) augmentation or reduction cystoplasty, and (6) laparoscopic exploration for pelvic malignancies.

Conclusion

Laparoscopic procedures in urology were initiated in the field of pediatric urology with the diagnostic localization and evaluation of nonpalpable testes. With the advancement of laparoscopic dissection techniques our surgical laparoscopic procedures have now extended to surgical management of high-lying abdominal testes with staged orchiopexy or orchiectomy. The various adult urologic laparoscopic procedures are now applicable for similar indications in the pediatric population. The progressive challenge of transformation to laparoscopic urology is perceptible in pediatric urology as much as in other spheres of urology. We must, however, exercise extra precaution during laparoscopy in children because of their small size and certain anatomic characteristics that are liable to result in injuries to the stomach, intestines, and urinary bladder. Careful anesthetic vigilance toward respiratory compromise and complications of hypercarbia should be emphasized from the onset of the procedure. Caution assumes extraordinary significance when pragmatic decision is poised between the extremes of safety and therapeutic excellence.

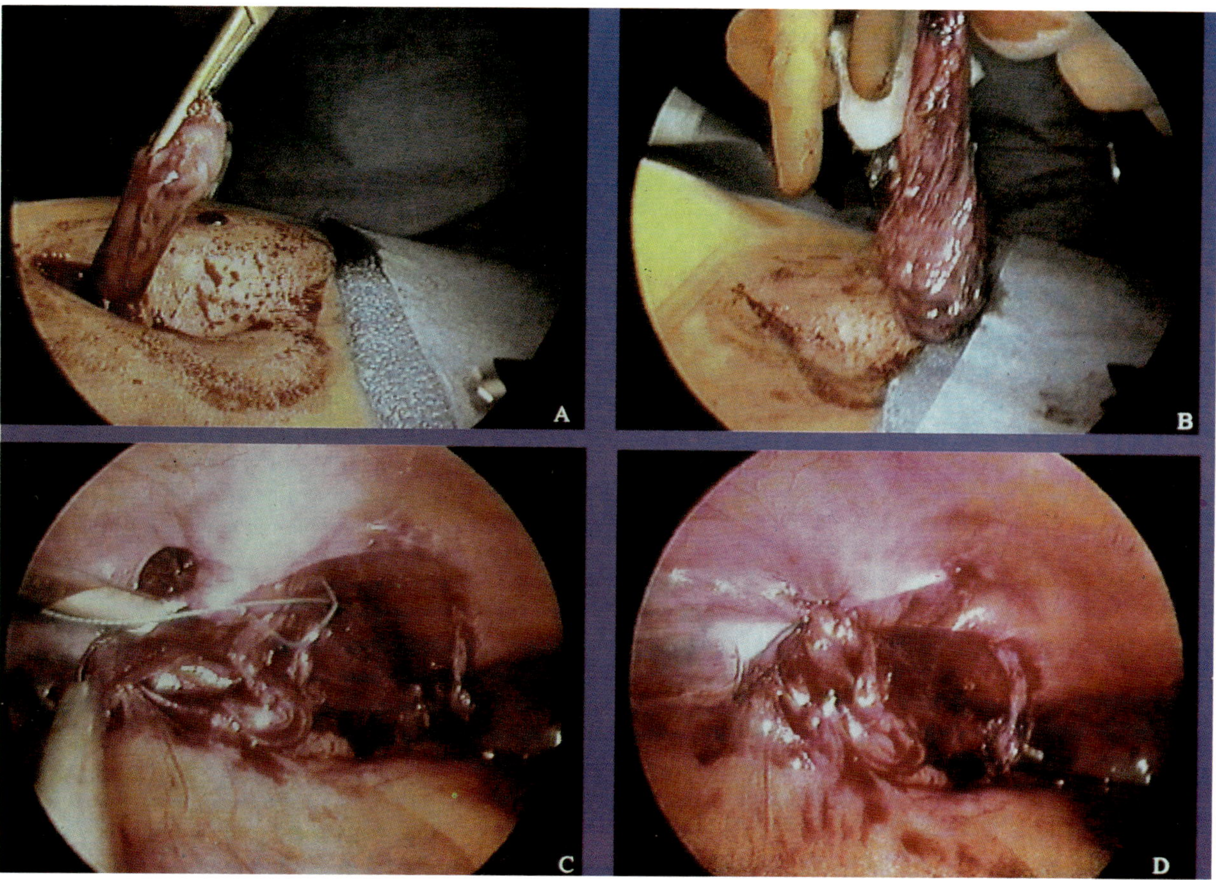

Figure 16-6 (*cont.*) (c) The testicle is delivered via one of the trocar sites and the defect can be closed in order to avoid a subsequent hernia. **(c)**

References

1. Cortesi N, Ferrar P, Zambarda E, et al: Diagnosis of bilateral abdominal cryptorchidism by laparoscopy. *Endoscopy* 8:33, 1976.
2. Uson AC: Laparoscopy for cryptorchidism (letter). *J Urol* 128:829, 1982.
3. Scott JES: Laparoscopy as an aid in the diagnosis and management of the impalpable testis. *J Pediatr Surg* 7:14, 1982.
4. Malone PS, Guiney EJ: The value of laparoscopy in localizing the impalpable undescended testis. *Br J Urol* 56:429, 1984.
5. Lowe DH, Brock WA, Kaplan GW: Laparoscopy for localization of non-palpable testes. *J Urol* 131:728, 1984.
6. Manson AL, Terhune D, Jordan G, et al: Preoperative laparoscopic localization of the non-palpable testis. *J Urol* 134:919, 1985.
7. Boddy SM, Corkery JJ, Gornal P: The place of laparoscopy in the management of the impalpable testis. *Br J Surg* 72:918, 1985.
8. Weiss RM, Seashore JH: Laparoscopy in the management of the non-palpable testis. *J Urol* 138:382, 1987.
9. Bloom DA, Ayers JWT, McGuire EJ: The role of laparoscopy in management of non-palpable testes. *J Urol (Paris)* 94:465, 1988.
10. Naslund MJ, Gearhart JP, Jeffs RD: Laparoscopy: Its selected use in patients with unilateral non-palpable testes after human chorionic gonadotrophic stimulations. *J Urol* 142:108, 1989.
11. Guiney EJ, Corbally M, Malone PS: Laparoscopy and the management of the impalpable testis. *Br J Urol* 63:313, 1989.
12. Das S: Laparoscopic evaluation of non-palpable testis. *Urology* 37:460, 1991.
13. Stephens FD: Fowler-Stephens orchiopexy. *Semin Urol* 6:103, 1988.

14. Bloom DA: Two-step orchiopexy with pelviscopic clip ligation of the spermatic vessels. *J Urol* 145:1030, 1991.

15. Pascual JA, Villanueva-Meyer J, Salido E, et al: Recovery of testicular blood flow following ligation of testicular vessels. *J Urol* 142: 549, 1989.

16. Ransley PG, Vordermark JS, Caldamone AA, et al: Preliminary ligation of the gonadal vessels prior to orchiopexy for the intraabdominal testicle: A staged Fowler-Stephens procedure. *World J Urol* 2:266, 1984.

17. Jordan GH, Robay EL, Winslow BH: Laparoendoscopic surgical management of the abdominal/transinguinal undescended testis. *J Endourol* 6:159, 1993.

18. Bogaert GA, Kogan BA, Mevorach RA: Therapeutic laparoscopy for intra-abdominal testes. *Urology* 42:2, 1993.

19. Krabbe S, Skakkeback NE, Berthelsen JG, et al: High incidence of undetected neoplasia in maldescended testes. *Lancet* 1:999, 1979.

20. Castilho LN, Ferreira U, Esteves SC, Valin C, Netto NR Jr: Laparoscopic orchiectomy. *J Urol* 145:206A, 1991.

21. Wolfman WL, Kreutner K: Laparoscopy in children adolescents. *J Adolesc Health Care* 5:261, 1984.

22. Steeno O, Knops J, Declerck L, et al: Prevention of fertility disorders by detection and treatment of varicocele at school and college age. *Andrologie* 8:47, 1976.

23. Oster J: Varicocele in children and adolescents: an investigation of the incidence among Danish school children. *Scand J Urol Nephrol* 5:27, 1971.

24. Okuyama A, Nakamura M, Naniki M, et al: Surgical repair of varicocele at puberty: Preventive treatment for fertility improvement. *J Urol* 139:562, 1988.

25. Zaontz MR, Firlit CF: Use of venography as an aid in varicocelectomy. *J Urol* 138:1041, 1987.

26. Kogan SJ: Prevention of persistent varicocele. *Soc Pediatr Urol Newsletter*, Feb 22: 6, 1984.

17

Retroperitoneoscopy

Durga D. Gaur

Introduction

Although the retroperitoneal organs are better exposed directly through a posterior approach, urologic laparoscopic surgeons initially took the transperitoneal route because retroperitoneoscopy in the past was not found to be satisfactory. This was mainly due to the dense retroperitoneal fat, which did not permit creation of a satisfactory pneumoretroperitoneum by pneumoinsufflation. Another contributory factor was the inadequate space available in the retroperitoneum for endoscopic manipulation. In addition, visibility due to overhanging fat and oozing blood was poor. These problems have mostly been solved by using the retroperitoneal balloon dissector cum expander previously described by the author.

Historical Aspects

When the word "laparotomy" was first introduced by Bryant[1] to describe the surgical exposure of the abdominal viscera, there was some criticism on the grounds that as *lapara* in greek means "flank," it should only be used for exposure of organs in that region. Therefore, a direct endoscopic exposure of organs in the lumbar region can etymologically be called retroperitoneal laparoscopy.

In 1969, Bartel performed the first retroperitoneoscopy with a mediastinoscope.[2] In 1974 Sommerkamp performed a renal biopsy with a semiopen technique using an illuminated lumboscope.[3] Pneumoinsufflation of the retroperitoneal space was first used by Wickham to perform a retroperitoneal endoscopic ureterolithotomy with a standard laparoscope.[4] Kaplan et al. attempted retroperitoneoscopy in dogs using nitrous oxide insufflation and were able to visualize most of the upper retroperitoneal structures.[5] Subsequently, Wickham and Miller reported on retroperitoneoscopy in cadavers using carbon dioxide insufflation but found the technique difficult due to their inability to create a satisfactory pneumoretroperitoneum.[6]

Hald and Rasmussen slightly modified the mediastinoscope and performed extraperitoneal pelvioscopy to investigate cases of bladder and prostatic cancer.[7] Mazeman and Wurtz further reported their experience of extraperitoneal pelvic lymphadenectomy using this direct vision pelvioscope.[8,9]

Eshghi et al. successfully used a laparoscope to monitor the percutaneous removal of a staghorn calculus in a pelvic kidney.[10] Weinberg and Smith performed a percutaneous nephrectomy in a pig by aspirating the renal parenchyma through a nephrostomy using an endoscopic ultrasonic aspirator (CUSA) after embolization of the artery and the vein.[11] However, at autopsy the renal pedicle was

TABLE 17-1 Indications for Retroperitoneal Laparoscopy

Procedure	No.
Renoscopy and renal biopsy	21
Para-aortic lymph node biopsy	3
Varicocelectomy	27
Ureterolithotomy	12
Pyelolithotomy	5
Nephrolithotomy	1
Nephrectomy	7
Adrenal exposure	3
Pelvic lymphadenectomy	3
Ligation of deep penile veins	2

still intact. Meretyk et al. reported the retrieval of a foreign body from the retroperitoneum through an established percutaneous track.[12] Although Clayman et al. performed a retroperitoneal laparoscopic nephrectomy early in their experience, they subsequently favored the transperitoneal approach.[13] With the author's recently described technique of retroperitoneoscopy using a balloon to expand the retroperitoneal space, new horizons have been opened in laparoscopic urology.[14]

Indications for Retroperitoneoscopy

The various retroperitoneal laparoscopic procedures performed at the Bombay Hospital Institute of Medical Sciences are shown in Table 17-1. However, any operation on the adrenals, kidneys, renal pelvis, ureter, urinary bladder, and prostate could become possible in the future with the development of newer laparoscopic instruments and bioadhesives.

Renoscopy and Renal Biopsy

Retroperitoneal laparoscopic renoscopy and renal biopsy is the procedure of choice where a percutaneous needle biopsy has failed[15] or in high-risk patients with hypertension, azotemia, or solitary kidneys.[16,17] It also has a place in developing countries, where computed tomography (CT) or ultrasound facilities may not be readily available.

Para-Aortic Lymph Node Biopsy

A para-aortic mass in the region of the renal hilum could be a contraindication for percutaneous needle biopsy, and in such a case a retroperitoneal laparoscopic approach may be of use. This technique has been utilized at our institution in patients with presumed tuberculosis and filariasis to establish a diagnosis.

Pelvic Lymphadenectomy, Bladder Neck Suspension and Varicocelectomy

Although these procedures are readily performed transperitoneally, in patients with pelvic adhesions the retroperitoneal approach may be a safer and better alternative. It may in fact be the approach of choice for laparoscopic bladder neck procedures.[18,19] While for varicocelectomy it may have a theoretical advantage. The risk of damaging the spermatic artery is less, since the ligation of the internal spermatic vein is done at a much higher level. Nevertheless, it has the disadvantages of difficult identification of the vein and unilateral exposure.

Lithotomy

Most stones in the upper urinary tract are best treated by extracorporeal shock-wave lithotripsy, ureteroscopy, or percutaneous lithotomy. Retroperitoneal laparoscopic nephrolithotomy, pyelolithotomy, and ureterolithotomy are viable alternatives for stones not amenable to these advances or if the technology is not accessible. It is indicated for large and hard stones in an extrarenal pelvis, impacted in the upper ureter, in a calyceal diverticulum, or in a dilated calyx with thinned out parenchyma.

Nephrectomy

Retroperitoneal laparoscopic nephrectomy is ideally suited for small, poorly functioning kidneys with lithiasis, recurrent infection, and/or hypertension.[20]

Adrenalectomy

The retroperitoneal approach provides good exposure of the adrenal gland after mobilization of the kidney, but as the space is limited, it may not be suitable for large adrenal masses.

Contraindications

As the balloon can only dissect and expand a virgin retroperitoneal space, the procedure is of limited value in patients with primary or secondary retroperitoneal fibrosis and previous retroperitoneal surgery. It is also contraindicated in patients with bleeding disorders and would be difficult in obese patients. In addition, large renal or adrenal masses should be considered a relative contraindication to this technique secondary to the limited space available in the retroperitoneum.

Retroperitoneal Surgical Anatomy

There are certain points unique to the surgical anatomy of the retroperitoneum that impact upon success in the laparoscopic approach.

1. The retroperitoneal fat is abundant up to the posterior axillary line. Therefore, the placement of the balloon for abdominal retroperitoneoscopy should not be anterior to this line in order to avoid the risk of tearing the peritoneum during initial digital and subsequent balloon dissection (Fig. 17-1).
2. Gerota's fascia is open caudally, which may allow the balloon to migrate inferiorly during its inflation. It is preferable to place the balloon deep to the fascia and directed toward the superior pole for better dissection of the kidney (Fig. 17-2).
3. The ureter and the internal spermatic vein lie between the peritoneum and an extension of the transversalis fascia. Consequently if the balloon has not been placed deep to the transversalis fascia, the abdominal ureter and the vein are not visible during retroperitoneoscopy and require a lengthy and difficult dissection for exposure.
4. The internal spermatic vein crosses the ureter anterolateral to medial at the level of L3. It is best identified at this juncture during retroperitoneoscopy. The inferior mesenteric vein lies medial to the left ureter at this level and can be seen after balloon dissection in thin patients. It must not be confused with a dilated internal spermatic vein (Fig. 17-3).

(a)

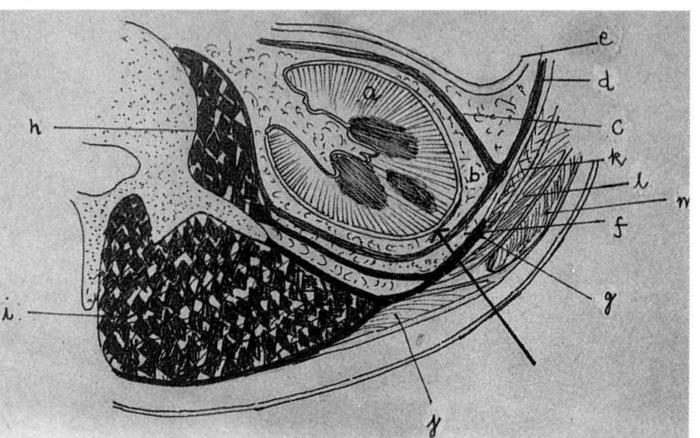

(b)

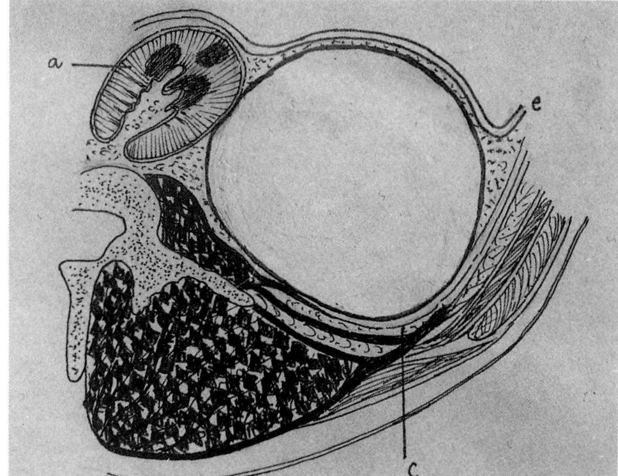

Figure 17-1 (a) Transverse section showing kidney (A), perirenal fat (B), Gerota's fascia (C), fascia transversalis (D), peritoneum (E), pararenal fat (F), lumbodorsal fascia (G), psoas (H), deep back muscles (I), latissimus dorsi (J), transversus (K), internal oblique (L), and external oblique (M). The arrow marks the route of balloon entry. (b) The balloon placed deep to Gerota's fascia has been inflated. The posterior peritoneum (E) has been lifted up, Gerota's fascia (C) has been disrupted, and the kidney (A) has been pushed anteriorly.

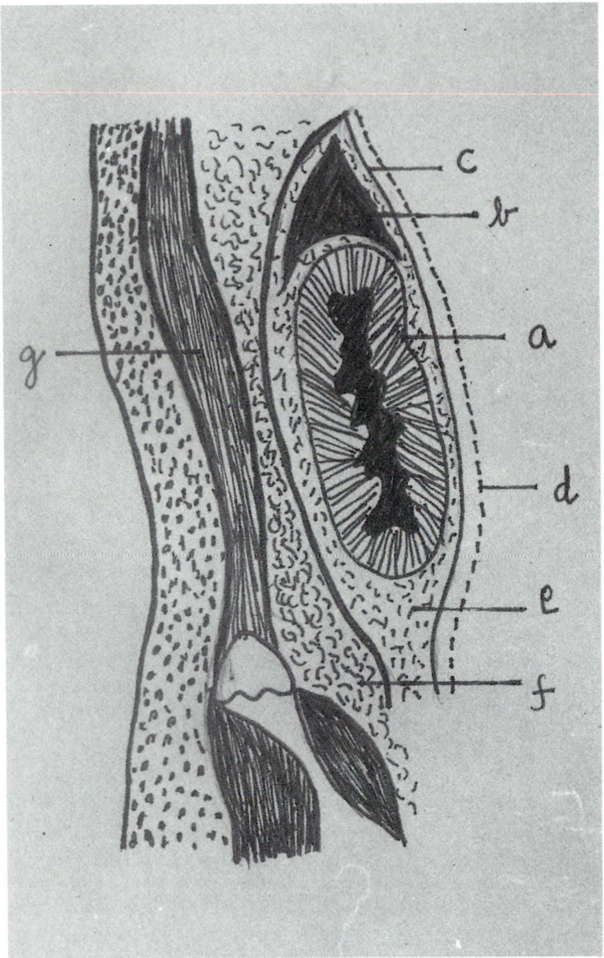

Figure 17-2 Sagittal section showing kidney (A), adrenal gland (B), Gerota's fascia (C), peritoneum (D), perirenal fat (E), pararenal fat (F) and muscles of the abdominal wall (G).

Necessary Equipment

Retroperitoneal Balloon Dissector cum Expander

This is the most important piece of equipment for retroperitoneoscopy. The original balloon (Fig. 17-4a) was a low-pressure balloon made with a red rubber catheter tied to varying lengths of a surgical glove. Several balloons have been developed for expansion of the retroperitoneal space and are available commercially (Fig. 17-4b). Since these balloons expand at a higher pressure, it is advisable to use fluid, not air, for inflation to avoid the risk of possible air embolism and visceral damage in the event or rupture. The degree of balloon distension depends upon the type of procedure to be performed (Table 17-2) and varies between 250 mL and 800 mL. For better dissection in the suprarenal area, a second balloon placed superiorly may be inflated to about 250 mL after the first one has been distended.

The Functions of the Balloon

1. Expands the retroperitoneal space to facilitate endoscopic manipulation (Fig. 17-1b).
2. Atraumatically dissects the retroperitoneal structures (Fig. 17-5).
3. Produces hemostasis.

The Retractable Endoknife

This instrument is reusable and accepts standard surgical blades (Cook Urological). The scalpel has

(a)

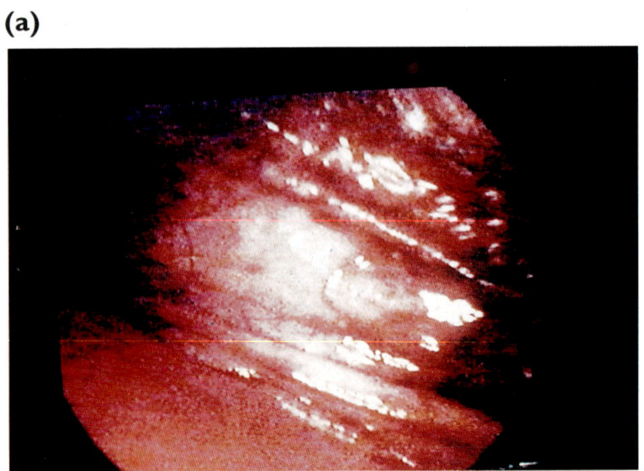

(b)

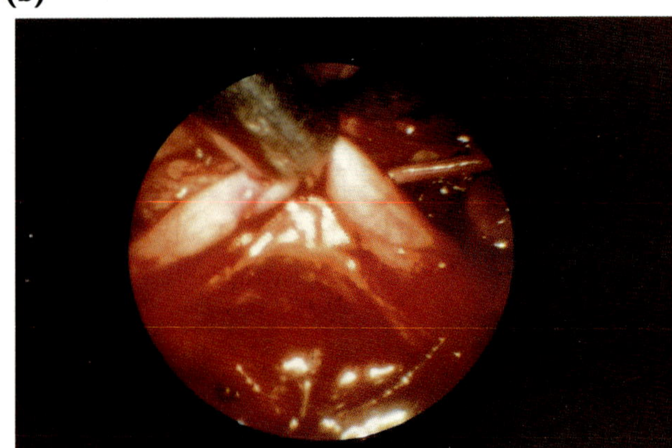

Figure 17-3 (a) Retroperitoneal laparoscopic view of the left abdominal retroperitoneum showing from top to bottom; the inferior mesenteric vein, the ureter, the internal spermatic vein, and the psoas. (b) View at a higher level showing the internal spermatic vein medial to the ureter.

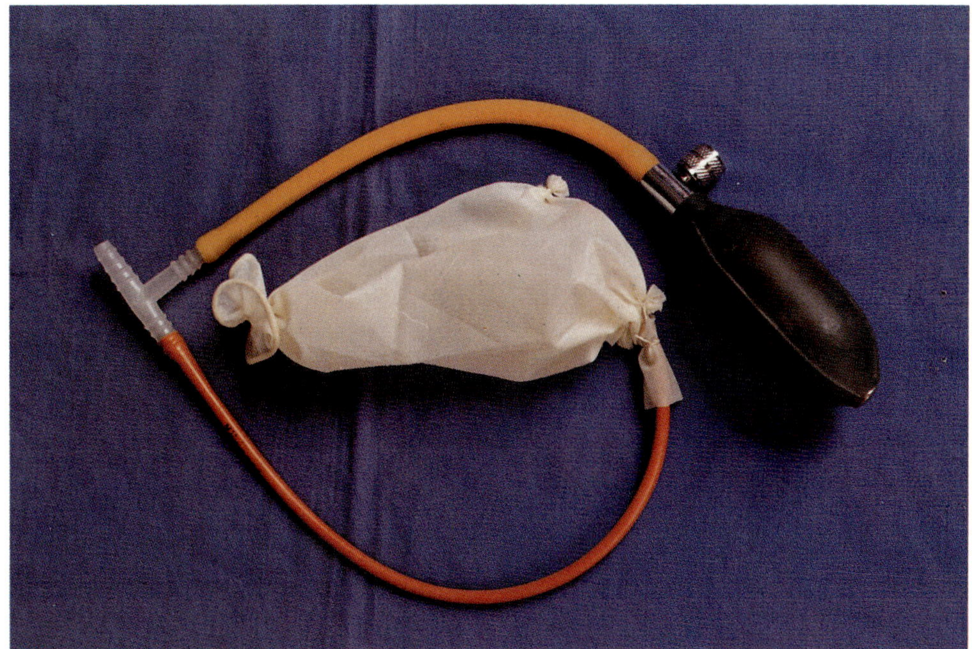

(a)

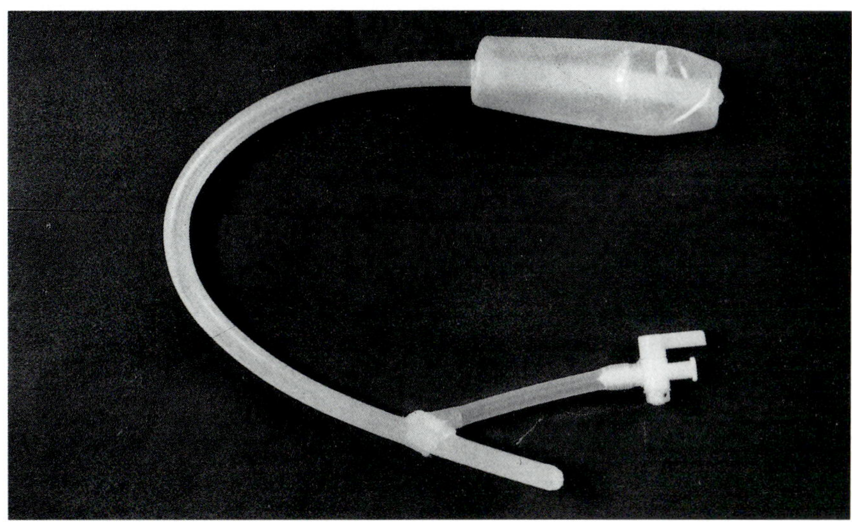

(b)

Figure 17-4 (a) The original balloon made of a red rubber catheter and surgical glove with pneumatic pump. (b) Gaur retroperitoneal balloon expander (Cook Urological).

TABLE 17-2 Balloon Distension Needed for Various Retroperitoneal Procedures

Procedures	Average Balloon Distension	No. of Pumpings (1 ≅ 35 mL)
Biopsy	250 mL	6 to 8
Renal		
Lymph node		
Lithotomy	750 mL	18 to 22
Uretero-		
Pyelo-		
Nephro-		
Varicocelectomy	600 mL	15 to 20
Nephrectomy	800 mL	20 to 25
Adrenalectomy		
Pelvic surgery	750 mL	18 to 22

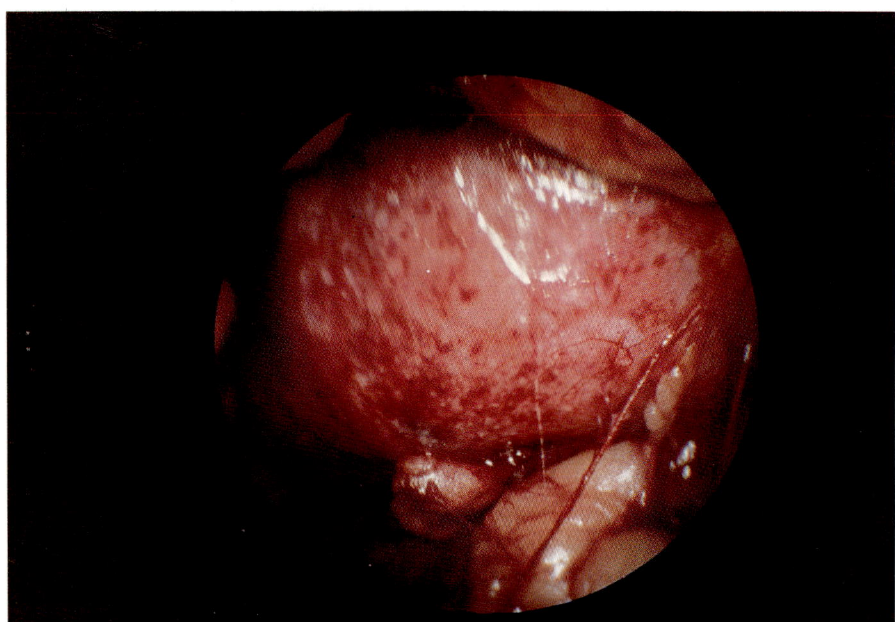

Figure 17-5 Neatly and atraumatically dissected kidney. Note that the capsular vessels have not been damaged by the balloon.

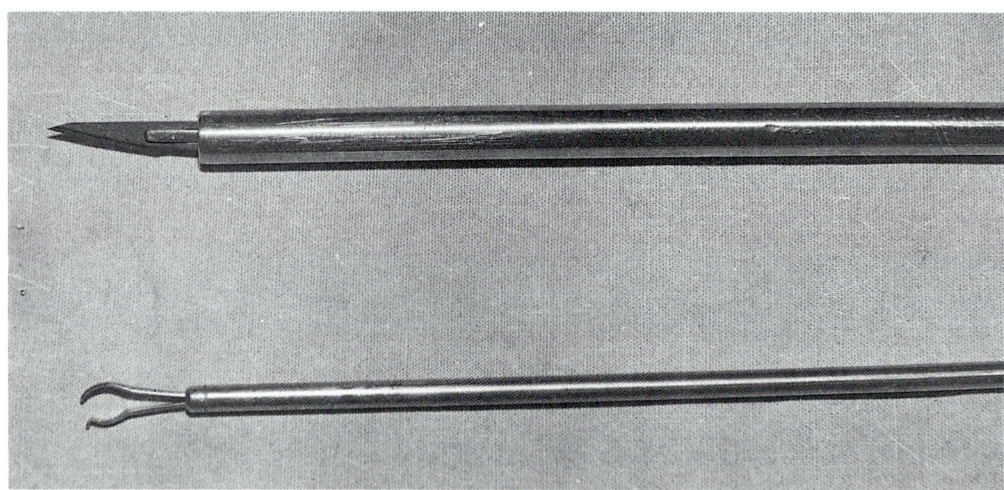

Figure 17-6 The retractable endoknife.

proven indispensable for endocavitary stone surgery (Fig. 17-6).

Other Instruments

The kidney dissector-retractor-ligator is of simple design, but useful for nephrectomy and pyelolithotomy (Fig. 17-7). Other modifications of existing surgical instruments are shown in Fig. 17-7.

Preoperative Preparation

Patients must receive informed consent. Except for the advisability of a mechanical bowel preparation because of the possibility that a distended colon might require greater insufflation pressure to keep the retroperitoneal space open, all other preparations are as described in Chapter 2.

Operative Procedure

Creation of Initial Retroperitoneal Space

The technique is slightly different for abdominal and pelvic retroperitoneoscopy, so it will be separately described.

Abdominal Retroperitoneoscopy

The patient is placed in a standard flank position. A subcostal line about 20 cm long is marked with the back of a knife to help in planning the trocar place-

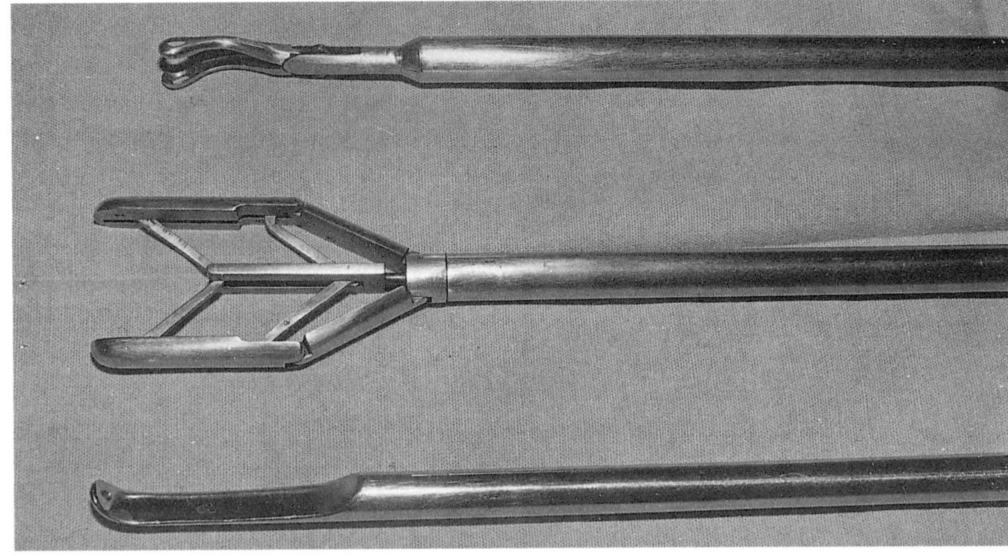

Figure 17-7 From top to bottom the endopyelolithotomy forceps, the retractor, and the multipurpose dissector-retractor-ligator.

ments. An incision 2 cm long is made at the center of the line and deepened by blunt dissection using a hemostat until resistance is felt at the transverse aponeurosis. This is pierced with a sharp thrust to create an entrance into the retroperitoneal space. A finger is then inserted into the retroperitoneum to bluntly dissect a space posteriorly.

The space is opened with small retractors, and the transversalis fascia is elevated with hemostats. The fascia is opened with scissors, and finger dissection is again performed to create a space between the fascia and the peritoneum. The balloon is then maneuvered into this space. To aid in maintaining the balloon in a desired position during inflation, the hemostats holding the edges of the cut fascia are not removed. For exposure of the kidney and the adrenal gland, Gerota's fascia is similarly grasped and incised with the balloon placed in the perirenal space.

Pelvic Retroperitoneoscopy

With the patient supine and a sandbag under the lumbosacral region a 2-cm incision is made in the suprapubic region. The incision is extended into the prevesical space, and the peritoneum is stripped away from the anterior wall of the bladder by blunt finger dissection. The balloon is then positioned in this virtual space.

Expansion and Dissection of the Retroperitoneal Space

The balloon is gradually inflated with sterile water or normal saline using a 50-mL syringe or squeeze pump similar to that found on a sphygmomanometer. The pump has proven preferable because it provides a better sensation of the expanding balloon (Fig. 17-8). With experience it is not mandatory to record balloon pressures. During the initial phase of the learning curve, however, monitoring the pressure provides assurance of expansion in the correct plane. As the balloon gradually expands, one can feel intermittent decreased resistance and occasionally hear the crackling sound of the breaking septae. After adequate inflation the balloon is left in place for 5 to 7 min to facilitate hemostasis. It is then deflated and removed.

The degree of distension of the balloon depends upon the type of operative procedure to be performed. Although Table 17-2 provides a rough guide for various retroperitoneal laparoscopic procedures, with experience one can judge the adequacy of the dissection by observing the bulging balloon in the abdomen. The balloon sometimes migrates away from the area to be explored due to the higher resistance offered by inflammatory adhesions in that area. This requires abdominal manipulation by applying counterpressure in the area of the unwanted migration .

Trocar Placement and Retroperitoneoscopy

A 10-mm trocar sheath without the obturator is inserted through the incision into the expanded retroperitoneal space, and the opening is made airtight with a mattress suture. The sheath is connected to an automatic insufflator, and the pressure is maintained between 10 and 30 mm Hg. One to three accessory

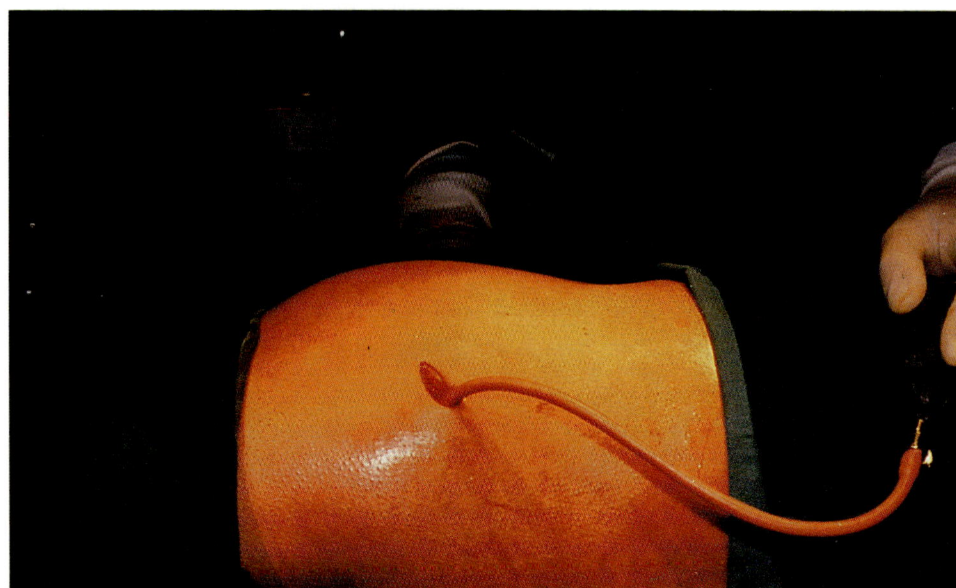

Figure 17-8 The balloon has been inflated in the retroperitoneal space. The bulge is clearly seen.

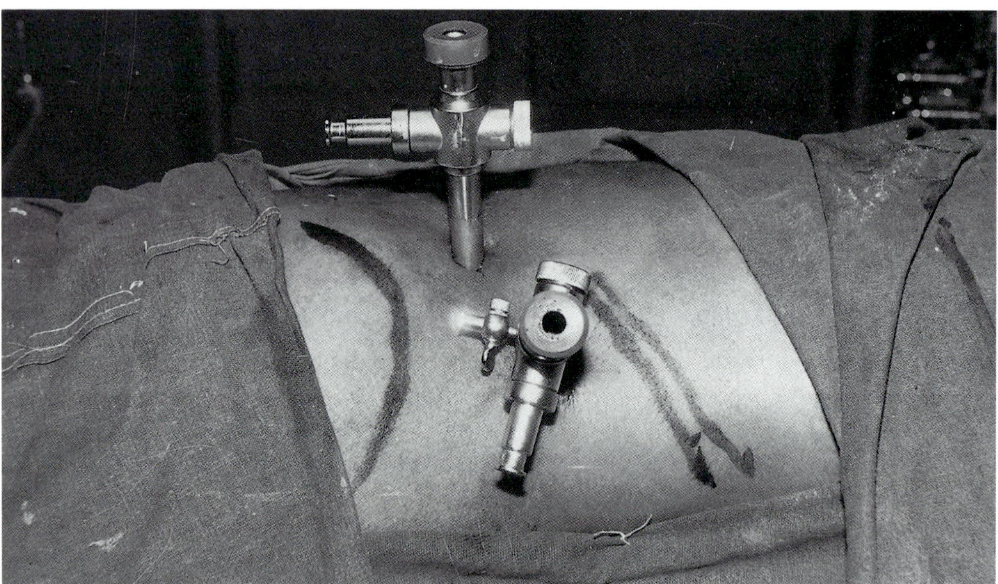

Figure 17-9 Trochar placement for varicocelectomy and ureterolithotomy. The iliac crest and the twelfth rib have been marked.

ports are then introduced under direct vision. For abdominal procedures two trocars are placed at each end of the marked subcostal line and the third above the iliac crest at the lateral border of sacrospinalis muscle. For pelvic procedures trocars are placed below the umbilicus and in the iliac regions.

Before the placement of any additional trocars a brief inspection with the telescope is performed to assess the quality of balloon dissection. If the area of interest has not been exposed properly, the balloon dissection is repeated, increasing the degree of inflation. However, this may not be possible in the presence of dense adhesions. The balloon dissection is considered satisfactory when one can clearly visualize the entire posterior surface of the kidney, the renal pelvis, the abdominal ureter, the internal spermatic vein, the iliac vessels, the urinary bladder, the prostate, the anterior vaginal wall, and the posterior abdominal muscles. In case of adhesions, these structures sometimes have to be further dissected endoscopically to be clearly identified.

Renoscopy and Renal Biopsy

The posterior surface of the kidney is inspected and a relatively avascular segment is selected. An adequate amount of tissue from the kidney is obtained

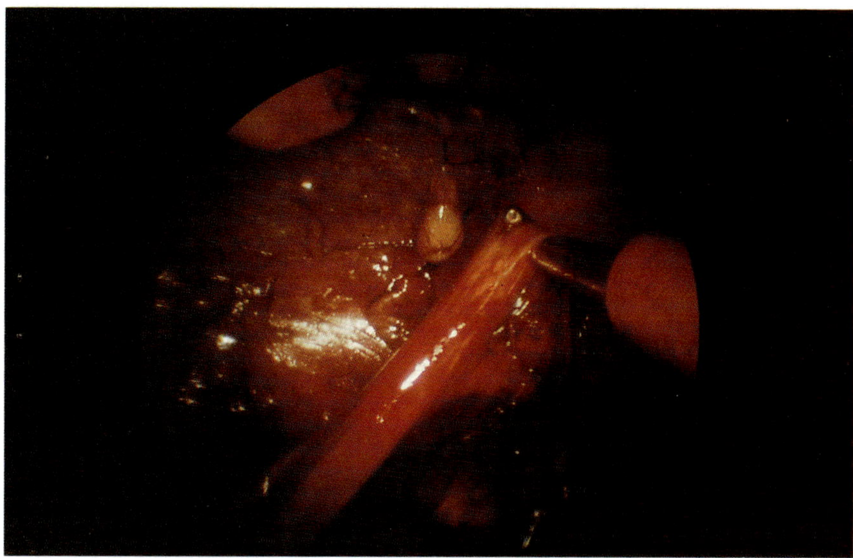

Figure 17-10 The internal spermatic vein has been dissected with a blunt hook.

by using a cup forceps through a 5-mm port placed at the renal angle. Hemostasis is established with laser or electrocoagulation using a suction electrode. The patient is discharged the same day without any drain, but sonography should be performed in selected cases 2 days later to detect any perinephric hematoma.

Varicocelectomy

This requires use of two accessory ports, one at each end of the marked subcostal line (Fig. 17-9). The internal spermatic vein is identified at the ureterovenous angle and should be traced to the internal ring for confirmation. It is dissected with a blunt instrument (Fig. 17-10), clip ligated, and divided. At this higher level multiple veins are less likely to be found. A drain is not required, and the patient can be discharged the same evening or the following day.

Ureterolithotomy

A calculus anywhere in the lumbar ureter can be easily removed using the same accessory ports as used for varicocelectomy. The ureteral identification is rarely a problem, as it is seen in most of the patients as soon as the telescope is inserted. If, due to improper balloon positioning or adhesions, the ureter has not been exposed, it should be endoscopically dissected around the calculus. An endo-Babcock and a hook are used for dissecting and mobilizing the ureter (Fig. 17-11). The dissection should be done from above downward so as not to dislodge the calculus accidentally. The stone can be identified by its bulge or by "feeling" it using the endo-Babcock to palpate the ureter. There is no need to stabilize the ureter if it is already fixed due to periureteritis. Under such circumstances the procedure can be done using only one 10-mm accessory port through the renal angle (Fig. 17-9). The retractable endoknife is introduced through the posterior port, and the blade is made to protrude only when one is ready to incise. The ureter is incised over the calculus, starting 5 mm proximally, while it is kept under mild stretch with the endo-Babcock placed just distal to the calculus through the anterior port. A curved dissecting forceps is used through the posterior port to loosen the calculus and deliver it into the retroperitoneum. A 10-mm cup forceps is used to grasp the stone via the posterior trocar so that it can be easily extracted. A large calculus may be removed through the 2-cm incision with a long hemostat under digital guidance. The ureteral incision is irrigated to flush out any loose residual fragments. Distal patency is tested through a curved flushing cannula. The incision in the ureter can be sutured, but we prefer to leave it open and drain it through one of the accessory ports. A double J stent is inserted cystoscopically to minimize urinary leakage. The patient is usually discharged the next day with the drain in place. Once drainage becomes negligible the drain is removed. The ureteral stent is discontinued 2 weeks later.

Nephrectomy

All three accessory ports previously described are used for a nephrectomy. If a proper balloon dissection has been done, the posterior surface of the kid-

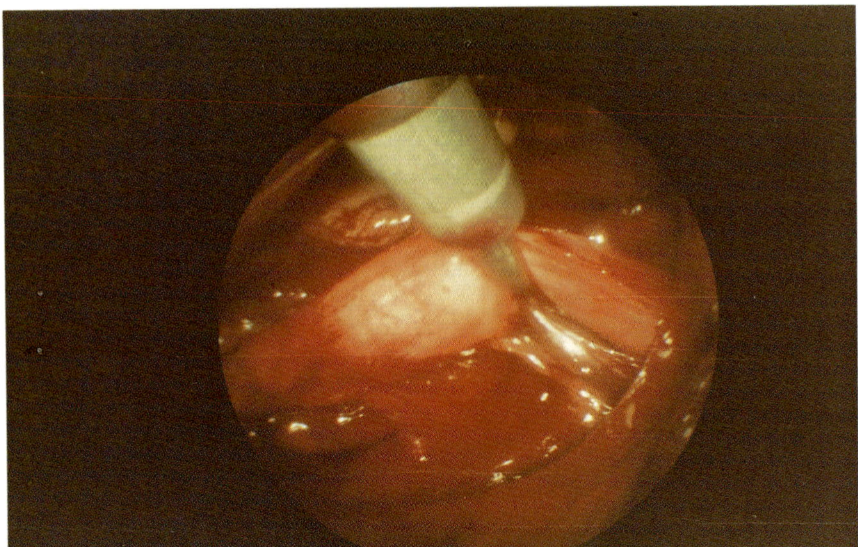

Figure 17-11 The ureter is dissected and grabbed above the calculus with and endo-Babcock.

ney, the renal pelvis, and the ureter are clearly visible. Otherwise the kidney is obscured by paranephric fat, requiring further endoscopic dissection (Fig. 17-12). Once the kidney is exposed the ureter is further dissected, mobilized, and divided between clips.

Next the posterior peritoneum is elevated with a retractor and dissected from the anterior surface of the kidney (Fig. 17-13). The kidney is then lifted by the proximal ureteral stump, and any adherent tissue between the pelvis and the posterior abdominal wall is divided to expose the renal pedicle. Further exposure is gained by exerting traction with the multipurpose instrument via the anterior port. This maneuver places the renal pedicle on stretch. Using a blunt dissector through the iliac port and a curved dissecting forceps through the posterior trocar, the pedicle is carefully dissected until the renal artery is exposed. If small, it is clip ligated and divided. Otherwise an endo-GIA may be employed. Alternative-

(a)

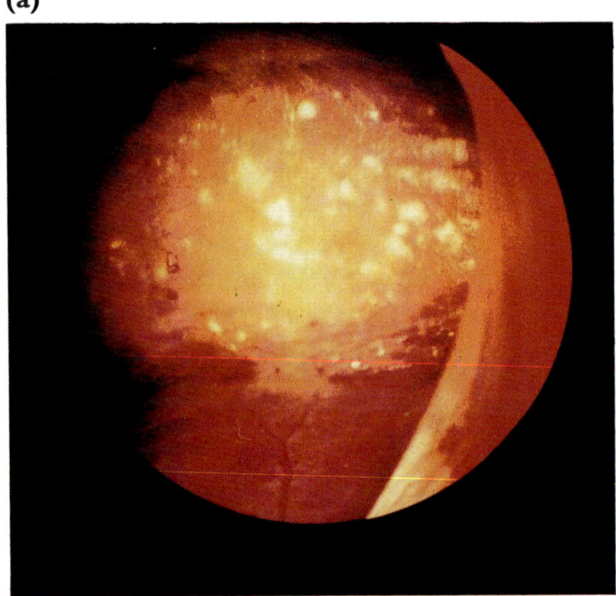

(b)

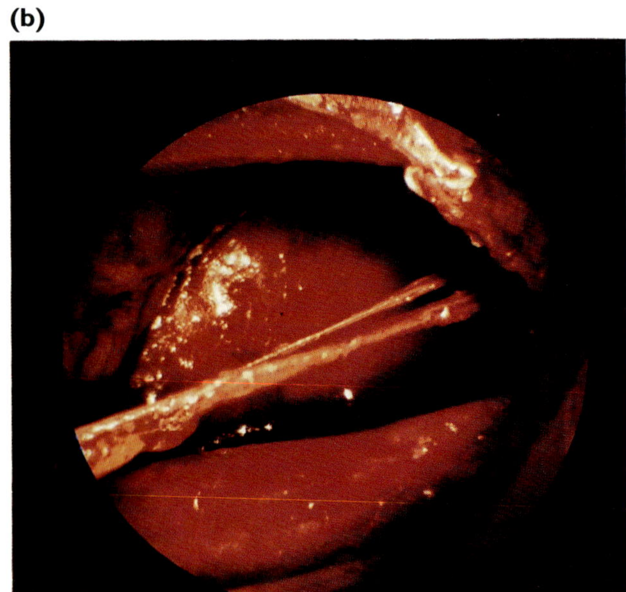

Figure 17-12 (a) Kidney covered with paranephric fat following balloon placement superficial to Gerota's fascia. The crescent of the lumbodorsal fascia and psoas muscle are clearly seen. (b) The fascia has been further dissected to expose the pyelonephritic kidney and psoas. A strand of uncut fascia is seen in the center.

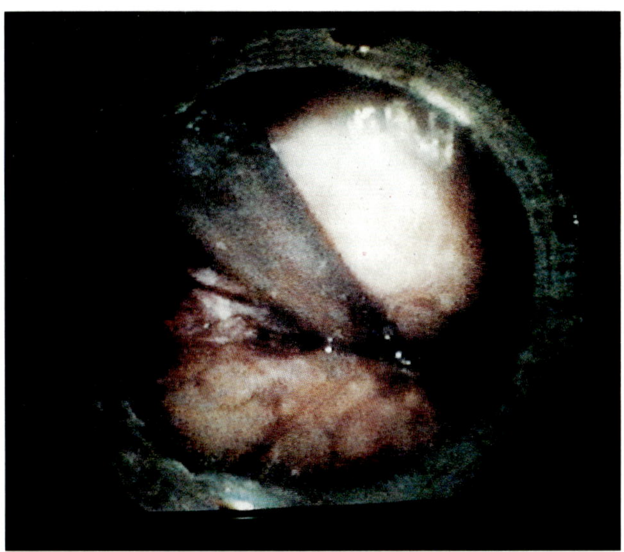

Figure 17-13 The anterior surface of the left kidney is being dissected at its lower pole using the multipurpose dissector.

ly, the multipurpose instrument may be used to ligate the renal pedicle (Fig. 17-14). After division of the artery the renal vein is similarly handled, freeing the kidney. Since this procedure is at present indicated only for benign atrophic renal units, it is not necessary to use an endocavitary bag or tissue morcellator. Instead the skin incision is enlarged by 1 cm, the opening stretched, and the kidney grasped with a sponge forceps under digital guidance and removed. The incisions are closed with absorbable sutures and drainage maintained for 24 h.[20]

Pelvic Retroperitoneoscopy

All four ports previously described are used for most pelvic procedures. Although the exposure is good, as in abdominal retroperitoneoscopy the working space is limited (Fig. 17-15).

Complications of Retroperitoneoscopy

To date retroperitoneoscopy has been performed safely with no major complications encountered. The minor complications discussed below are mostly operator related and can be prevented with experience.

Peritoneal Tear

A peritoneal tear can occur during digital dissection of the retroperitoneal space, overenthusiastic balloon distention, or if rupture of the balloon occurs during dissection of the retroperitoneal structures. This may lead to poor expansion of the retroperitoneal space secondary to leakage of CO_2 into the peritoneum. When faced with this dilemma during a short procedure, one may continue after placing a Veress needle in the peritoneal cavity as a vent. Otherwise the procedure should be converted to a standard open operation.

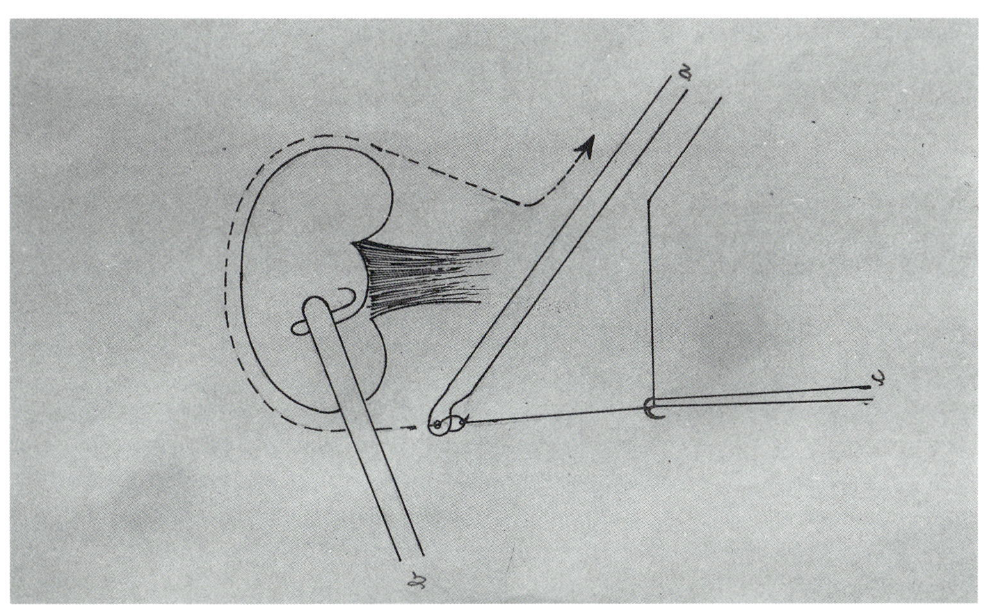

Figure 17-14 Multipurpose instrument being used as ligature carrier, by moving it along the dotted line. The kidney is maneuvered by holding the proximal ureter through the anterior port, while the ligature is opened up with a hook through the iliac port.

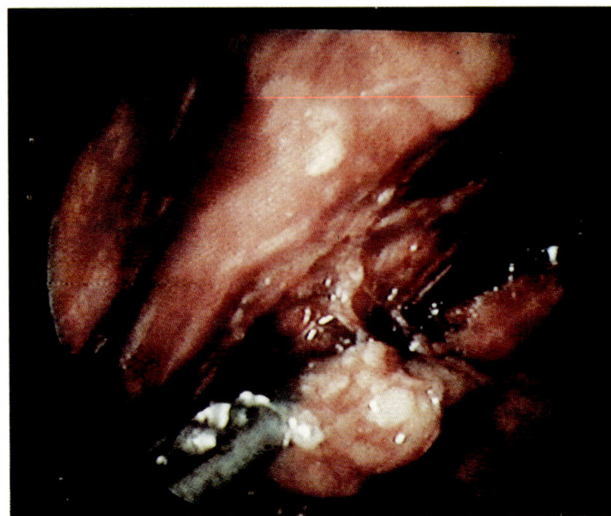

Figure 17-15 Lymph nodes in the left paravesical space being picked up with a dissecting forceps. The superior ramus of the left pubic bone is clearly seen.

Surgical Emphysema

Surgical emphysema occurs secondary to leakage of the gas around the initial trocar and is often due to a superficially placed mattress suture. The emphysema can sometimes extend from the scrotum to the face. It usually subsides within a few hours but can be eliminated by squeezing the gas out through the 2-cm incision at the conclusion of the procedure.

Primary Hemorrhage

Primary hemorrhage is most often encountered during renal biopsy, nephrolithotomy, pyelolithotomy, or nephrectomy and usually must be controlled by open surgery. Digital pressure through the 2-cm incision after packing with ribbon gauze can sometimes control the bleeding, and thereafter it can be clip ligated. Venous bleeding can also be controlled by reinserting the balloon and inflating it, but one should be careful not to occlude the vena cava on the right side.

Secondary Hemorrhage

In my experience secondary hemorrhage has usually occurred in dialysis patients following a renal biopsy.

Paralytic Ileus

The most likely etiology of paralytic ileus is the presence of blood in the retroperitoneum. The only patient who had this complication in our series was diagnosed to have widespread tuberculosis. Treatment should be conservative with nasogastric suction and parenteral fluids. Nevertheless, associated abdominal pathology may require more specific intervention.

Prevention of Other Possible Complications

1. *Air embolism* was a possibility during our initial experience secondary to rupture of the balloon. We now advocate use of fluids for inflation to avoid this disastrous possibility.
2. *Visceral damage* is another possible complication. The colon is at risk of injury during placement of the anterior trocar. It is difficult to distinguish if the path of the trocar is through the extraperitoneal fat or the colon. To prevent injuring the colon, the trocar should be placed under digital guidance. After removing the telescope and the cannula, the index finger is introduced into the retroperitoneal space and the colon is bluntly peeled from the abdominal wall. Trocar puncture is then done directly over the finger, which guides the trocar safely into the retroperitoneal space. The duodenum is at risk on the right and requires a similar approach.

Summary

Retroperitoneoscopy using the balloon technique is a safe, simple, and minimally invasive procedure for exposing the retroperitoneal organs from the subdiaphragmatic region to the pelvis. Though it provides a fast and reasonably good exposure of these organs, it has some limitations. The space may not be adequate for endoscopic manipulation in patients with large renal or adrenal masses, and the procedure is not advisable in patients with obesity, bleeding disorders, or retroperitoneal fibrosis.

The exploitation of the balloon in medicine is not new, but its use for expanding and dissecting the retroperitoneal space for performing retroperitoneoscopy is a completely new concept. With the passage of time, wider applications of this technique are likely to surface.

References

1. Bryant T: *Pract Surg* 1:630, 1878.
2. Bartel M: *Zdl Chir* 94:377, 1969.
3. Sommerkamp H: Lunboscopic: ein neues diagnostisch-therapeutisches prinzip der Urologie. Acta Urol 5:183, 1974.
4. Wickham JEA: The surgical treatment of renal lithiasis. In: *Urinary Calculus Disease*. Edited by Wickham JEA. New York, Churchill Livingstone, p 145, 1979.
5. Kaplan LR, Johnston GR, Hardy RM: Retroperitoneoscopy in dogs. *Gastrointest Endosc* 25:13, 1979.
6. Wickham JEA, Miller RA: Percutaneous Renal Access. In: *Percutaneous Renal Surgery*. Edited by Wickham JEA. New York: Churchill Livingstone, chap 2, p 33, 1988.
7. Hald T, Rasmusen F: Extraperitoneal pelvioscopy: A new aid in staging of lower urinary tract tumors. A preliminary report. *J Urol* 124:245, 1980.
8. Mazeman E, Wurtz A, Sauvege L, Rousseau O: Extraperitoneal pelvioscopy in the evaluation of lymph node extension of prostatic cancer. In: *Prostate Cancer*. Edited by Murphy GP, Küss R, Khoury S, Chatelain C, Denis L. New York: Alan R. Lis, Inc, part B, p 49, 1986.
9. Wurtz A: L'ensdoscopie de l'espace retroperitoneal: Techniques, resultats et indications actuelles. *Ann Chir* 43:475, 1985.
10. Eshghi AM, Roth JS, Smith AD: Percutaneous transperitoneal approach to a pelvic kidney for endourological removal of a staghorn calculus. *J Urol* 134:525, 1985.
11. Wienberg JJ, Smith AD: Percutaneous resection of the kidney: Preliminary Report. *J Endourol* 2:355, 1988.
12. Meretyk S. Clayman RV, Myers JA: Retroperitoneoscopy: Foreign body retrieval. *J Urol* 147:1608, 1992.
13. Clayman RV, Kavoussi LR, Sopa NJ, Albala DM, Figenshau RS, Chandhoke PS: Laparoscopic nephrectomy: Review of the initial 10 cases. *J Endourol* 6:127, 1992.
14. Gaur DD: Laparoscopic operative retroperitoneoscopy: Use of a new device. *J Urol* 147:1137, 1992.
15. Diaz-Buxo JA, Donadio JF Jr: Complications of percutaneous renal biopsy and analysis of 1000 consecutive biopsies. *Clin Nephrol* 4:221, 1975.
16. Levy AS, Madrio MP, Perrone RD: Laboratory assessment of renal disease. In: *The Kidney*. Edited by Brenner BM, Rector FC Jr. Philadelphia: WB Saunders 4th ed, chap 22, p 950, 1991.
17. Dodge WF, Daeschner CW Jr, Brennan JC, Rosenberg HS, Travis LB, Hoppes HC: Percutaneous renal biopsy in children. 1. General considerations *Pediatrics* 30:278, 1962.
18. Polascik TJ, Moore RG, Rosenberg MT, Kavoussi LR: Comparison of laparoscopic and open retropubic urethropexy for treatment of stress urinary incontinence. *Urol* 45:647, 1995.
19. McDougall EM, Klutke CG, Cornell T: Comparison of transvaginal versus laparoscopic bladder neck suspension for stress urinary incontinence. *Urol* 45:641, 1995.
20. Gaur DD, Agarwal DK, Purohit KC: Retroperitoneal laparoscopic nephrectomy: Initial case report. *J Urol* 149:103, 1993.

18

Laparoscopic Retroperitoneal Lymph Node Dissection

Raul O. Parra

The gold standard for appropriately staging clinical stage 1 nonseminomatous testicular carcinomas remains a retroperitoneal lymphadenectomy (RPLND). Anatomic advances and improvements in surgical technique have made possible the select preservation of the sympathetic nerves and plexus responsible for emission and ejaculation, markedly improving the quality of life of the young men most frequently afflicted by this malignant process. Nevertheless, approximately 70 percent of stage 1 patients undergoing a RPLND will be found to have negative lymph nodes and still must bare the possible morbidity and cosmetic insult of a laparotomy.[1,2]

With the intent of minimizing morbidity and based on the assumption that available effective *cis*-platinum-based chemotherapy would rescue relapsers, surveillance protocols were instituted. Results from several large centers reveal a relapse rate of close to 30 percent with 7 percent of those patients dying from their recurrence despite rescue chemotherapy.[1] In addition, surveillance protocols subject the patients to an extremely rigid and costly follow-up regimen which is difficult to adhere to and employ outside of specialized centers.

The advent of advanced laparoscopic techniques and instrumentation have made possible access to the retroperitoneal structures in a reliable and safe way.[3] It is obvious that if an endocavitary retroperitoneal dissection can be safely performed with results similar to an open modified dissection, patients could be surgically staged yet take advantage of the faster convalescence offered by laparoscopic surgery.

Indications

The only appropriate candidate for a laparoscopic RPLND as an alternative to a standard open dissection is a patient with a clinical stage 1 non-seminomatous testicular tumor who is clearly aware of the potential limitations and risks of this novel technique. We do not consider this option on any patient suspected to have positive nodes based on findings on computed tomography or the presence of persistently elevated tumor markers.

Patient Preparation

No special preparation is required other than a mechanical bowel preparation to decompress the intestines, thus facilitating intraoperative exposure. The patient is typed and crossed for two units of blood, however, autologous donation is preferable. A broad spectrum antibiotic (usually a cephalosporin) is administered 1 h before the procedure and continued for two additional doses after surgery.

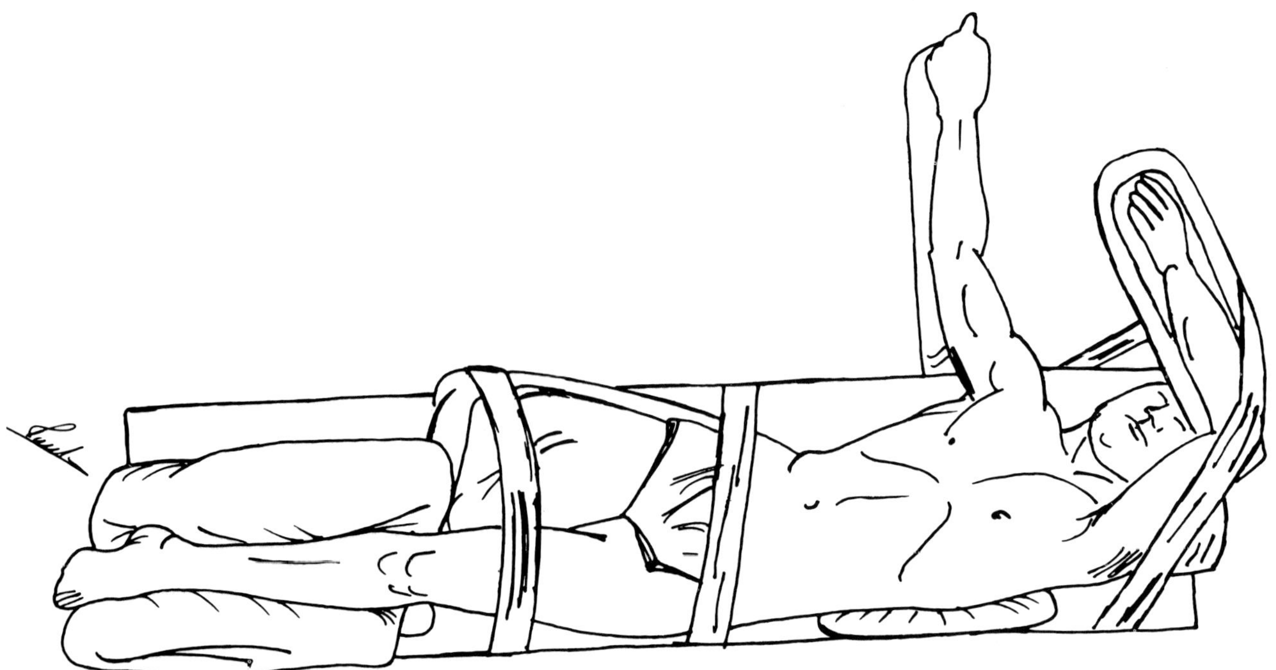

Figure 18-1 The patient is placed in a posture similar to that for a thoracoabdominal approach to the kidney with the ipsilateral side rotated 30 to 45 degrees and the arm placed across the chest.

Surgical Technique

Patient Positioning

After adequate anesthesia is induced, a nasogastric tube and urethral catheter are placed. The patient is positioned in a semiflank posture of 45 degrees with the break just above the iliac crest. The contralateral leg is flexed 90 degrees at the knee and about 30 degrees at the hip. The ipsilateral leg lies straight over the top, and a pillow is placed between the legs for padding. The ipsilateral arm is brought across the chest and supported by a Krauss stand. The table is then fully flexed and the patient secured with heavy adhesive tape (Fig. 18-1).

Pneumoperitoneum and Trocar Location

Access for establishment of the pneumoperitoneum and trocar placement is all done with the patient in the position just described. The pneumoperitoneum is obtained according to the surgeon's choice. We prefer an open technique because of its ease and safety and because it provides quick filling of the peritoneal cavity.

The number of trocars and their location varies among different authors. The arrangement I have found most useful is demonstrated in Fig. 18-2. All trocars are at least 10 mm in diameter offering flexibility in the number and size of instruments that may be utilized. In addition to the umbilical port uti-

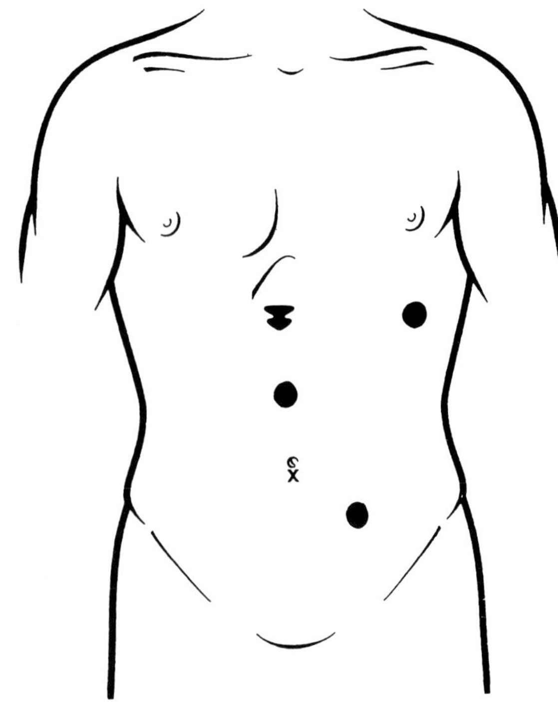

Figure 18-2 Trocar configuration utilized for left-sided laparoscopic lymph node dissection.

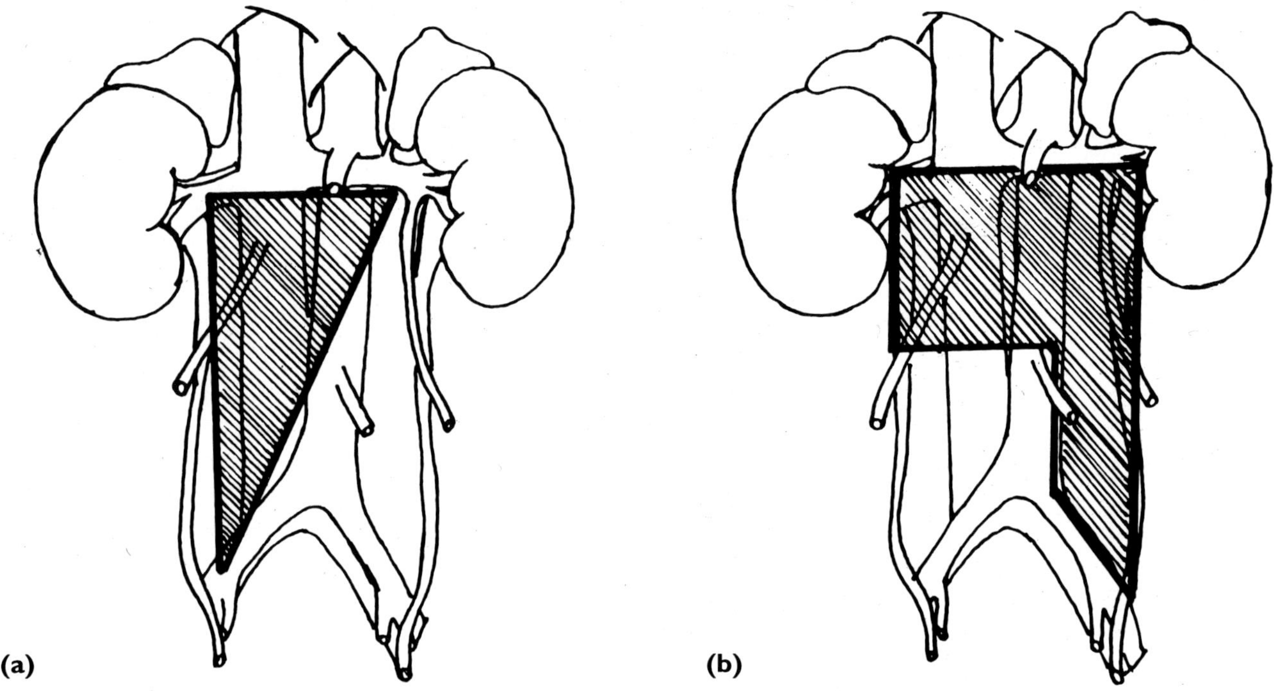

Figure 18-3 (a) Template for right-sided dissection. (b) Template for left-sided dissection.

lized for introduction of the laparoscope at least three more trocars are required. Two working ports are placed, one 3 to 4 cm above the umbilicus and the other along the midclavicular line approximately at McBurney's point. The third trocar is placed in the mid-axillary line at the level of the twelfth rib to introduce a retractor to displace the liver, spleen, or other upper quadrant viscera. An additional port is often necessary at a subumbilical location in the midline in order to retract the bowel medially.

Margins of Dissection

We believe that in order to be worthwhile this procedure must be a true dissection, not simply a nodal sampling procedure. Therefore, a template pattern was adapted from those already proven in open dissections (Fig. 18-3).

Dissection

Exposure is obtained by incising the line of Toldt of the corresponding side of dissection all the way from the iliac bifurcation past the splenocolic or hepatocolic flexure. This maneuver is aided by grasping the colon with endo-Babcock graspers and retracting medially placing the pericolic tissues under tension and facilitating their dissection with the endoscopic scissors (Fig. 18-4). Continued traction on the colon together with blunt dissection exposes the retroperitoneum and the great vessels covered by the lymphatic tissues. On the left side the inferior mesenteric artery is discernible coursing in an acute angle towards the mesentery. This serves as an important landmark, since the aortic dissection should not extend below this level in order to avoid damage to the hypogastric plexus.

The ureter is identified at the level of the iliac bifurcation and fully mobilized to the renal pelvis. Next we dissect the spermatic cord from the internal ring to its draining point—either on the renal vein or inferior vena cava depending on whether the left or right side is being operated upon (Fig. 18-5). The spermatic vessels are then clipped and the cord removed through one of the trocar sites.

If a left retroperitoneal dissection is being performed the adventitial tissue overlying the aorta at the take-off of the inferior mesenteric artery is grasped with nontraumatic endoscopic forceps and a window created with the scissors until the aortic

(a) (b)

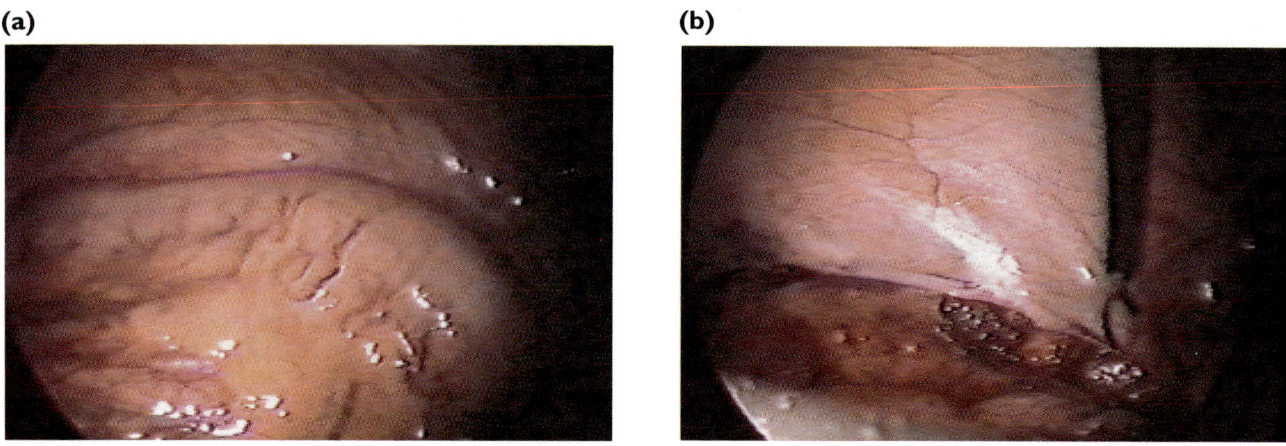

Figure 18-4 (a) The left colon is visualized as well as the line of Toldt. (b) The left peritoneal reflection is opened throughout its entire length.

wall is visualized. The lymphatic package is then split in the middle to the level of the renal vein (Fig. 18-6).

The lateral lymph tissue located between the aorta and the left ureter is then dissected beginning at the renal pedicle. The nodal package is grasped superiorly and with a combination of sharp and blunt dissection freed from the surrounding tissue in a caudad direction (Fig. 18-7). The interaortocaval nodes are removed next by carefully dissecting the

(a) (b)

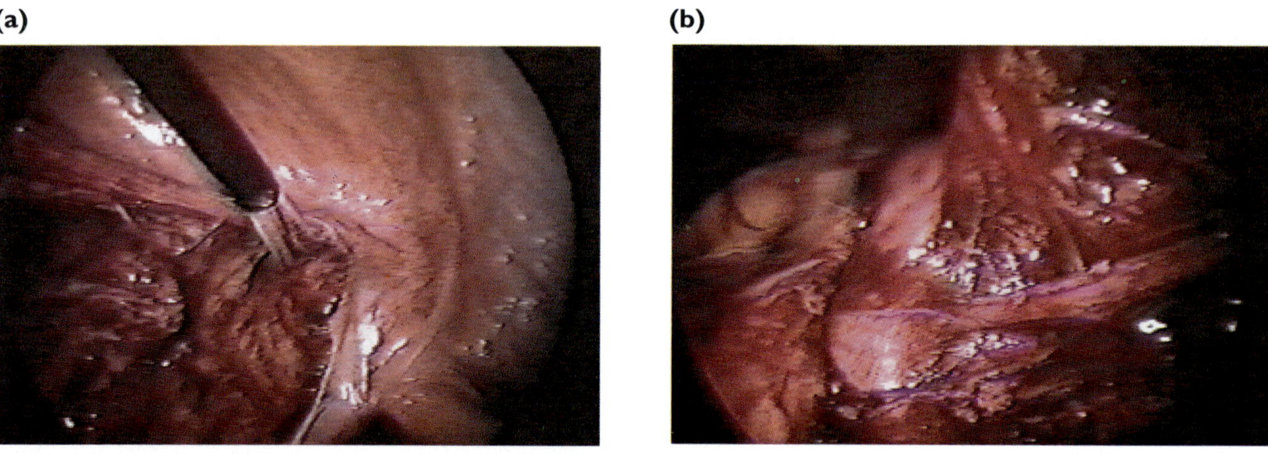

(c)

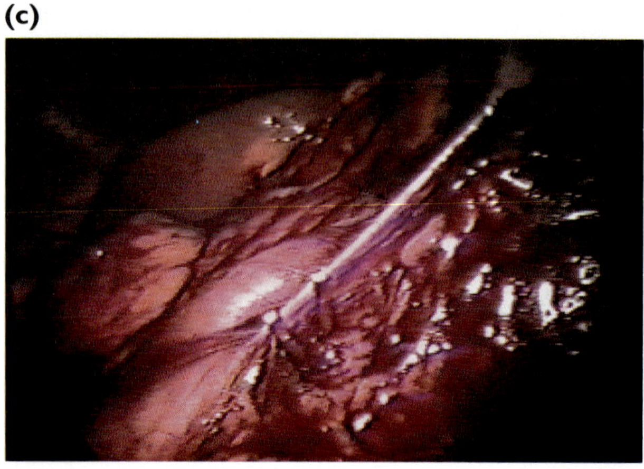

Figure 18-5 (a) Left spermatic cord is totally mobilized and excised at the internal ring. (b) The entrance of the left gonadal vein to the renal vein is demonstrated. (c) The gonadal vein is divided and the entire spermatic cord removed.

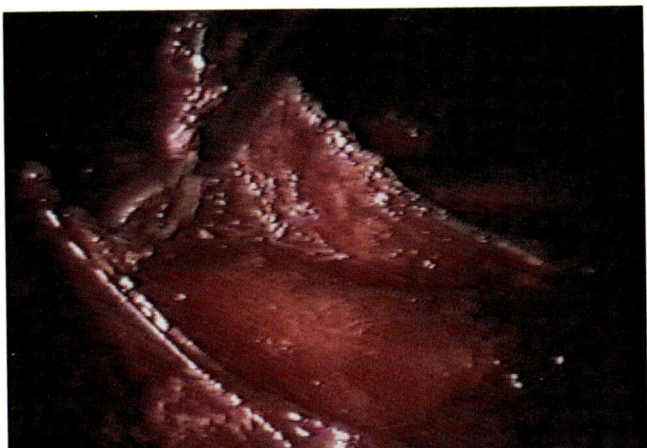

Figure 18-6 The technique of dissection of the aortic and periaortic nodal packets is demonstrated. The tissues are split in the middle following the principle of split and roll described by Donahue.

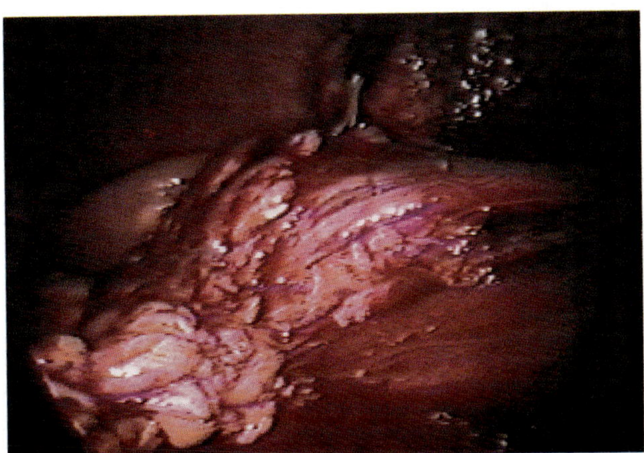

Figure 18-7 The Hilar nodal packet is being dissected.

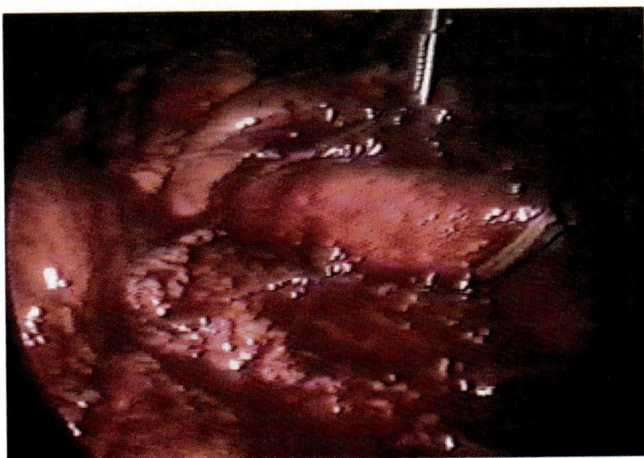

Figure 18-8 The aortic dissention has been completed and the interaortal tissue is clearly seen.

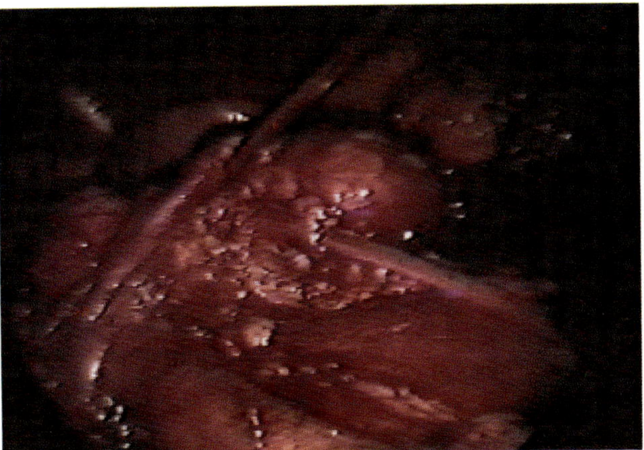

Figure 18-9 The completed dissection is demonstrated.

left renal vein, again working in a caudad direction, until the anterior spinal ligament is identified. The nodal bundle must be maintained under tension so that a cleavage plane between the medial vena caval and aortic borders is established (Fig. 18-8). Any lumbar vessels encountered are clipped and divided. We have found the use of an endoscopic vein retractor quite helpful during this part of the procedure to adequately expose the posteromedial aspects of the great vessels. The aorta, periaortic, and interaortocaval regions are cleanly dissected and the nodal tissues extracted (Fig. 18-9). Finally, the colon is brought over the left retroperitoneum and tacked to the divided parietal peritoneum edge with either a regular endoscopic clip applier or an automatic endoscopic hernia stapler in order to retroperitonealize the area of dissection. If instead, the operation is being done for a right-sided tumor, the dissection commences at the aortic bifurcation medial to the ureter and includes the tissues in the interaortocaval and aortic regions. The rest of the technical aspects of the procedure are similar to that for a left-sided dissection.

Postoperative Care

The nasogastric tube is removed in the recovery room and the urethral catheter once the patient is fully awake. A clear diet is instituted on the first postoperative day and advanced as tolerated. Most patients can be discharged by the third day and resume regular activities a week later. Follow-up is the same as for any other patient treated for a testicular neoplasm.

Results and Comments

To date a total of eight retroperitoneal node samplings or dissections have been reported in the literature, with several more surely having been performed without subsequent documentation.[3,4,5,6,7] The number of lymph nodes retrieved has ranged between 3 and 29. However, those reported by Kavoussi should be considered nodal sampling procedures, since only 3 and 7 nodes were retrieved respectively in the two patients in which they were able to complete the procedure successfully. In a third patient the operation could not be completed as planned due to bleeding. Operative time, when reported, has ranged from 5 to 10 h with relatively few postoperative complications. Our experience has been quite encouraging with a total of 25 nodes obtained in our first patient. The operative time was 2 h and 40 min. The patient was discharged on the third postoperative day and was able to return to regular activities within 6 days, maintaining antegrade ejaculation.

Rassweiler has amassed the largest experience to date.[8] In his series of 14 consecutive patients undergoing a laparoscopic retroperitoneal dissection, including postchemotherapy and stage 2 patients, no complications were encountered and a dissection comparable to an open procedure was accomplished.

The assimilation of the laparoscopic retroperitoneal lymph node dissection by the urologic oncology community will be difficult, with detractors citing the possibility of an incomplete dissection and the long operative time required as drawbacks. However, there is no denying the fact that patients will certainly benefit from the rapid convalescence offered by a laparoscopic approach.

References

1. Ritchie JP: Neoplasms of the testis. In: *Campbell's Urology* 6th Ed. Edited by Walsh PC, Retik AB, Stamey TA, Vaughn ED Jr. Philadelphia: W.B. Saunders, vol. 2, chap. 30, pp 1222–1263, 1992.
2. Donohue JP, Foster RS, Rowland RG, Bihrle R, Jones J, Grier G: Nerve sparing retroperitoneal lymphadenectomy with preservation of ejaculation. *J Urol* 144:287–292, 1990.
3. Hulbert JC, Fraley EE: Laparoscopic retroperitoneal lymphadenectomy: New approach to pathologic staging of clinical stage 1 germ cell tumors of the testis. *J Endourol* 6(2):123–125, 1992.
4. Rukstalis DB, Chodak GW: Laparoscopic retroperitoneal lymph node dissection in a patient with stage 1 testicular carcinoma. *J Urol* 148:1907–1910, 1992.
5. Rassweiler J, Henkel TO, Potempa DM, et al: Transperitoneal laparoscopic nephrectomy: Training, technique, and results. *J Endourol* 7:505–516, 1993.
6. Stone NN, Schlussel RN, Waterhouse RL: Laparoscopic retroperitoneal lymph node dissection in stage A nonseminomatous testis cancer. *Urol* 42:610–614, 1993.
7. Capelouto CC, Kavoussi LR: Laparoendoscopic surgery of the genital tract. *Atlas Urol Clin North Am* 1(2):93–101, 1993.
8. Rassweiler J, Henkel T, Tschda R, Junemann K, Alken P: Modified laparoscopic retroperitoneal lymphadenectomy for testicular cancer—the lessons learned. *J Urol* 151:499A, 1994.

19

Technique of Radical Perineal Prostatectomy in Combination with Laparoscopic Pelvic Lymphadenectomy

Raul O. Parra
Marceliano Garcia Perez
M. Pilar Laguna
Santiago Isorna

The advent of laparoscopic lymphadenectomy has revitalized the perineal approach to the radical excision of the cancerous prostate. Disinterest in the radical perineal prostatectomy arose from the morbidity associated from the separate abdominal incision required to perform a staging node dissection, the high incidence of impotence, and the lack of training of current urologists in the perineal technique. Nevertheless, a radical perineal prostatectomy when applied in conjunction with an endocavitary pelvic node staging offers a seemingly less morbid alternative in select patients undergoing surgical treatment of prostate cancer.

Historical Development

The first recorded surgical removal of prostatic tissue must be considered incidental. In A.D. 25, Celsus removed part of a prostate through a curved perineal incision while attempting to extract a stone presumably located in the bladder.[1] Other reports of similar accidental procedures followed in the ensuing centuries. It was not until the 1800s that, as a consequence of better anatomopathological descriptions of the prostate and its afflictions together with the availability of anesthesia, the first crude prostatectomies were performed. Billroth in 1867 must be credited with the first planned prostate excision for the cure of prostate cancer. Throughout this century renowned surgeons such as Lagenbuch, Demarquay, Leisrink, and others attempted with an array of different techniques to remove the diseased gland. Unfortunately, results were less than satisfactory, with most cases resulting in what must be considered subtotal prostatectomies secondary to limited surgical access and significant bleeding, which in essence resulted in blind operations.[1] The twentieth century brought significant advances in anatomic knowledge and instrumentation, which led the way to the establishment of direct vision anatomic prostatectomies. Proust in 1901 was the first to perform a perineal prostatectomy via a median incision entirely under direct vision.[1] However, Young must be considered the pioneer of the procedure. He improved the technique by introducing instruments of his own design and applied sound oncologic principles—simultaneously removing the seminal vesicles, ampulla, and surrounding periprostatic fascia—for the first time, making the surgery potentially curative for patients with prostate cancer.[2] Further refinements such as the direct vesico-urethral anastomosis promulgated by Wildbolz[1] and the subsphincteric modification of Haim and Belt helped establish the radical perineal prostatectomy as the surgical procedure of choice for clinically localized prostate cancer until supplanted by the retropubic approach in the 1970s. Three relevant points contributed to this: (1) The importance of a staging lymphadenectomy became obvious, making the retropubic operation more attractive by avoiding the second incision necessary in the perineal approach; (2) the contributions of Walsh paved the way to a more anatomic procedure significantly reducing blood loss, incontinence, and impotence[3,4,5] and (3) the lack of training of most modern-day urologic surgeons in perineal approach.

Recent developments in endocavitary surgery, in particular the laparoscopic staging of the pelvic lymph nodes, now obviates the need for a separate abdominal incision while potentially reducing postoperative discomfort.[6] In addition, anatomic principles learned from the retropubic experience have also been applied perineally, with the resultant preservation of the erectile nerves and maintenance of potency[7] (Table 19-1).

Pertinent Anatomic Points

Paramount to the performance of a successful radical perineal prostatectomy is an understanding of the different fascial layers enveloping the prostate and seminal vesicles and their relationship to the rectum and other perineal structures.

Neurovascular Bundles

The autonomic nerves innervating the bladder, prostate, rectum, and urethra are derived from the pelvic plexus located in the retroperitoneum with nerves originating from spinal cord segments S2–S4. The prostatic cavernous branches course on the dorsolateral aspect of the prostate immediately outside the prostatic capsule and within the lateral

TABLE 19-1 Historical Landmarks in the Development of Perineal Prostatectomy

Contribution	Surgeon	Year
BLIND TECHNIQUES		
First perineal lithotomy	Ammonius Lithotomus	460–357 B.C.
Curved perineal incision for lithotomy; incidental partial removal of the prostate	Celsus	A.D. 25
Incidental excision of a prostatic lobe during perineal lithotomy	Covillar	1639
First perineal prostatectomy	Guthrie	1834
First perineal prostatectomy for carcinoma	Billroth	1867
Transrectal prostatectomy	Demarquay	1873
Finger enucleation via median perineal urethrotomy	Gouley	1873
Curved incision used for excision of prostate cancer and urethral reconstruction	Leisrink	1882
Ischiorectal prostatectomy	Dittel	1890
Assisted perineal prostatectomy by a second abdominal incision used to depress the prostate	Bryson	1899
Prostate pulled into perineum by a balloon inflated in the bladder	Syms	1900

TABLE 19-1 *(continued)*

Contribution	Surgeon	Year
DIRECT VISION TECHNIQUES		
Prostatectomy via a median perineal incision; special perineal table, prostatic tractor, and lobe enucleator used	Proust	1901
Conservative perineal prostatectomy: curved or inverted Y incision, preservation of veru montanun and ejaculatory ducts; introduction of special instruments	Young	1903
Radical perineal prostatectomy; concomitant removal of seminal vesicles, ampullae of the vas, and fascia	Young	1905
Preservation of structures around sphincter; urethra anastomosed to the vesical neck	Wildbolz	1906
Hemostatic bag for perineal approach	Davis	1924
Control of bleeding by suture obliteration of prostatic fossa	Gibson	1928
Exposure of the prostate between external anal sphincter and rectal wall	Haim	1936
Standardization of subsphincteric approach	Belt	1939
MODERN-DAY CONTRIBUTIONS		
Nerve-sparing technique for radical perineal prostatectomy	Weldon	1988
Laparoscopic lymphadenectomy introduced	Shuessler	1991
Laparoscopic lymphadenectomy best when combined with a perineal prostatectomy	Parra	1993

pelvic fascia, with branches to the prostate perforating the fascia and penetrating the substance of the gland. The nervi erigenti continue on the lateral surface of the membranous urethra and then traverse the urogenital diaphragm and reach the corpora cavernosa, coursing behind the dorsal penile artery and nerve.

Fascial Layers

The areolar tissue layer between the posterior surface of the prostate and rectal wall, better known as Denonvillier's fascia, is the most important anatomic landmark in the performance of a radical perineal prostatectomy. Erroneously this structure has been described as being composed of two layers, anterior and posterior. Tobin and Benjamin[8] have clearly demonstrated that Denonvillier's fascia is a single membrane formed by the fusion of the peritoneum in the pelvic cul de sac, which, as with other embryonic fusion of mesothelial intestinal surfaces, eventually becomes adherent, regresses, and disappears, leaving only the underlying connective tissue as a fibrous film intimately adherent to the dorsal prostatic capsule. This true Denonvillier's fascia is the one imprecisely labeled the anterior layer. On the other hand the so-called posterior layer is in reality the ventral rectal fascia, which separates the anterior rectal wall from the posterior aspect of the prostate covered by Denonvillier's fascia.

Immediately underneath the endopelvic fascia lies the pelvic fascia, which embryologically is mesenchymal in origin and surrounds the bladder, prostate, and rectum. The portion of pelvic fascia covering the anterolateral prostate is called the lateral pelvic fascia, which is continuous and fuses posteriorly with Denonvillier's and the ventral rectal fascia. It is within the lateral pelvic fascia that the cavernous nerves course in a dorsolateral direction with respect to the rectum, continuing caudally onto the lateral surface of the membranous urethra. Consequently, as elegantly described by Weldon, a vertical incision made on the ventral rectal fascia all the way to the proximal membranous urethra will avoid damage to the nervi erigenti.

Indications

Indications for a laparoscopic pelvic lymphadenectomy will not be addressed in detail here, since they have already been covered in Chap. 10. Briefly we recommend an endocavitary staging aside from cases considered for perineal prostatectomy or radiotherapy in the following circumstances:

Prostate specific antigen levels >20 ng/mL.

Poorly differentiated tumors (Gleason Score ≥7).

Clinical Stages B2 or C.

Combinations of the above parameters.

On the other hand our decision to perform a radical perineal in lieu of a retropubic prostatectomy relies on the following criteria:

Patients previously staged laparoscopically found to have negative lymph nodes.

Impotent men.

Obese patients.

Patients with previous lower abdominal surgery involving the perivesicular and periprostatic area.

Patients with vascular grafts in the pelvic region.

Patients with stage A tumors, especially if an aggressive transurethral resection was performed. Identification between the prostatic apex and urethra is often difficult in such cases via the retropubic route but considerably easier to discern perineally.

Individuals electing the procedure after informed consent.

Patients with well to moderately differentiated tumors (Gleason Score <7) and PSAs <10 ng/mL.

Contraindications

Most patients considered surgical candidates must also be considered good candidates for a radical perineal prostatectomy. However, in certain circumstances this technique is not indicated:

Patients with physical disabilities making it impossible to place them in stirrups (hip contractures and/or unstable hip replacements).

Previous perineal or rectal surgery (except abdominal perineal resection) .

Prostate gland volumes over 70 grams; large prostates can be difficult to remove, possibly leading to increased intraoperative bleeding and positive surgical margins.

Patients with severely impaired pulmonary function.

Patient Preparation

Bowel Preparation

We believe that a thorough bowel cleansing is necessary because of the slight increase in the risk of rectal injury with the perineal approach.

Day Before Surgery

Clear liquid diet.

GOLITELY 2–4 L.

Erythromycin/Neomycin base 1 g by mouth at 1300, 1500, and 2100.

Day of Surgery

A broad spectrum cephalosporin plus clindamycin 600 mg 2 h before surgery.

Patient Positioning

Immediately after completing the laparoscopic staging lymphadenectomy the patient is placed in an exaggerated lithotomy position and the area prepped in the standard fashion (Fig. 19-1). A sterile disposable O'Connell TUR drape is routinely used, which allows the surgeon to manipulate the rectum during the dissection if necessary.

Instrumentation

Few special instruments are truly required. We routinely only employ the following:

A curved Lowsley tractor.

A Young tractor.

Two narrow Deaver retractors.

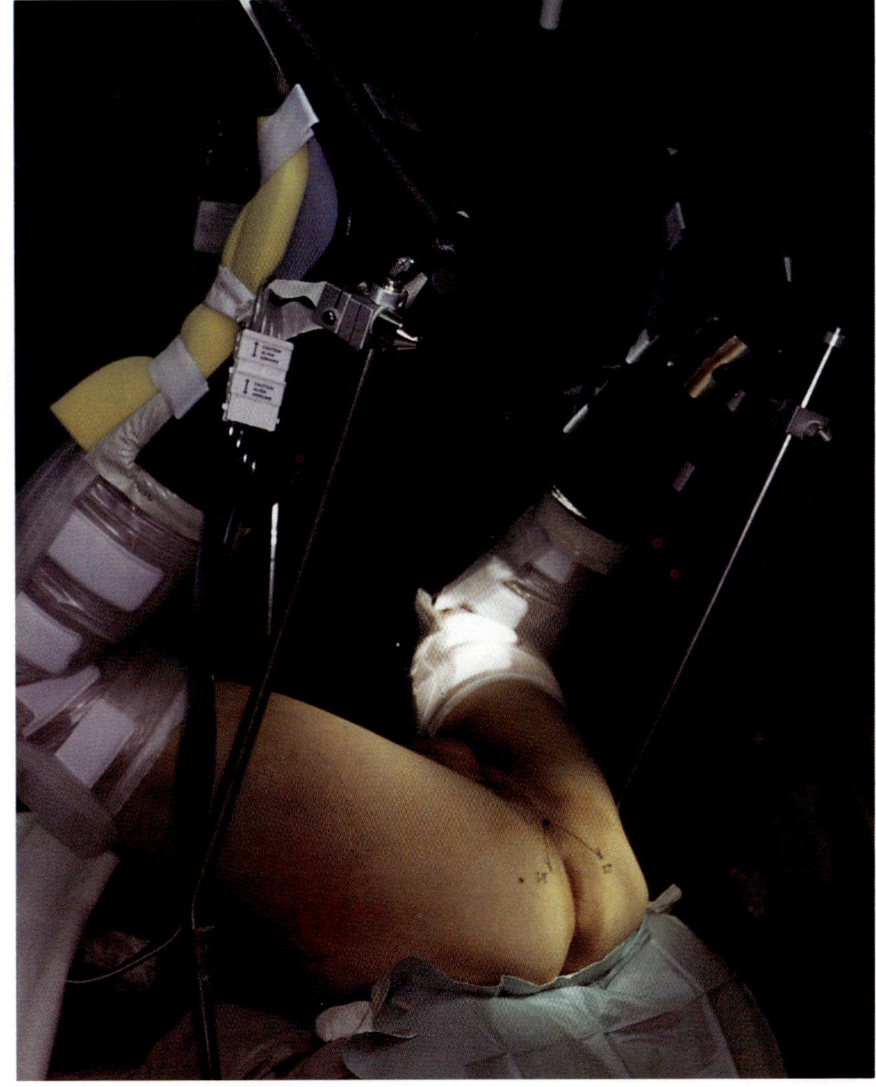

Figure 19-1 In preparation for surgery, the patient is placed at the edge of the table with the legs in Allen stirrups in an exaggerated dorsolithotomy position. Note the sequential pneumatic stockings used to minimize the risk of deep venous thrombosis.

Surgical Technique

After the curved Lowsley tractor is passed per urethra into the bladder (Fig. 19-2), a skin incision is made approximately 1.5 to 2 cm above the anal verge extending from ischial tuberosity to ischial tuberosity (Fig. 19-3). The underlying subcutaneous adipose tissue and superficial fascia are divided with electrocautery to the level of the deep aponeurosis which covers the gap between the rectum and the ischial tuberosities. Care is taken not to include the central perineal tendon within this subcutaneous tissue dissection (Fig. 19-4). The next step consists of developing the ischiorectal fossae bilaterally. This is accomplished by digitally creating the virtual space between the prostate and ischial rami (Fig. 19-5). Once the ischiorectal spaces are fully developed, the lateral aspects of the prostate and ischium can be readily palpated allowing the surgeon to encircle the central perineal tendon with the index finger (Fig. 19-6a). The tendon can then be divided with the aid of electrocautery (Fig. 19-6b). This maneuver exposes the rectourethralis muscle, which extends between the rectum and the bulbourethralis muscle. The rectourethralis is variable in its development, often consisting of a distinct muscular band that must be divided sharply (Fig. 19-7). Other times, however, this muscle is less well developed, appearing instead as a thin sheath of muscular fibers covering the posterior prostate and Denonvillier's fascia (Fig. 19-8). A finger in the rectum often aids in the performance of this maneuver by facilitating proper identification of the anterior rectal wall.

After division of the rectourethralis muscle, blunt dissection with a moist sponge allows development of the plane between the rectum and Denonvillier's fascia clearly exposing Denonvillier's fascia overlying the prostate, the so-called pearly gates (Fig. 19-9). A midline vertical incision is made on the ventral rectal fascia from the membranous urethra to the

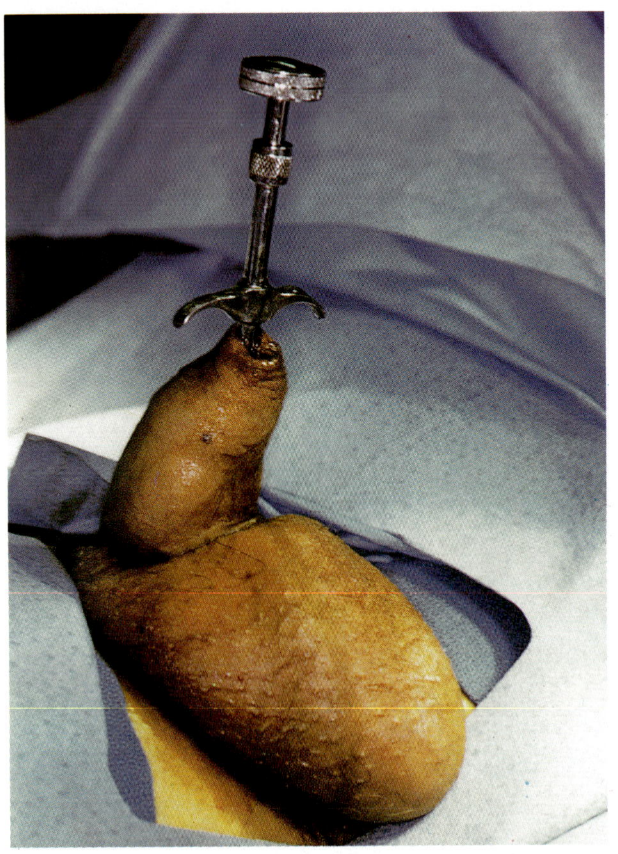

Figure 19-2 The curved Lowsley tractor is in place. Manipulation of this instrument will facilitate exposure of the prostate.

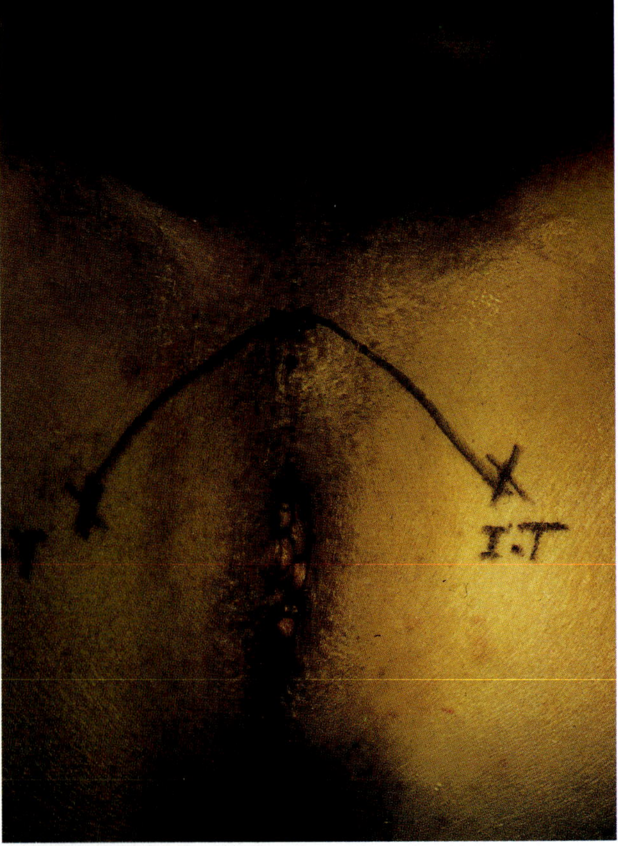

Figure 19-3 The skin incision extends between both ischial tuberosities, approximately 1.5 to 2 cm above the anal verge.

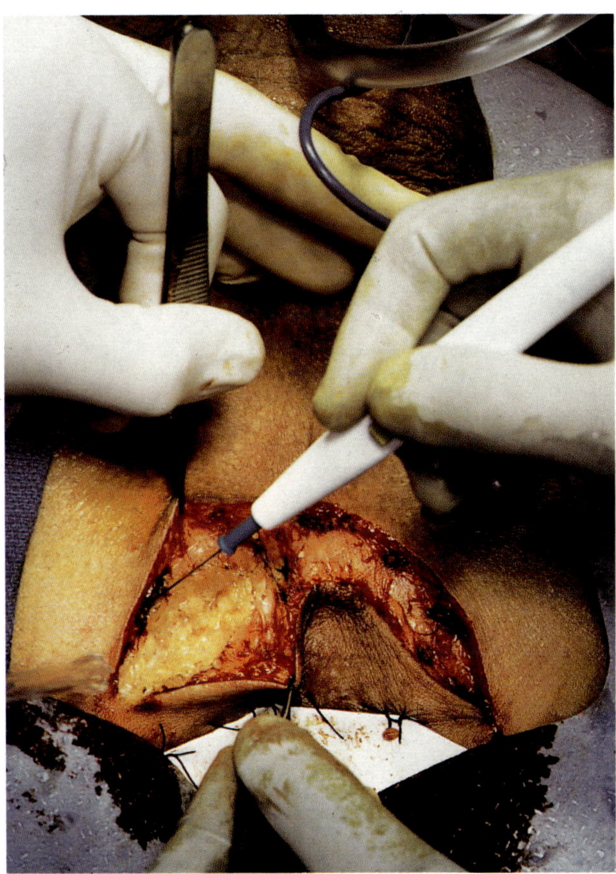

Figure 19-4 Following the skin incision, the subcutaneous adipose tissue is incised with electrocautery. Care is taken to preserve the central perineal tendon.

base of the prostate. A cleavage plane is then developed between the prostatic capsule, the wall of the membranous urethra and the fascia by gently dissecting with the tips of the scissors (Fig. 19-10). Next the urethra is encircled with a right-angle clamp, carefully excluding the fascia containing the cavernous nerves as they course to the urogenital diaphragm. Once isolated, the urethra is secured with a vessel loop. These last two steps are perhaps the most important if a nerve sparing prostatectomy is contemplated. If a wider excision is dictated by the patient s clinical stage or if potency is not an issue the dissection is carried out outside of the pelvic fascia. However, the nerve-sparing modification demands an intrafascial enucleation.

The posterior urethral wall is now sharply divided with a scalpel at the level of the prostatic apex until the Lowsley tractor is visualized (Fig. 19-11). At this time the curved tractor is removed and the anterior urethral wall is tented up by the vessel loop and transected. A straight Lowsley or Young tractor is then passed into the bladder through the open prostatic urethra.

Manipulation of the tractor draws the prostate caudally toward the incision, allowing dissection of the anterior surface of the prostate. This plane of dissection must be developed beneath the anterolateral pelvic fascia so that the puboprostatic ligaments

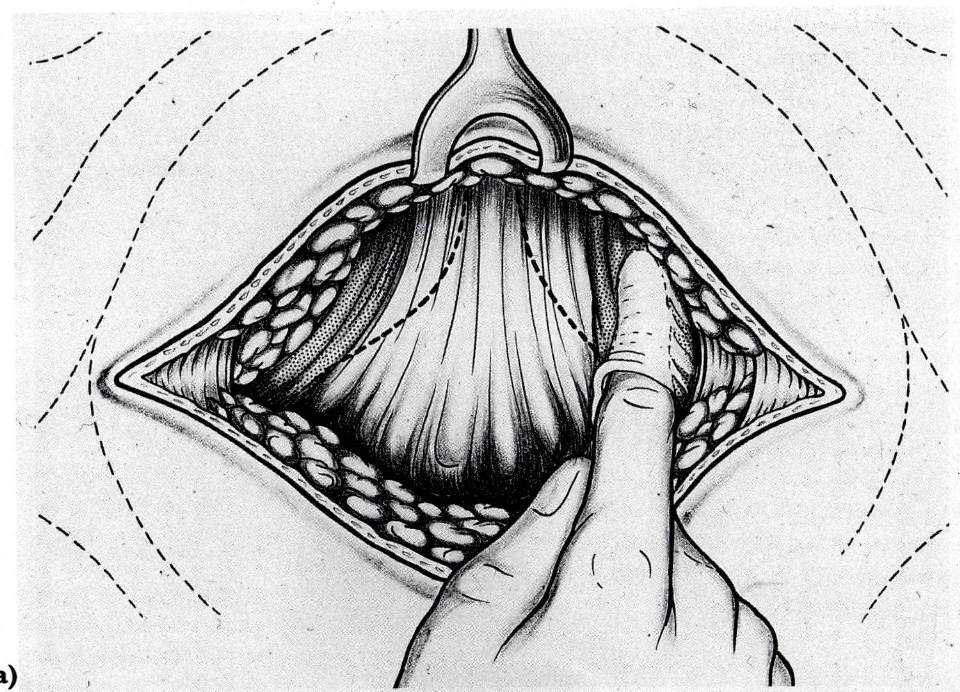

Figure 19-5 (a) The ischiorectal fossa is developed by blunt digital dissection. If the proper plane is entered, the urethra with the Lowsley tractor inside and the lateral aspect of the prostate can be palpated medially and the ischion laterally.

(a)

(b)

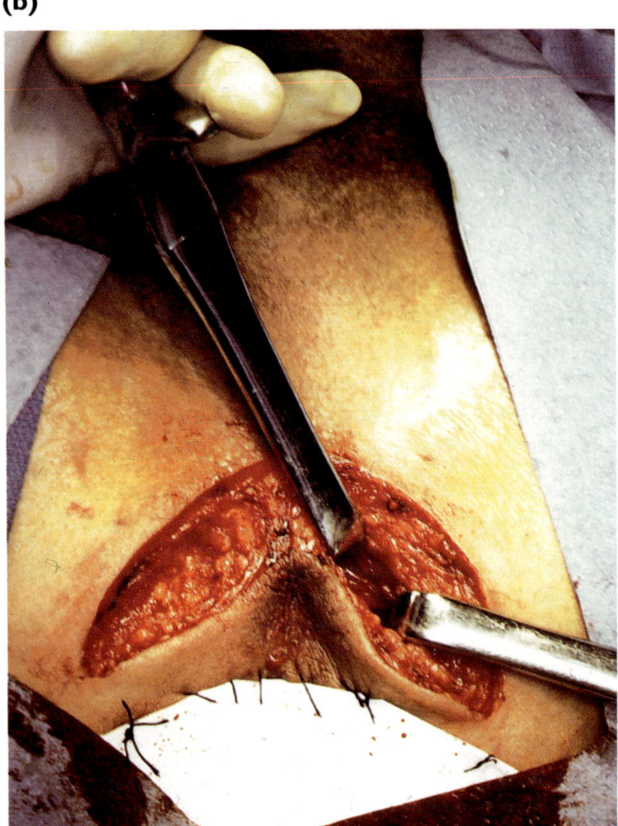

Figure 19-5 (b) The left ischiorectal fossa has been developed.

and the dorsal venous complex remain anteriorly, avoiding the risk for troublesome bleeding. I find that placing a narrow Deaver retractor with a moist gauze immediately over the severed urethral stump not only offers enhanced exposure during this part of the operation but also provides hemostasis by tamponading any small vessels from this area (Fig. 19-12).

Palpation of the open blades of the straight tractor helps identify the bladder neck. The dissection can then proceed from medial to lateral so that as much of the circular fibers of the bladder neck as possible can be preserved. If there is suspicion of tumor extension wider resection of the vesical neck should be undertaken (Fig. 19-13). Once the bladder neck is open the tip of the suction cannula is introduced into the bladder and its contents drained. The trigone is then transected, taking care to avoid the ureteral orifices. Placing an Allis clamp on the lower lip of the trigone and lifting it while pulling on the tractor facilitates the next step, creation of the plane between the bladder base, seminal vesicles, and

(a)

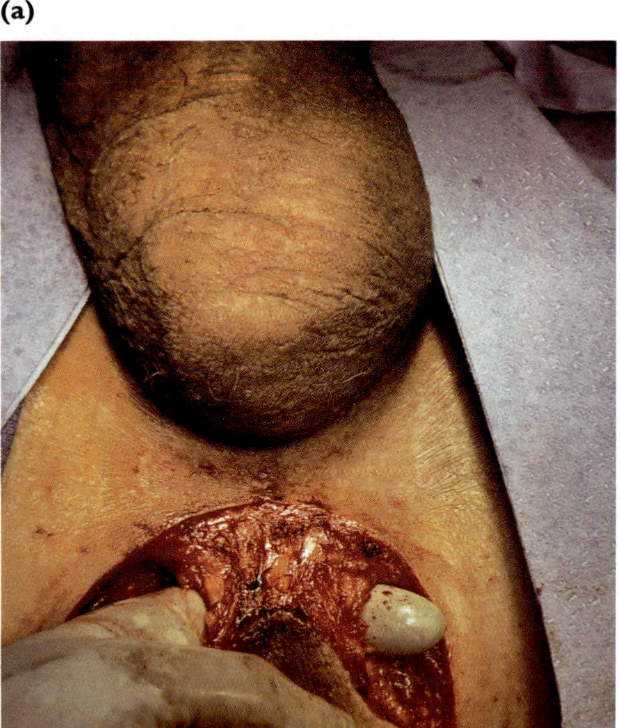

(b)

Figure 19-6 (a) The central perineal tendon has been isolated and encircled with the index finger. (b) The central perineal tendon is divided with electrocautery. The index finger protects the rectum from possible injury.

(a)

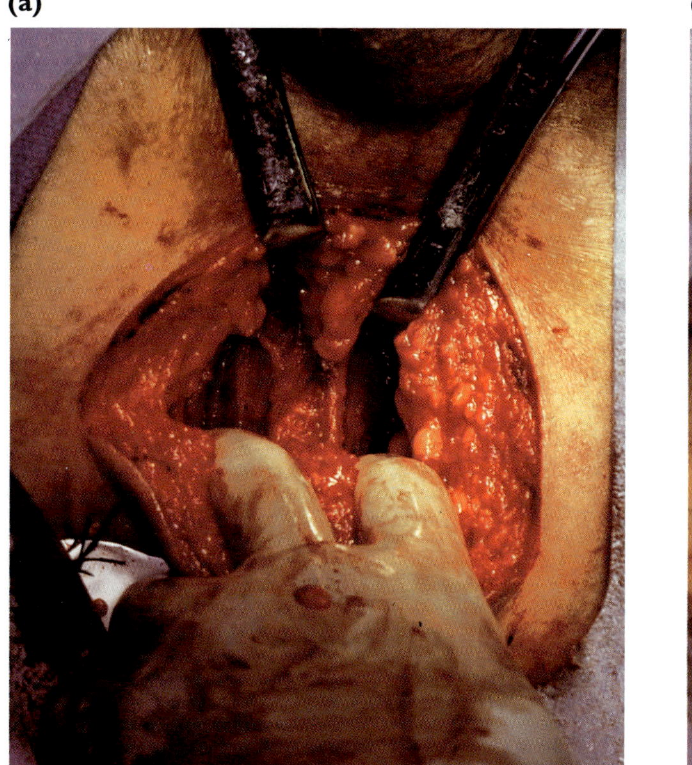

(b)

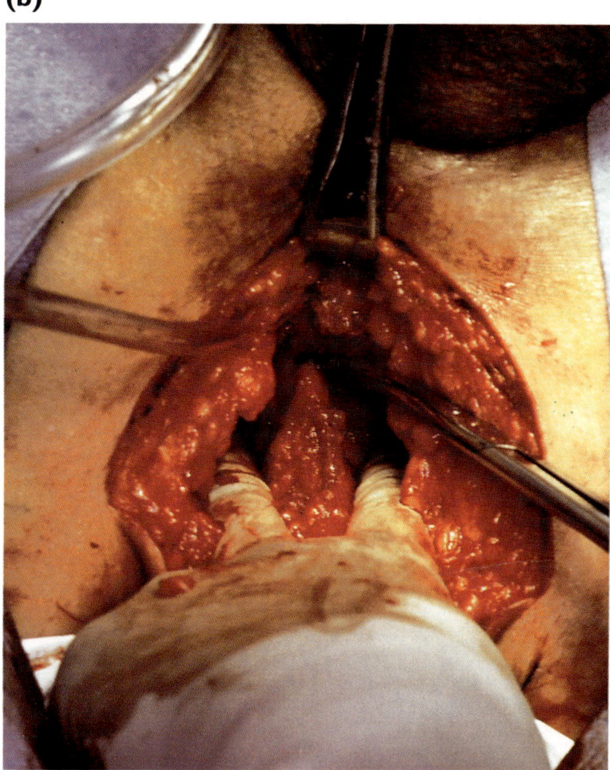

Figure 19-7 (a) Once the central tendon is divided, the rectourethralis muscle is exposed. This muscle extends between the rectal wall and the urethral bulb and can be varied in its presentation. (b) Division of the rectourethralis muscle is done sharply away from the rectum. If necessary a finger can be inserted in the rectum to assist in this maneuver.

ampulla. The narrow Deaver is now repositioned so that it pulls on the bladder superiorly, clearly exposing the ampulla, seminal vesicles, and vascular pedicles (Fig. 19-14). Hemoclips or ligatures are then used to control the vascular pedicles, leaving the prostate attached only by the ampulla and seminal vesicles (Fig. 19-15). By dividing the ampullae next, the small seminal vesicle pedicles can be clipped and transected, and the specimen removed.

If necessary the bladder neck is reconstructed in a tennis racket fashion with a running 3-0 polyglycolic acid suture to approximately a 20 to 22 French diameter. The bladder mucosa is then everted with interrupted 3-0 chromic to minimize the incidence of postoperative anastomotic strictures.

The vesicourethral anastomosis is performed with 3-0 polyglycolic acid sutures The stitches are first passed outside in through the margins of the urethral stump starting at the anterior edge and continuing circumferentially. The anterior bladder neck is then anastomosed to the anterior urethral border by passing the first two anteriorly placed sutures from the inside to the outside of the bladder. These are tied and a 20 or 22 French catheter passed into the bladder and the balloon inflated. The remaining sutures are passed and tied as described above and the anastomosis completed (Fig. 19-16).

A Penrose drain is positioned near the suture line and brought out through a separate stab wound. Closure is accomplished by reconstructing the perineum as anatomically as possible. The levator ani muscles and the central perineal tendon are reapproximated with 2-0 polyglycolic acid suture The skin is closed with a subcuticular 4-0 PGA suture and a sterile dressing applied.

Postoperative Care

Most patients are able to tolerate a full liquid diet the evening of surgery and a regular diet by the next day. The drain is usually removed 24 to 48 h postoperatively, and patients are normally discharged on the third or fourth day after surgery, although some

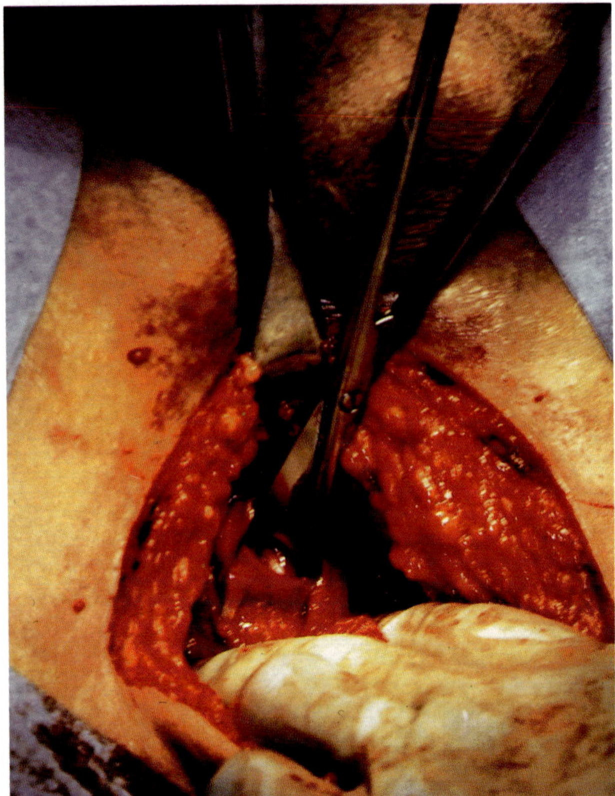

Figure 19-8 In this case the rectourethralis is not as well developed, instead it appears as a thin sheath of tissue immediately over Denonvillier's fascia.

can be released sooner. Oral antibiotics are administered until the catheter is removed. The patients are also discharged on stool softeners and a nonsteroidal analgesic. A cystogram is obtained 10 days after surgery, and if no extravasation is evident the catheter is removed.

Complications

Intraoperative

Bleeding

Venous bleeding can occur during the dissection of the anterior prostate following division of the urethra if the wrong plane is entered. This problem can be avoided by maintaining the dissection below the anterolateral pelvic fascia, thus avoiding the dorsal venous plexus. If bleeding does occur, sutures can be placed in a figure eight fashion to occlude the open venous channels, but it is often best to simply tamponade the problem area with a narrow Deaver retractor and continue the operation. Oozing from the bladder neck and seminal vesicles area is to be expected, and in the majority of cases ceases once the prostate is removed .

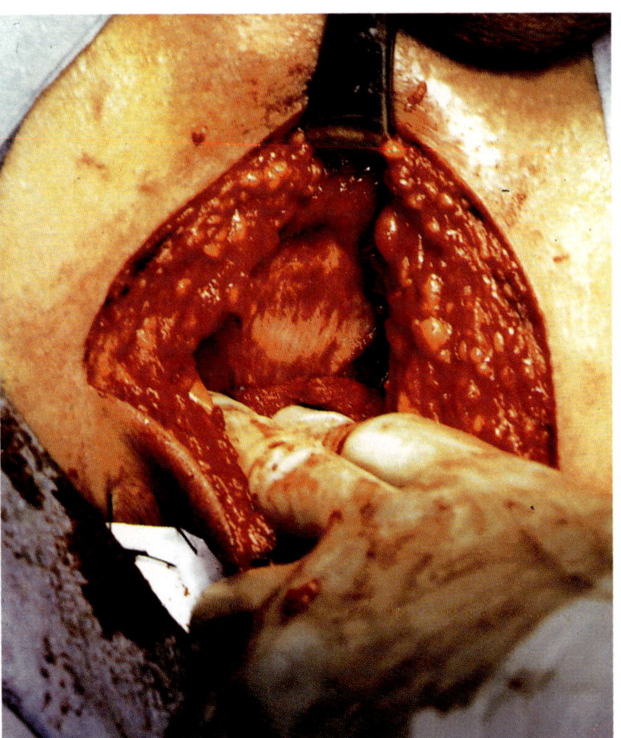

(a)

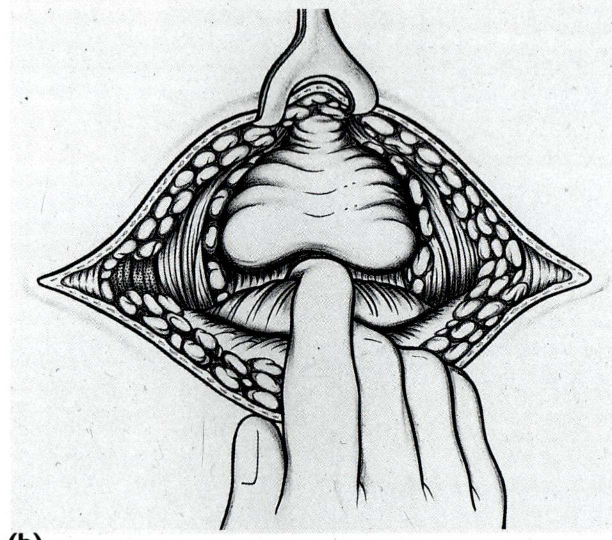

(b)

Figure 19-9 (a & b) Following the division of the rectourethralis muscle, blunt dissection with a moist sponge allows exposure of Denonvillier's fascia, also called the "pearly gates."

Disruption of the Bladder Neck

Entering the incorrect plane of dissection during the posterior transection of the prostate from the trigo-

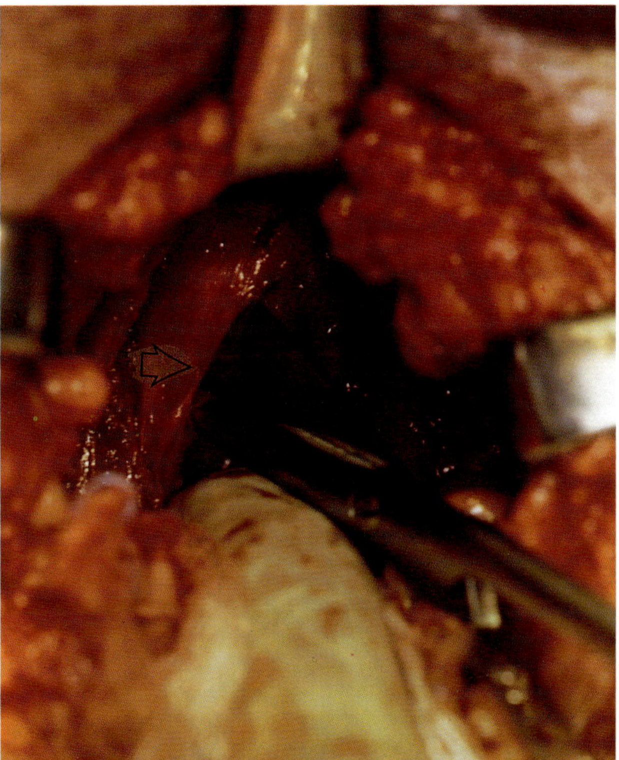

Figure 19-10 After incising the fascia vertically with a scalpel, if preservation of the neurovascular bundles is desired, the plane between it and the prostatic capsule is developed. Arrow points to the lateral pelvic fascia.

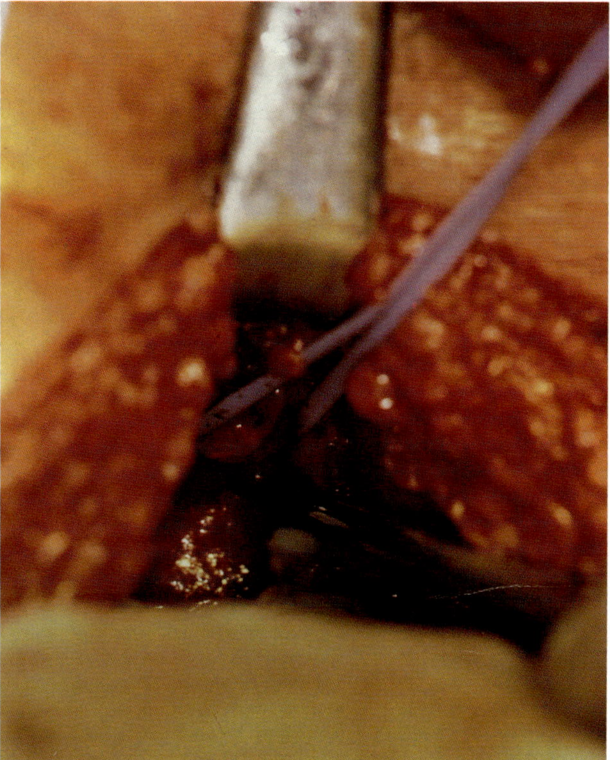

Figure 19-11 After the urethra has been isolated, it is divided until the tractor is visualized. The curved tractor is then removed, after which the anterior urethral wall can be divided.

nal musculature can create disruption of the bladder neck. The resultant thinning and tearing of the detrusor muscle can make identification of the ureteral orifices difficult. If this problem is encountered, reconstruction of the bladder neck is best accomplished by imbricating the detrusor muscle posteriorly and not attempting to incorporate the mucosa in the suture line. If possible an attempt should be made to catheterize the ureters to help in their identification.

Rectal Injury

If a bowel prep was instituted preoperatively and the injury is immediately recognized, the prostatectomy is completed as planned and a primary repair in two layers carried out. The first layer incorporates the serosa and muscularis as well as the mucosa, utilizing a running 3-0 PGA suture. The second consists of an interrupted 3-0 silk serosal imbricating Lembert suture. Drainage and antibiotic therapy is maintained for 7 days. A cystogram is performed to ascertain that an anastomotic colovesical fistula has not developed. If the cystogram is normal the drain is removed and routine postoperative care continued. If the bowel was inadequately prepared or a bowel prep not employed and/or the injury is substantial, a diverting colostomy with a Hartman s pouch must be done in order to ensure proper healing.

Postoperative Complications

Fistula

Leakage of urine from the incision is often due to a fistulous tract originating from the urethrovesical anastomosis as a result of disruption of one of the sutures or premature catheter removal. This problem often first becomes evident when the patient experiences seepage of urine from his wound when he voids. Management consists of replacement or continuation of the urethral catheter until the leakage stops.

Strictures

Stenosis of the vesicourethral anastomosis usually presents with the gradual onset of a diminished urinary stream accompanied by other symptoms of bladder outlet obstruction. The etiology is commonly scar tissue formation, which usually responds to

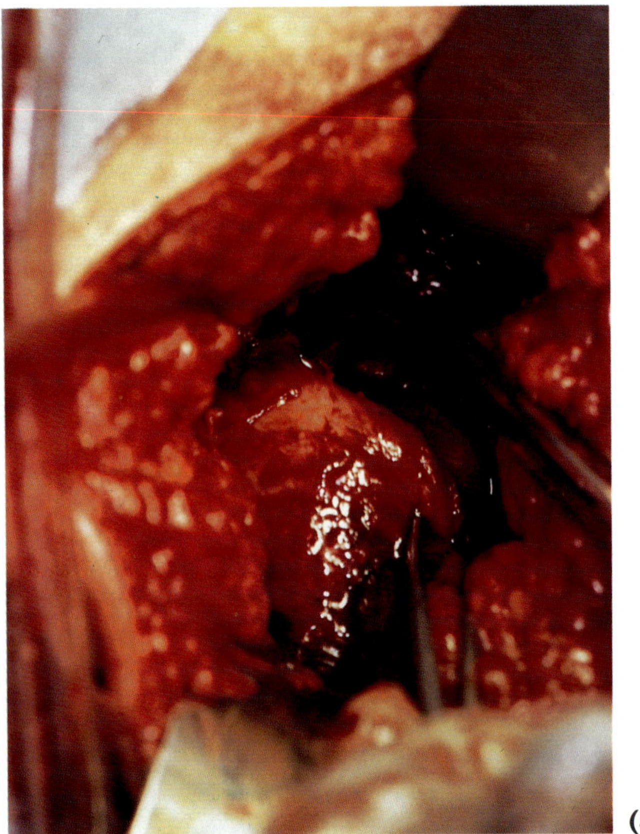

(a)

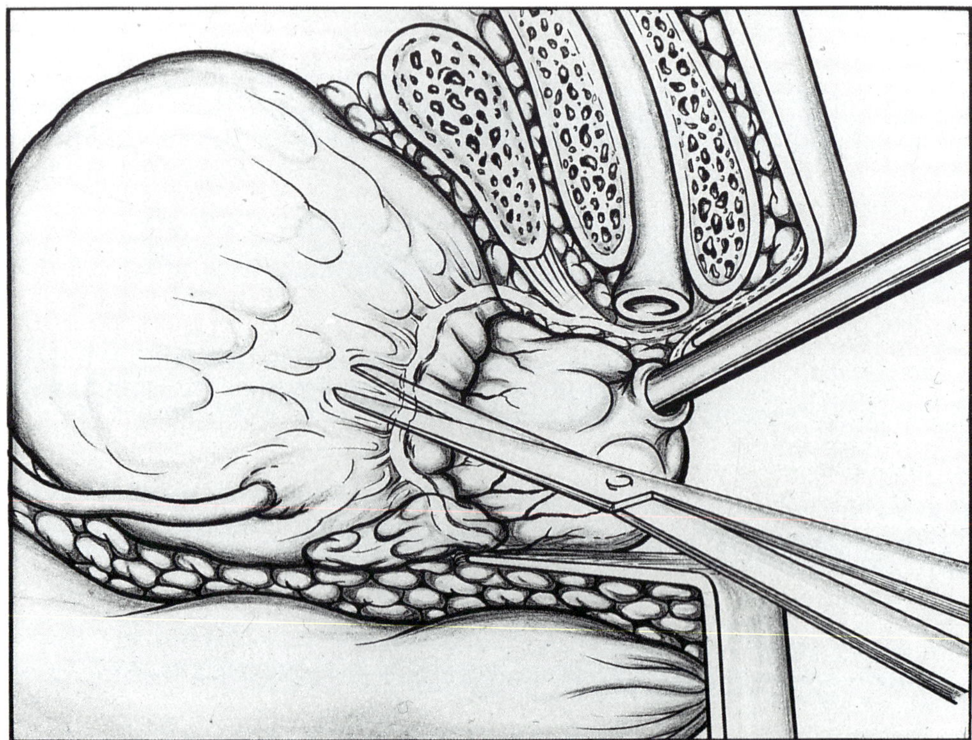

(b)

Figure 19-12 (a & b) A straight Lowsley tractor has been inserted into the bladder. Traction on it pulls the prostate towards the surgeon, allowing dissection of the anterior prostate and bladder neck. This dissection must be kept close to the prostate in order to avoid entering the venous plexus or injuring the neurovascular bundles.

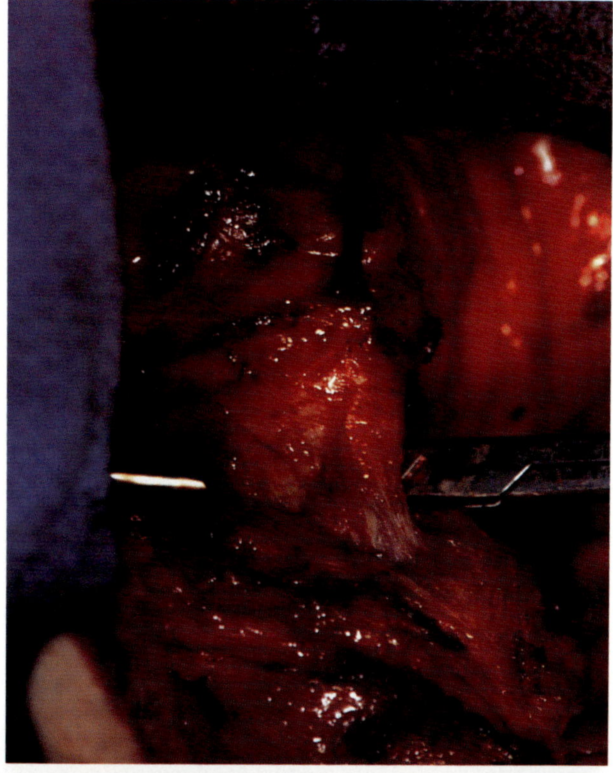

(a)

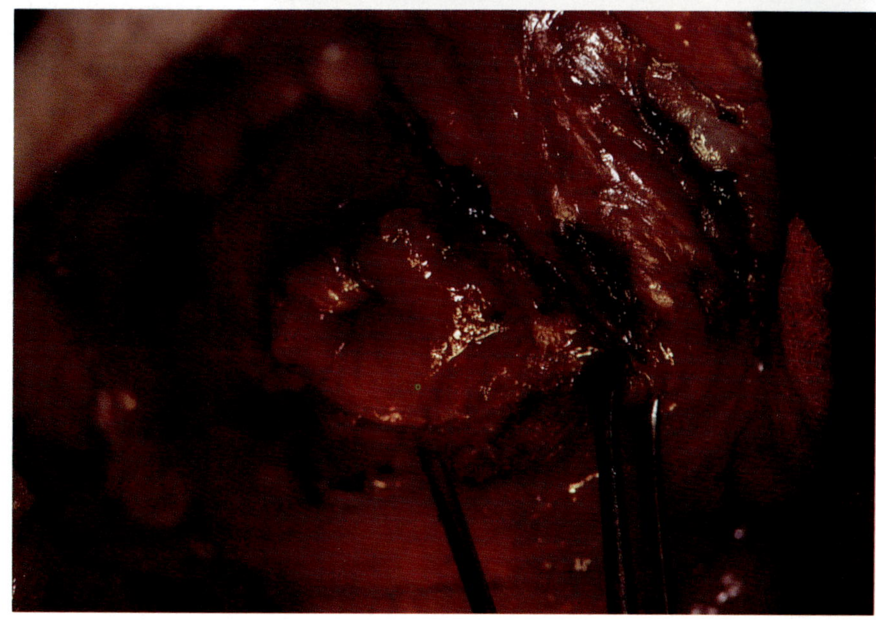

(b)

Figure 19-13 (a & b) In selected patients the bladder neck dissection can be carried out so that the fibers can be preserved, allowing for a more anatomic reconstruction.

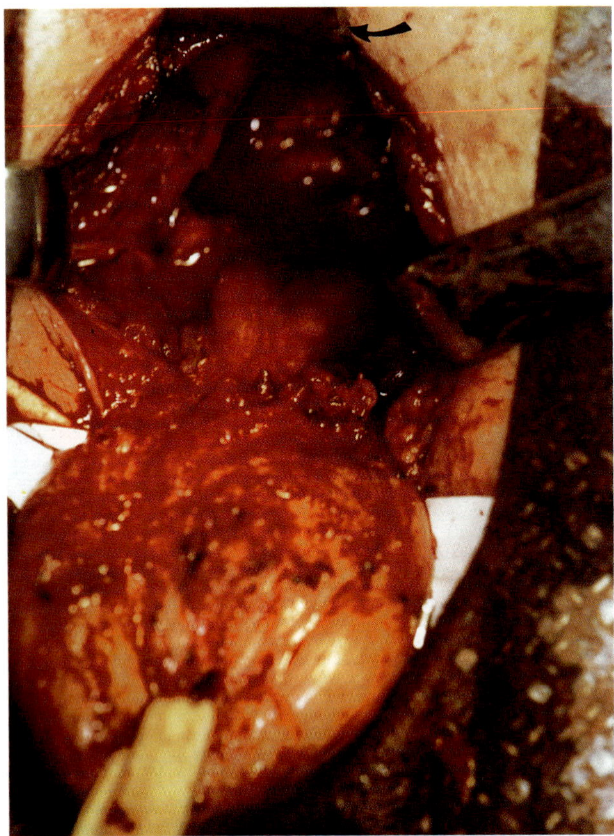

Figure 19-14 Following division of the bladder neck and trigones, the plane between the bladder, ampulla, and seminal vesicles is developed. A narrow Deaver is used to retract the bladder cephalad, which provides better exposure (arrow).

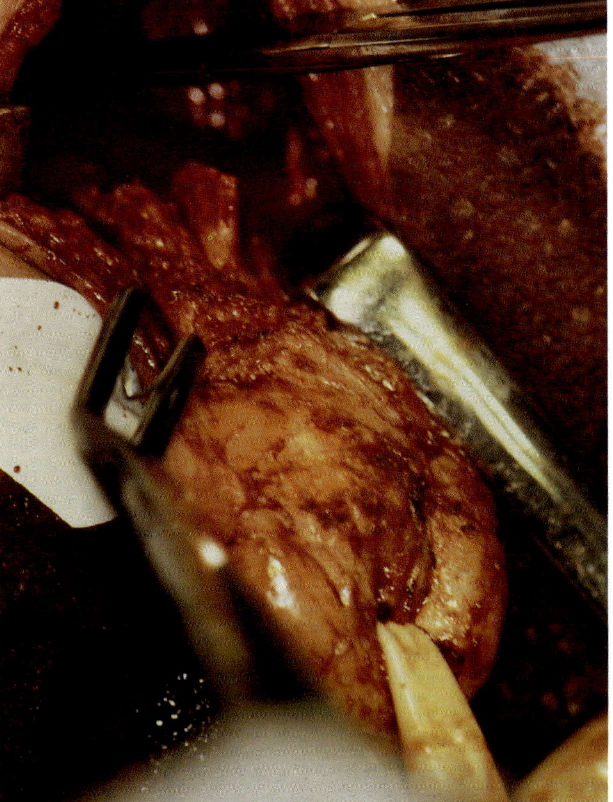

Figure 19-15 The prostatic vascular pedicles are hemoclipped or ligated, which will allow control of the seminal vesicles and removal of the specimen.

dilation. If the stricture reoccurs promptly following dilation, particularly in the presence of an abnormal PSA level, a local recurrence must be suspected and corroborated with transrectal ultrasound and biopsy of the anastomotic area. We routinely attempt to evert the bladder mucosa so that good mucosa to mucosa coaptation is achieved decreasing the probability of this complication.

Late Complications

Impotence

Despite application of the anatomic nerve-sparing technique herein described, some patients still suffer erectile dysfunction. The incidence of this detrimental complication is considerably less when the nerve sparing technique is applied to well-selected patients. Potency rates of 56 and 77 percent have been reported by both Weldon and Frazier independently.[7,9] Our overall experience in men with at least a year of follow-up reveals a potency rate of 30 percent. However, in a selected group of younger, potent patients, 51 percent maintained full or partial erections adequate for intercourse.

Incontinence

The return of urinary continence following a radical perineal prostatectomy is a gradual process. Most patients will have full return of sphincteric control by 6 months, with very few experiencing permanent incontinence. In our series we have not encountered any patient with total incontinence and only 5 percent have suffered from stress incontinence.

Careful attention to detail during the apical dissection is paramount in order to avoid inadvertent damage to the striated sphincter. Once the urethra has been identified and isolated it must be transected close to the prostatic apex, taking care not to extend the dissection cephalad across the bulbocavernosus muscle and striated sphincter. Likewise meticulous technique must be used in the reconstruction of the bladder neck and performance of the

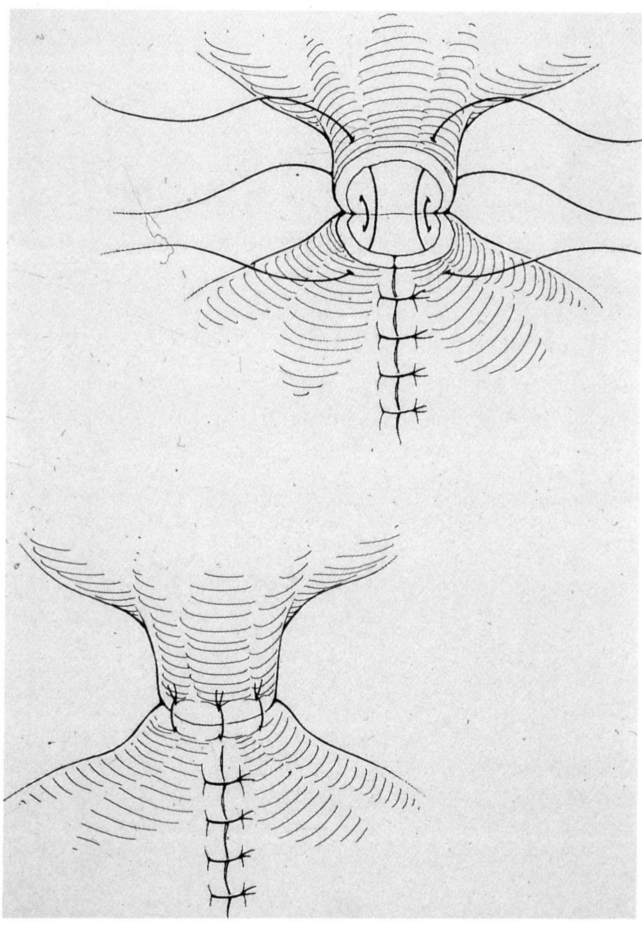

Figure 19-16 Technique of vesicourethral anastamosis.

anastomosis, since the development of a scarred anastomotic area can render the sphincter mechanism incompetent, leading to incontinence.

Conclusions

The refinements in surgical technique here described together with the laparoscopic staging of the pelvic lymph nodes have rekindled interest in the radical perineal prostatectomy. Without doubt the application of these innovations offers a potentially less morbid curative treatment to patients with localized prostate cancer.

References

1. Weyrauch HM: Perineal Prostatectomy In: *Surgery of the Prostate*. Edited by Weyrauch HM. Philadelphia: WB Saunders, chap 10, p 172–228, 1959.
2. Young HH: The early diagnosis and radical cure of carcinoma of the prostate: Being a study of 40 cases and presentations of a radical operation which was carried out in four cases. *Bull Johns Hopkins Hosp* 16:315–321, 1905.
3. Walsh PC, Donker PJ: Impotence following radical prostatectomy: Insight into etiology and prevention. *J Urol* 128:492–497, 1982.
4. Walsh PC, Lepor H, Eggleston JC: Radical prostatectomy with preservation of sexual function: Anatomical and pathological considerations. *Prostate* 12:187–199, 1983.
5. Walsh PC, Quinlan DM, Morton RA, Steiner MS: Radical retropubic prostatectomy: Improved anastomosis and urinary continence. *Urol Clin North Am* 17:679–684, 1990.
6. Parra RO, Andrus C, Boullier JA: Staging laparoscopic lymph node dissection: Comparison of results with open pelvic lymphadenectomy. *J Urol* 147:875–878, 1992.
7. Weldon VE, Tavel FR: Potency-sparing radical perineal prostatectomy and anatomy, surgical technique and initial results. *J Urol* 140:559–562, 1988.
8. Tobin CE, Benjamin JA: Anatomical and surgical restudy of Denonvillier's Fascia. *Surg Gynecol Obstet* 80:373–388, 1945.
9. Frazier MA, Roberston JE, Paulson DF: Radical prostatectomy: The pros and cons of the perineal versus retropubic approach. *J Urol* 147:888–890, 1992.

20

Laparoscopic Bowel Surgery

Jorge Cueto Garcia
Alejandro Weber Sanchez
Raul O. Parra

Introduction

At present, the application of laparoscopic surgical techniques upon the intestinal tract has limited application in urology. Nevertheless, a basic understanding of the surgical principles involved is important for the urologist involved in advanced laparoscopic surgery of the genitourinary tract. This chapter will specifically deal with laparoscopic techniques employed for handling intestinal segments that are potentially useful in reconstructive laparoscopic urology.

Patient Preparation

Routine preoperative measures are the same as for any other procedure already described in this text. A mechanical bowel preparation is instituted the day prior to surgery together with prophylactic antibiotics. If manipulation of the large bowel is planned, oral erythromycin and neomycin preparations are administered to reduce fecal bacterial counts.

Small Bowel Surgery

Laparoscopic techniques upon the small intestines can be of interest to the urologic surgeon in three circumstances: (1) Postoperative bowel obstruction, (2) Harvesting a segment for either an ileal conduit or augmentation cystoplasty, and (3) Other reconstructive procedures such as harvesting the appendix for a Mitrofanoff procedure.

Diagnosis and Management of Bowel Obstruction

Suffice it to say from the outset that only in selected cases will laparoscopy be indicated in this setting. However, when small bowel obstruction is suspected following a cystectomy or other intraperitoneal urological procedures, laparoscopy can be employed as an alternative to open laparotomy. The most important consideration prior to initiating such a procedure is the anticipation of dilated loops of bowel susceptible to injury during access. Therefore the open technique of entry into the peritoneal cavity described repeatedly in this book is highly recommended. Once access has been gained, a thorough inspection is performed, taking care to maximize patient positioning by the use of the Trendelenburg and lateral decubitus postures as circumstances mandate. In addition, such maneuvers facilitate displacement of the dilated loops of bowel, allowing the safe introduction of the accessory trocars under direct vision. Fig. 20-1 demonstrates the recommended positioning of these ports. Any adhesions encountered are lysed (Fig. 20-2). The bowel is run and the peritoneal cavity copiously irrigated. Discovery of significant spillage of intestinal contents, indicative of perforation or severe enterotomies too large to be adequately repaired intracorporeally, mandates conversion to an open laparotomy.

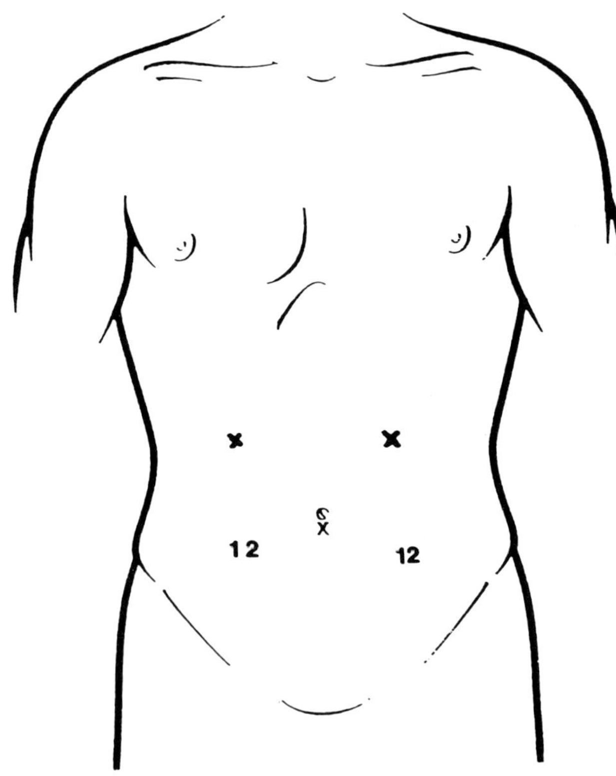

Figure 20-1 Location of trocars for bowel surgery.

Laparoscopy has proven useful in urology in the management of bowel obstructions following endocavitary procedures. Several case reports have recently appeared in the literature emphasizing the potential for loops of bowel to become entrapped in an improperly closed trocar site. Kreutzer and colleagues reported on the successful treatment of two patients in whom a bowel obstruction ensued following a laparoscopic pelvic lymph node dissection.[1] In both individuals small bowel and/or omentum was discovered incarcerated through the fascial defect of a port site. Repeat laparoscopy and atraumatic manipulation of the bowel assisted by external pressure on the trocar site resulted in a favorable resolution of the problem, avoiding the morbidity of a laparotomy.

The typical presentation of this phenomenon involves a patient who returns 3 to 5 days after an uneventful laparoscopic procedure with symptoms and signs of abdominal obstruction. Occasionally the involved trocar site may have a palpable, exquisitely tender mass. Repeat laparoscopy performed through fresh abdominal sites can reveal the incarcerated bowel loops within the fascial opening. Manipulation of the bowel by exertion of careful traction toward the abdominal cavity with an atraumatic forceps with simultaneous manual external pressure disincarcerates the involved viscera (Fig. 20-3). The fascial defect is then properly closed under visual laparoscopic control.

Laparoscopic Ileal Conduit: Harvesting of a Bowel Segment and Anastomosis

Indications

Clearly, the performance of a laparoscopic ileal conduit is indicated in a limited number of well-selected patients. It is our belief that the best indication is in an individual needing urinary diversion for a benign condition such as neurogenic bladder or fistulae in whom a concomitant cystectomy is not required.[2]

Technique

Trocar placement and location is as depicted in Fig. 20-1. It is important to bear in mind that the endoscopic stapling device requires a 12-mm port for its introduction. We believe that at least two of the trocars must be 12 mm in diameter to provide enough flexibility for the surgeon to perform the anastomosis efficiently. It is preferable to place one of these large trocars in the right lower quadrant so that the future stoma site can be created in its place.

Patient positioning and induction of the pneumoperitoneum does not differ from that already described for an intraperitoneal procedure elsewhere in this book. The procedure begins with localization of the ureters. If necessary, this can be assisted by prior ureteral catheterization. The ureters are usually most easily found at their crossing over the iliac bifurcation. If required, colonic mobilization is performed to adequately visualize this area bilaterally. Bowel mobilization is more frequently required on the left, since the sigmoid often overlies the iliac bifurcation. Once the ureters are isolated, an endoscopic Babcock clamp or an umbilical tape is used to surround the ureter and place it under tension. With the ureter under traction, a combination of

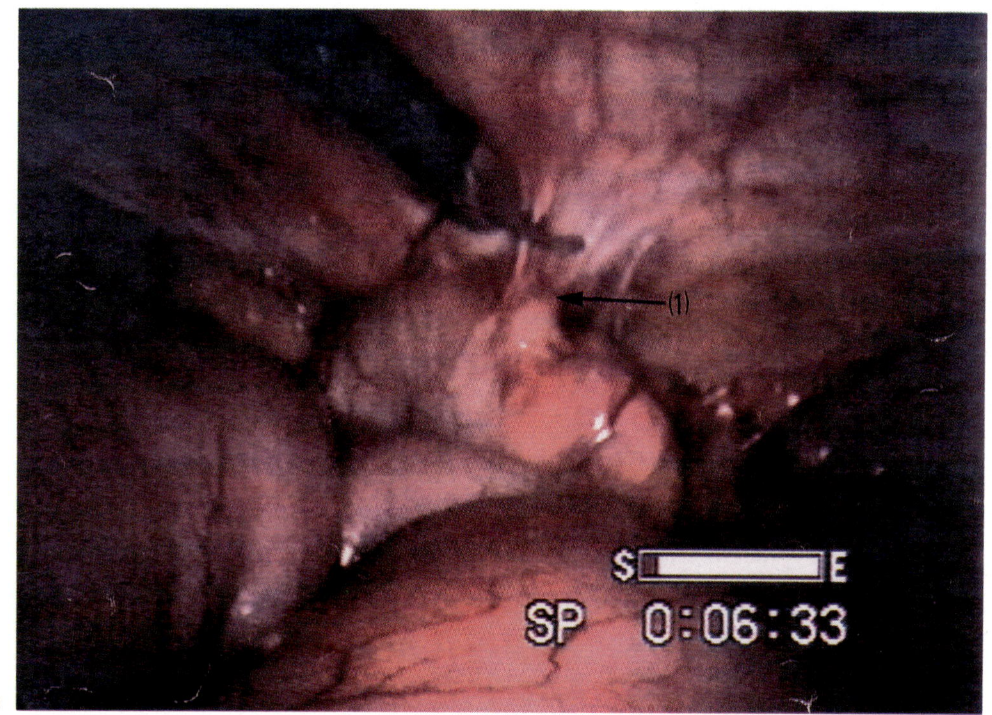

(a)

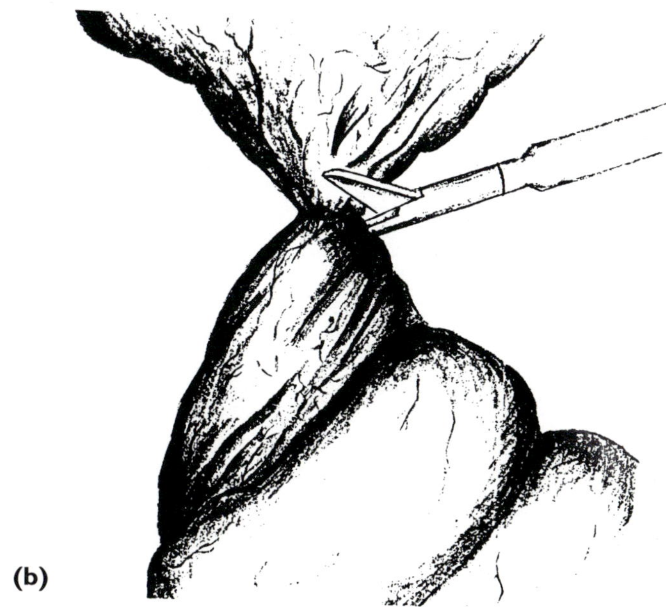

(b)

Figure 20-2 (a & b) Adhesiolysis in a case of small bowel obstruction secondary to adhesions.

sharp and blunt dissection is utilized to free the ureter as far as possible into the pelvis, where it is clipped and transected.

The sigmoid colon is then grasped with an endo-babcock clamp to place its mesentery under tension, and a tunnel is created at the level of the sacral promontory by blunt dissection with an atraumatic instrument. The left ureter is then brought across to the right side, taking care not to cause any kinking or ureteral angulation.

Once the ureters have been prepared, bowel is inspected and a segment of distal ileum selected for the conduit. We have found that partially deflating the abdominal cavity to approximately 8 to 10 mm of Hg aids greatly in determining the length of bowel required to construct the ileal conduit. The next step of the operation involves the transection and anastomosis of the bowel. This can be accomplish either entirely intracorporeally or extracorporeally. In the former technique the endo-GIA stapler

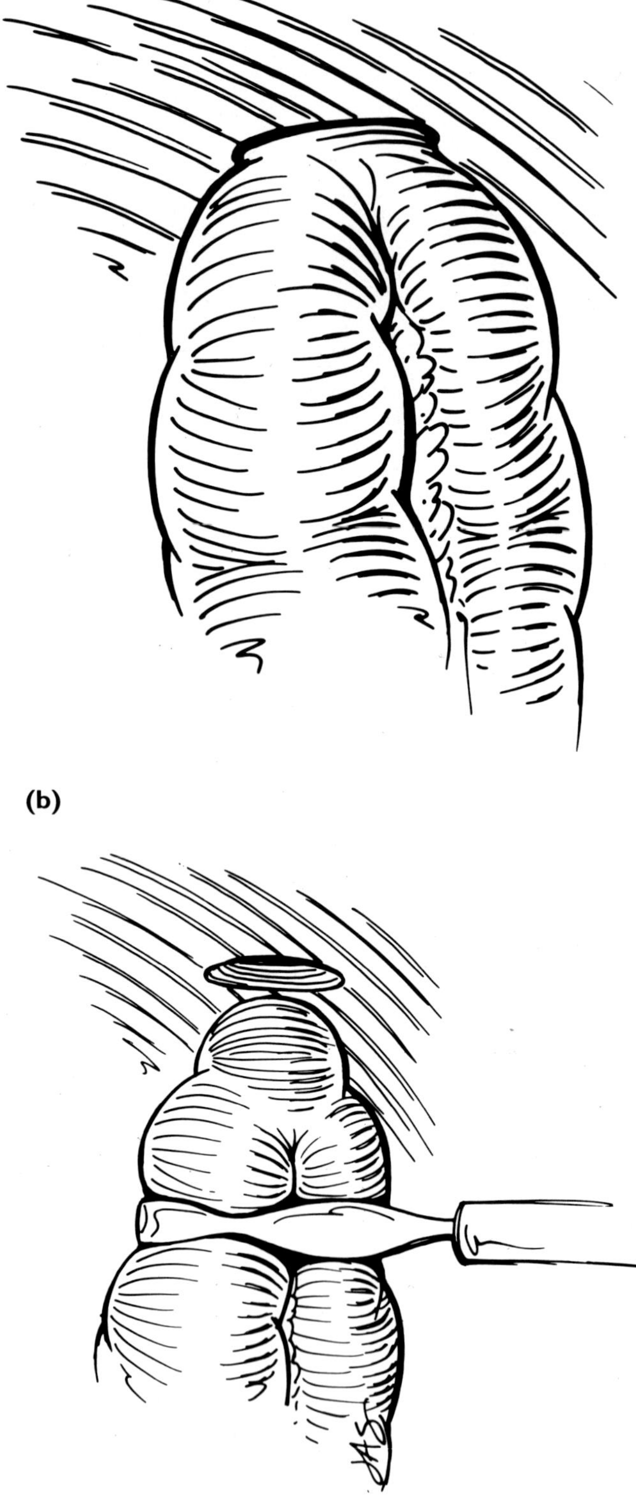

Figure 20-3 (a) Laparoscopic view of small bowel and fascial defect of previous trocar site. (b) By exerting traction on the bowel combined with external pressure, the herniated viscera can be disincarcerated.

is introduced and placed across the antimesenteric border at the distal end of the selected bowel segment and fired (Fig. 20-4a).

Following transection of the bowel, the stapler is reintroduced across the mesentery in line with the previous cut and fired again (Fig. 20-4b). The process is then repeated on the proximal end of the conduit, and the bowel and mesentery inspected for bleeding and viability. Depending upon the mobility attained in the loop, it may be necessary to fire the endo-GIA one more time across the mesentery of the distal end in order to obtain the flexibility necessary to reach the abdominal wall. Bowel continuity is then established by means of a functional side to side anastomosis performed by creating enterotomies in the antimesenteric borders of distal and proximal ileal ends. The jaws of the endo-GIA stapler are then introduced through these openings and the stapler fired (Fig. 20-4c). Finally, the open ends of the anastomosis are closed by additional firings of the endo-GIA stapler.

The ureteroileal anastomosis are performed by intracorporeal suture techniques. After spatulation of the ureter, the ureteral wall is anchored to a selected site in the ileum with a suture of 4-0 polyglycolic acid loaded in an RB-1 needle. A small enterotomy is made and a mucosa-to-mucosa anastomosis performed with the same suture material. This anastomosis can be done in a running or interrupted fashion, with the former technique being perhaps less time-consuming. Regardless of the suture method employed, if the placement of a ureteral stent is desired, this must be done before completing the anastomosis. This is accomplished by bringing the distal end of the ileum through the 12-mm right lower quadrant trocar site, excising the staple line, and passing a cystoscope to the anastomotic site. A guidewire is passed to the corresponding collecting system and a single J urinary diversion stent fed over the wire to the renal pelvis. Following completion of the anastomosis, the stoma is matured in the standard fashion. A suction drain is then placed in the area of the ureteroileal anastomosis and brought out through the contralateral lower quadrant trocar site. The procedure is terminated just like any other laparoscopic intervention.

The extracorporeal technique offers several advantages over the intracorporeal method described above. It offers the surgeon the opportunity to employ standard open techniques in a more

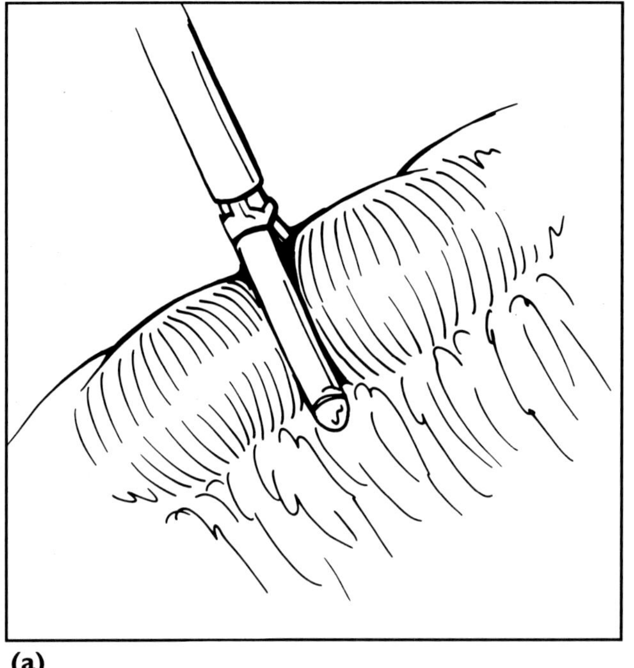

(a)

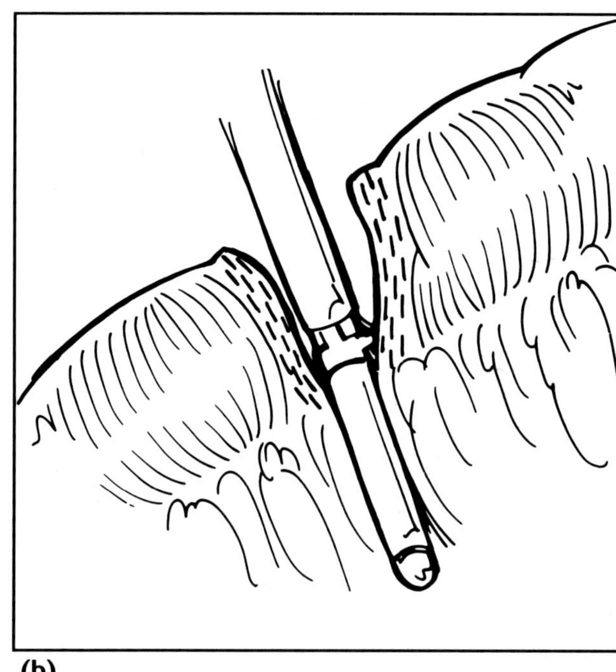

(b)

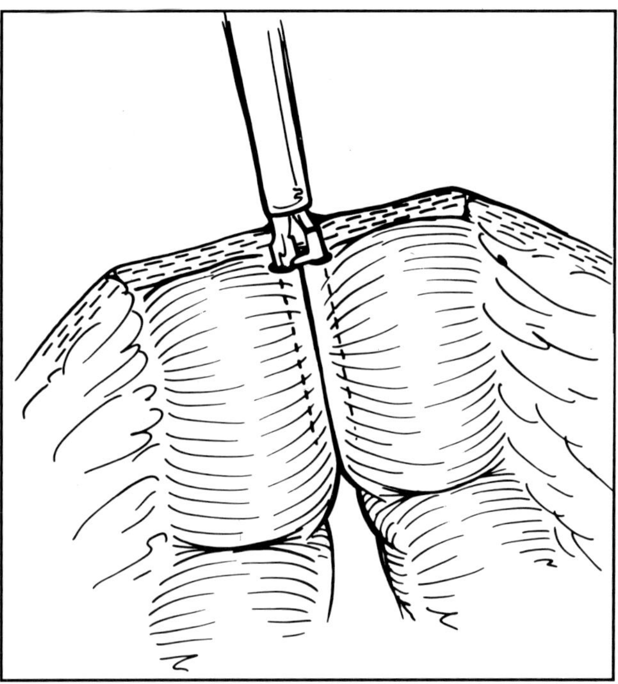

(c)

Figure 20-4 (a) The endo-GIA stapler is placed across the antimesenteric border of the bowel and fired. (b) After division of the bowel, a second and sometimes third firing of the stapler is preferred for transection of the mesentery. (c) Two small enterotomies are made at the antimesenteric ends of the bowel and a functional side-to-side anastomosis created with the endo-GIA stapler.

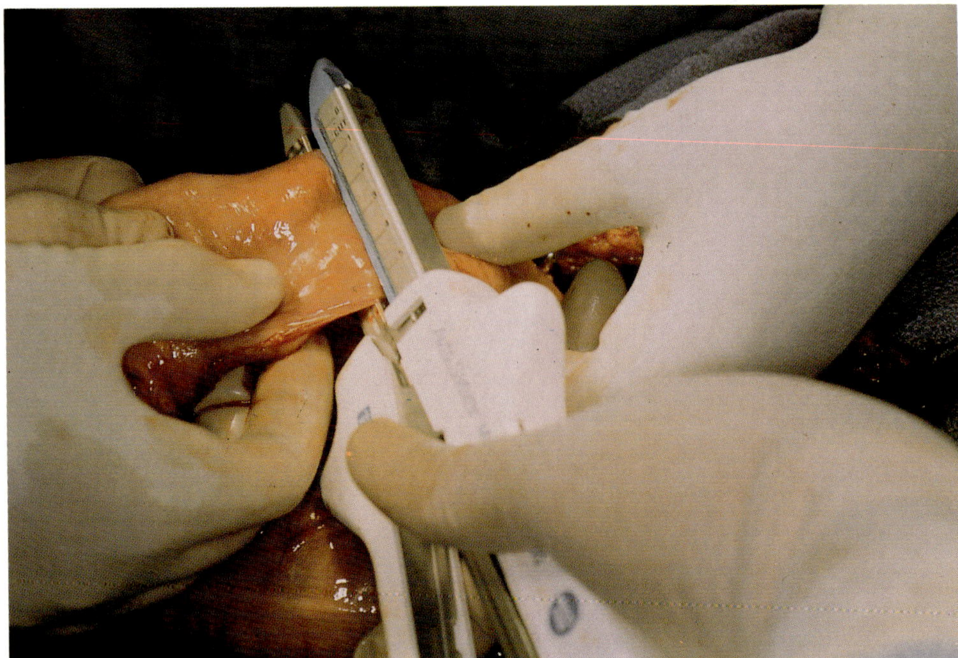

(a)

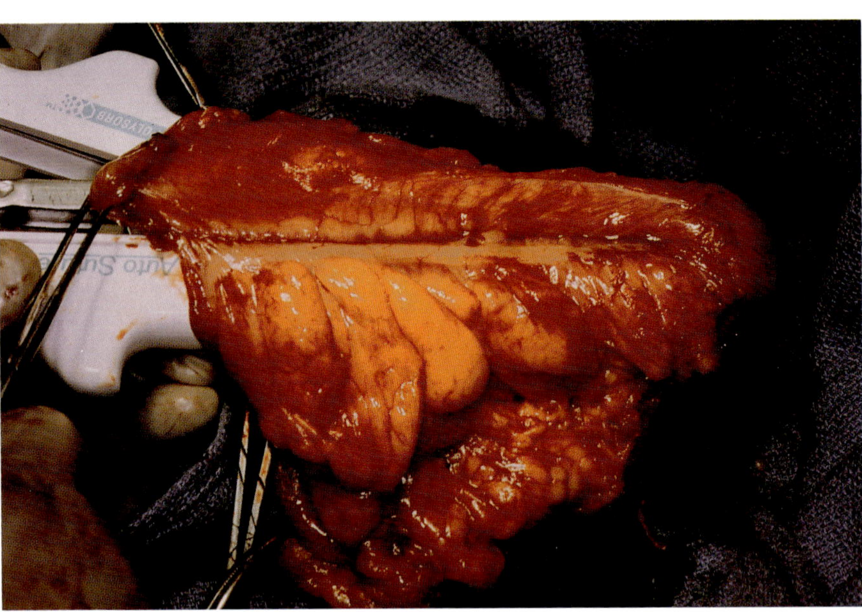

(b)

Figure 20-5 (a) Extracorporeal bowel anastomosis: After the selected bowel segment is exteronized, bowel division is carried out with the GIA stapler. (b) Extracorporeal side to side bowel anastomosis.

controlled environment. The placement of staples and sutures can be accomplished more quickly and with more precision. Once an appropriate segment of bowel has been chosen laparoscopically, it is brought out through the right lower quadrant 12-mm trocar site. Bowel division, anastomosis, and mesenteric defect repair is then performed with staples and sutures just as if an open operation were being conducted (Fig. 20-5). The anastomosed bowel is replaced in the peritoneal cavity and the ileal segment and ureters exteriorized. The ureteroileal anastomosis is completed in a Bricker fashion, placed intra-abdominally, and the stoma matured. Postoperative care in either case is identical to that of the open counterpart.

Other Applications

Laparoscopic Appendectomy

This procedure is being routinely performed by our colleagues the general surgeons. Although it is unlike-

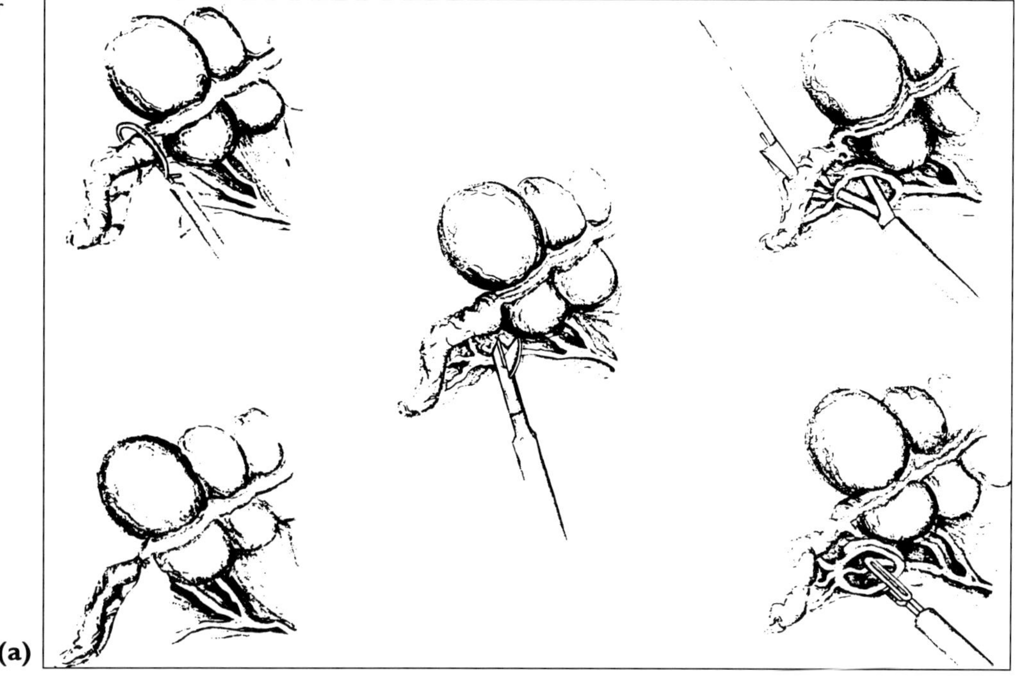

Figure 20-6 Technique for laparoscopic appendectomy. (a) Harvesting the appendix with preservation of the arterial supply.

ly that the occasional urologic laparoscopist will be involved with its use, those interested or engaging in more advanced laparoscopic reconstructive techniques might find it useful. In fact, a laparoscope-assisted Mitrofanoff procedure has already been accomplished,[3] and it is likely that other skilled and adventurous laparoscopists will expand on the procedure. The intracorporeal technique for harvesting the appendix is depicted in (Fig. 20-6). Alternatively these steps can be simplified by the use of the endo-GIA linear stapler.

Bladder Augmentation

A technique similar to that described for obtaining a bowel segment for construction of an ileal conduit is all that is required, the length of bowel necessary varying according with the individual patient's anatomy or condition being treated. Anastomosis of the bowel to the bladder would require extensive use of the intracorporeal suturing technique described in Chap. 7.

Conclusions

At this time the application of laparoscopy in the intestinal tract for urologists inspires little interest. However, as more sophisticated instrumentation is developed and the time required for the performance of these complex procedures is shortened more interest in their application in reconstructive laparoscopic surgery is likely to emerge.

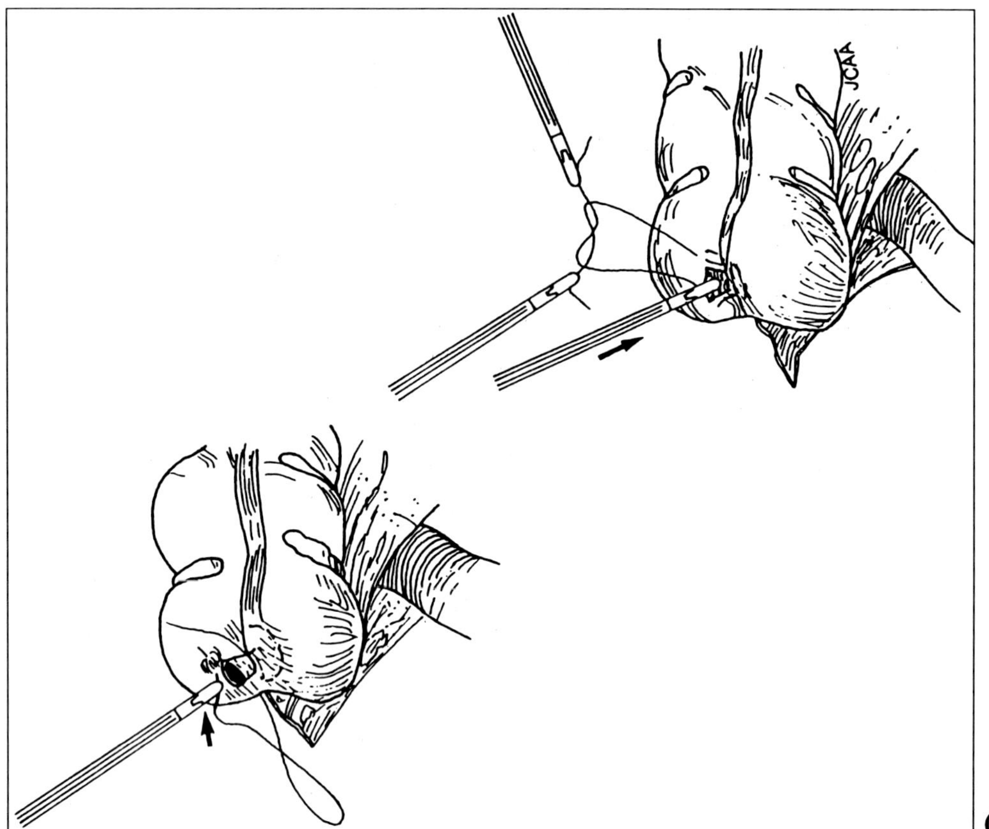

(b)

Figure 20-6 Technique for laparoscopic appendectomy. (b) Closure of the cecal defect with intracorporeal suturing technique.

References

1. Kreutzer ER, Lerner SE, Kahan NZ, Melman A: Laparoscopic treatment of small-bowel obstruction following laparoscopic lymphadenectomy. *Urology* 44(5):768–770, 1994.

2. Kozminski M, Partamian K0: Case report of laparoscopic ileal loop conduit. *J Endourol* 6:147–150, 1992.

3. Jordon GH, Winslow BH: Laparoscopically assisted continent catheterizable cutaneous appendicovesicostomy. *J Endourol* 7:517–520, 1993.

INDEX

Index

Page numbers followed by f denote figures.
Page numbers followed by t denote tables.

D

N

O

P

V

W

Y

ISBN 0-07-048580-1